Deaf Children in China

Deaf Children in China

Alison Callaway

Gallaudet University Press
Washington, D.C.

Gallaudet University Press
Washington, DC 20002

© 2000 by Alison Callaway.
All rights reserved. Published 2000
Printed in the United States of America

Library of Congress Cataloging-in-Publication Data

Callaway, Alison.
    Deaf children in China / Alison Callaway.
      p. cm.
    Originally presented as the author's thesis (Ph.D. — Bristol University).
    Includes bibliographical references and index.
    ISBN 1-56368-085-8
    1. Deaf children — China.   2. Deaf children — China — Family relationships.   3. Hearing impaired children — China — Family relationships.   I. Title.

HV2888.C35 2000
362.4'2'083951 — dc21   99-088446

∞ The paper used in this publication meets the minimum requirements of American National Standard for Information Sciences — Permanence of Paper for Printed Library Materials, ANSI Z39.48-1984.

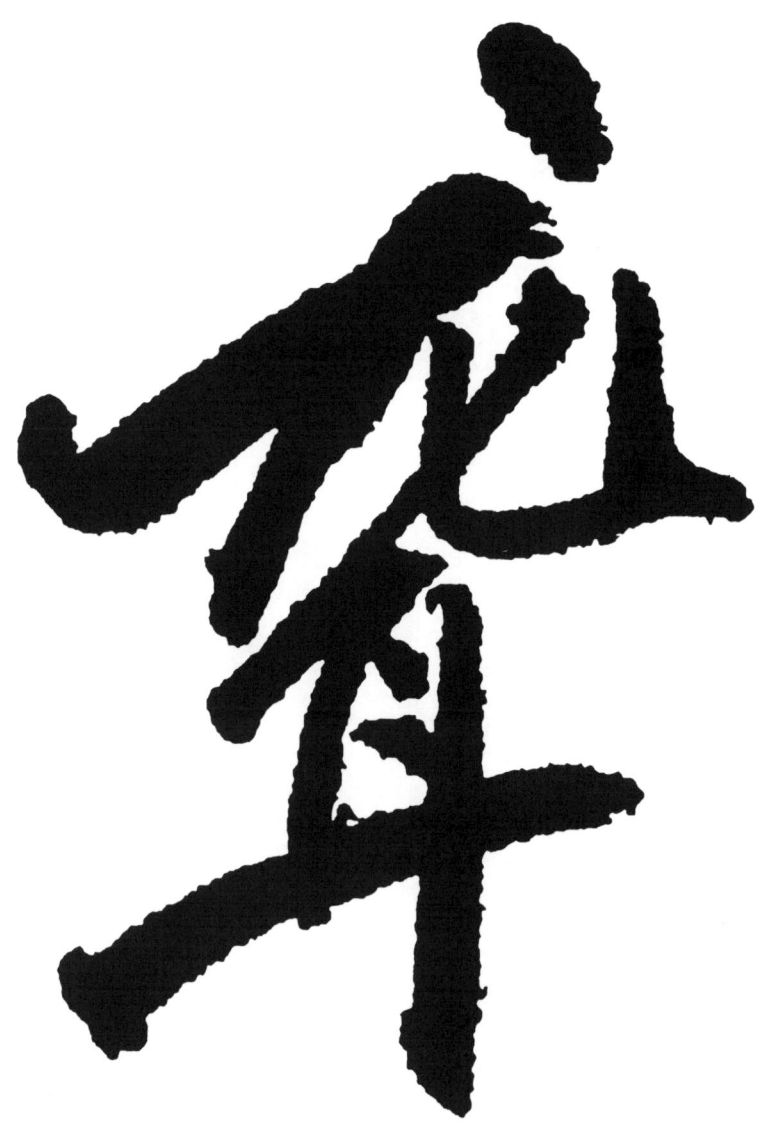

The Chinese character for "deaf" includes the character for "dragon"; thus the animal in Chinese culture that symbolizes success, outstanding achievement, and leadership is embedded and perpetuated in the written language in the concept of deafness; phonetically the two words are the same.

Contents

	Acknowledgments	ix
1	Introduction	1
2	The Chinese Family and the Deaf Child	11
3	Deafness in China	48
4	The Role of Professionals and Parents in the Education of Deaf Children	93
5	Urban Families with Deaf Children	122
6	Letters to Zhou Hong	198
7	Conclusions	253
	Appendix: Interview Questionnaire	267
	Notes	277
	References	287
	Index	307

Acknowledgments

Many people contributed information, help, and advice during the preparation of the material for this book. I would particularly like to thank the following:

The parents and teachers in China who contributed their views and experiences to this research; in Nanjing, Wu An'an, director of the Social Welfare Division of the Amity Foundation, who facilitated my fieldwork, and Zhou Hong, principal of the rehabilitation center for deaf children whose parents agreed to be interviewed for this research; in Beijing, Wan Xuanrong and Liang Wei at the China Research and Rehabilitation Center for Deaf Children; in London, Edmond Tang at the China Desk of the Council of Churches for Britain and Ireland; and in Oxford, Hui Li, Zhu Buxian and Deng Ziwan, Zhang Manhua, Zhuang Yaqin, Zhang Zhichao, Fan Jinping, and Zhang Wenli for assistance with documentary sources, interpretation of data, and discussion of aspects of Chinese life and culture;

My academic advisors Jim Kyle (director, Centre for Deaf Studies, University of Bristol) and Alys Young, and colleagues and staff at the Centre for Deaf Studies, especially Clark Denmark and Jennifer Ackerman for their advice on a joint project with Nanjing Deaf School;

Cheung Suk-chong, Diana Martin, and Elvire Roberts, who read and commented on drafts of my work; Mary Plackett at the library of the RNID in London, for help obtaining source materials, especially concerning the first school for the deaf in China; Ruth Baker, for her advice on key initial contacts; and Patricia Potts at the Open University for useful discussions.

This research was supported by a studentship from the Economic and Social Research Council. The first year of my research, and my first field trip to China, was supported by grants from the Great Britain–China Educational Trust, the A. H. F. Barbour's Trust for China Mission, the Methodist Church, and the Alice Horsman Travelling Fellowship awarded by Somerville College, Oxford.

My especial thanks to my family for their support over the last four years.

Deaf Children in China

CHAPTER ONE

INTRODUCTION

My interest in China began in the early 1980s. After qualifying as a doctor in Britain and practicing for several years as an ear, nose, and throat specialist, I went to China in 1983 with my five-year-old Chinese son to teach at a medical college in Chongqing, a large city on the Yangtse River in Sichuan province. I spent two years there, during which time I learned to speak Chinese. Having a preschool-age child to look after brought me in contact with Chinese mothers with children of the same age, and through these friendships I could not help but absorb many Chinese ideas and attitudes about bringing up children. On returning to Britain I kept up my Chinese by teaching it in evening classes, and I did some interpreting and translation work as well.

In 1993 I started research on the topic of deaf children and their families in China at the Centre for Deaf Studies at Bristol University. This subject was really a kind of drawing together and synthesis of my previous professional and personal experiences. I was fortunate to be based in the Centre for Deaf Studies, as it is one of the key centers in the United Kingdom for research on sign language and deaf issues; it has also initiated a comprehensive bilingual/bicultural program for preschool-age deaf children in the Bristol area. Because of my medical training I already had an understanding of medical and audiological aspects of deafness, but in studying for a Ph.D. at Bristol I began to consider educational issues more closely and to take into account the value systems underlying them. Deaf cultural perspectives and the philosophy of sign bilingualism in deaf education have significantly influenced my approach to exploring the circumstances of deaf children and their families in China.

The bilingual/bicultural approach to the education of deaf children values children's deaf identity, involves deaf adults, and promotes the use of sign language as a first language for communication and learning at home and at school. I subscribe to these basic principles and believe that deaf children, particularly those with profound or severe hearing loss, ideally should have access to a bilingual program. The views of a researcher are likely to color his or her research to some degree, and while I have aimed for a factually accurate and balanced account, my perspective on the education of deaf children has probably influenced to some extent the choice of topics included for discussion and the focus of the discussion—for example, the exploration of the status of sign language in China in chapter 3 and the discussion of the development of educational options for deaf children in chapter 7.

For my fieldwork in China I planned to interview parents of deaf children, and so I prepared a questionnaire before my trip to China at the end of 1994. The actual circumstances of these interviews and the information provided by the parents are presented in chapter 5. During my stay in China I was given a large collection of letters written by Chinese parents of deaf children. They were addressed to Zhou Hong, who at the time was principal of a preschool for deaf children; he is also the parent of a deaf child and he has gained national acclaim for his success in teaching her. The letters conveyed so much information about the parents' experiences and concerns for their children that I decided to examine them systematically; this evidence and its analysis, which provides a second angle on my primary area of research, are presented in chapter 6. I discovered that the interviews and the letters complement each other, in ways I describe more fully at the end of this chapter.

I began my research with these questions: What is the experience of Chinese parents of preschool-age deaf children? What are their attitudes toward their child's deafness? and What courses of action do they follow in response to it? I hoped to find out how Chinese parents felt when they first suspected their child might be deaf, how they reacted to the diagnosis of deafness in their child, who they looked to for support, and what state services were available to them. I wanted to ascertain the parents' method of communication with their child at home, their attitudes toward the use of sign language, and their views on their child's education and future. My aims were to obtain as full a picture as possible of parents' experiences with their deaf children and, even more important, of how they interpreted those experiences and understood the implications of having a son or daughter who was deaf. All these factors—

the parents' experience, their attitudes toward their child's deafness, and their resultant behavior—would strongly influence the development of the deaf child and affect his or her future, particularly through the parents' choice of educational options.

In preparing for the interviews with parents, I was particularly careful to ensure that the issues covered were actually relevant to their situation. It would be pointless to ask a set of questions developed with Western families in mind, as I might miss areas that were crucial to Chinese parents; an inappropriate framework of assumptions and values could easily lead to misunderstanding. A failure to appreciate the surrounding context would not only affect the nature of the information I obtained but would also make it difficult for me to interpret it accurately and sensitively. It therefore seemed essential to gain a detailed understanding of the social, political, and cultural factors affecting Chinese families with deaf children: I wanted as far as possible to understand the key issues as respondents themselves perceived and expressed them (in anthropological terms, an "emic" perspective), rather than as they were shaped by the emphases and biases of my own culture (an "etic" perspective).

The first step was to use information from statistical and documentary sources to establish the social and cultural context of Chinese families with deaf children. The family is a particularly strong institution in Chinese society. I had to take into consideration its role and functions, as well as evaluate the very significant impact of the government's birth control policies on family structure and values. I examined studies of child socialization in China, including research on the behavior of only children, an area of concern now that the majority of urban couples have only one child. I collated information on the medical and rehabilitation services available to Chinese families and on the status of deaf people and sign language in China, and I collected and reviewed articles and papers that presented the views of Chinese professionals on the rehabilitation of deaf children and on parents' role in their children's education. This essential background information is presented in chapters 2 to 4.

Throughout the book, I use terminology that reflects professional usage in China: for example, "rehabilitation," which is not commonly used now in the United States or the United Kingdom in the context of preschool interventions for deaf children, is used here because it is a literal translation of the Chinese term, and its connotations are integral to Chinese concepts of special education.

Using evidence obtained from these sources, I identified a number of key issues affecting the experience of Chinese parents with deaf children that could be covered in the interviews. The support of grandparents and other family members, the implications for parents of having a deaf child when only one child is permitted, parents' preoccupation with finding a medical cure, the availability of hearing aids and professional support, and social attitudes toward deafness and deaf people were among the issues that were clearly very relevant to these parents.

I also consulted Western studies concerning deaf children and their families. One in particular, Susan Gregory's study (1976) based on interviews with 122 English mothers of deaf children under the age of six, was especially useful; her interviews covered many aspects of life with a deaf child, including development of language and communication, social behavior, play, and education. Some areas, such as parents' attitudes toward discipline and the use of sign/gesture at home, were incorporated into the questionnaire for Chinese parents; this allowed some useful if tentative comparisons to be made between the responses of Chinese parents and those of English ones.

There have been many Chinese surveys of deaf children in the last ten years: several of the most important are referred to in chapters 3 and 4. These are closely related to planning and monitoring the levels and effectiveness of rehabilitation services, and thus they focus on the quantifiable: typically, the population of deaf children in a given area, causes of deafness, levels of hearing aid use, access to rehabilitation facilities, and the number of deaf children who are able to enter mainstream schooling after speech training in the preschool period. On the whole, Chinese surveys do not inquire into parents' views and attitudes, perhaps because Chinese professionals assume they understand these and do not believe that special investigation is merited. With these Chinese surveys in mind, I also considered it important to obtain extensive basic information concerning the deaf children in the families I interviewed—cause of deafness, age at diagnosis, hearing aid use—since all these factors affect the course and nature of intervention and provide essential context. Ultimately, out of the 133 questions posed, 106 questions sought straightforward, factual information and 27 asked parents for their views, attitudes, reactions, or perceptions concerning a particular issue.

Personal accounts by parents of deaf children reveal in great detail their experiences at the various stages following the diagnosis of deafness in their child. Western parents of deaf children who have provided such accounts include Thomas and James Spradley (1978), Marcia Forecki (1985), Pauline Shaw (1985), Lorraine Fletcher (1987), and Kathy Robinson (1991). Of several articles I read relating the experiences of Chinese parents, I was particularly struck by an account by Zhou Hong, later principal of the nursery school for deaf children where I carried out my research, of bringing up his deaf daughter (Oblau 1993). He offers a vivid firsthand description of his persistent visits to one doctor after another and his search for a medical cure following the diagnosis of his daughter's deafness. This and other sources detailing the same pattern of parental behavior underlined the importance of questioning the parents on their consultation of doctors and the various medical treatments they tried for their child.

I considered incorporating a control group of Chinese families with preschool-age hearing children in the research design, but I was uncertain that I would be able to obtain access to such a group. As a result, I decided to focus on interviews with families with deaf children only. For information concerning the experiences and attitudes of parents with hearing children, I relied on documentary sources (see chapter 2); I also could draw on my own experience bringing up a preschool-age child in China. Still, a key question to keep in mind when analyzing the data is whether comments by the parents interviewed and by the parents who wrote the letters to Zhou Hong are particular to their experience as parents of deaf children or could also have been made by parents of hearing children; in most cases the answer is clear or can be deduced from the context.

Through contacts with a Chinese nongovernmental organization, the Amity Foundation, I was able to arrange visits to a rehabilitation center the foundation sponsors for preschool-age deaf children in Nanjing, a large city in eastern China. The principal of the center, Zhou Hong, and the senior teacher asked the parents or grandparents of the fourteen children attending the nursery school if they were willing to be interviewed: they all agreed. The interviews were conducted in November and December 1994 (I was in China from October to December 1994, and made further visits in 1996, 1997, and 1998); a detailed account of the circumstances under which the interviews were carried out is given in chapter 5.

I was in fact able to interview parents on a one-to-one basis in their own homes. There is no doubt I was fortunate to have this opportunity to talk with parents, as many social science researchers, especially when on short research visits to mainland China, find it difficult to get past official frameworks and institutions and arrange less formal, person-to-person interviews. Everything in these circumstances depends on personal contacts and the willingness of individual officials or professionals to facilitate and support an outside research initiative.

In addition to the interviews with parents of children at the center in Nanjing, I sought out as many other parents with deaf children as possible, although these interviews were not easy to arrange. Ultimately, five additional parents were interviewed in the city and seven in the countryside. Most of their children were older than the children in the preschool. Furthermore, the circumstances of the interviews varied—particularly in the countryside, where respondents were not interviewed on a one-to-one basis, the prepared interview questions had to be set aside in favor of a less structured conversation, and an interpreter was used because the local dialect was very different from the standard Chinese spoken in Nanjing. Nevertheless, these interviews provided very useful information: they enabled me to assess the representativeness of the views of the nursery school parents, affirmed the importance of certain key themes, and introduced more nuance into the picture.

Besides interviewing parents, who were the main focus of my study, I also talked with teachers, administrators, and staff at preschool rehabilitation centers and deaf schools in Beijing, Chongqing, and Nanjing. A morning spent at the Hexagon Well Primary School in Nanjing, which had accepted five deaf children into its first-year class, was particularly informative: the children themselves gave their views on their experience in school, and their teachers were also very helpful. I was also able to travel to the northern part of Jiangsu province to find out about some of the facilities for deaf children there, both in the town of Yancheng and in the surrounding countryside.

Certain problems are characteristic of all cross-cultural research. My knowledge of Chinese and my personal experience of living and working in China were useful in developing an understanding of the issues I was investigating; the background documentary study undertaken before the field research was also helpful in this respect.

Nevertheless, I am not Chinese—I am still essentially a cultural outsider and thus must address the question of the extent to which any outsider can accurately, sensitively, and fairly interpret data embedded in a cultural context in which he or she is a nonnative. For example, I became aware that my own attitudes toward deafness and deaf people, reinforced in the academic center in the United Kingdom where I was based, may have led me to assume that respondents in China had similar views and to underestimate how incapacitating and undesirable the Chinese perceive deafness to be (a perception that is of course common in other countries and cultures as well). After informally discussing the topic with several Chinese colleagues, I realized that I had to be more careful in interpreting evidence concerning attitudes toward deafness in China—without going to the other extreme and finding prejudice when there was little evidence for it. In general, I approached my research knowing I must be always cautious, cross-check the evidence, and be aware of how my own beliefs and attitudes might affect my interpretation of data.

At the same time, one can also argue that the position of a cultural outsider has certain advantages, as Kleinman and Lin (1981) maintain in their discussion of social research in Chinese communities. What the insider may take for granted, as natural or inevitable occurrences, can appear striking to the researcher who has experience of alternative cultural practices with which to contrast them. For example, it seemed very significant to me that parents of deaf children met only when convened by nursery school staff: they had no organized cooperative or mutual support system independent of educational institutions. Yet a Chinese researcher familiar with this cultural pattern might well have passed it over as unexceptional (conversely, a Chinese researcher studying deaf children and their families in Western countries would probably perceive phenomena and patterns of behavior that would be invisible to native observers).

The reliability and validity of research findings must be evaluated. In addition, it is necessary to assess their generalizability—the extent to which findings from the research sample or samples can be assumed to be true of other similar populations. The key question here is how applicable the findings from the interviews and letters are to other families with preschool-age deaf children in China. The question arises with particular force for the study, based on in-depth interviews with parents because it involved a relatively small number of respondents.

In quantitative as well as qualitative research, the reliability of the results depends both on an appropriate and systematic research design and on its careful implementation. These should be described, so that the methodology of the study becomes transparent and open to evaluation by others. For this reason, I have detailed how information was acquired so that readers can assess whether it was obtained systematically and carefully and is therefore likely to be reliable. Establishing the reliability of factual information may be relatively straightforward, but information about people's attitudes has to be assessed differently: views and opinions are liable to vary, affected both by time and by circumstances (in particular, who is speaking to the respondent). Again, a systematic, consistent, and transparent research methodology tends to strengthen the credibility of findings concerning attitudes and experiences: in this case, in analyzing both the interviews and the letters we must consider specific contexts—for example, the relationship between the respondent and the interviewer or between the writer and the recipient of the letters. These issues are discussed further in chapters 5 and 6.

Data are considered "valid" if they accurately represent social reality. Validity is often associated with qualitative research, which focuses on the meanings of, connections between, and explanations for social phenomena rather than simply enumerating features of social life. It is possible to obtain very informative and valid data through qualitative studies with relatively small samples (Haralambos and Holborn 1991). Ideally, a study should give the researcher insight into the social reality or realities of the respondents as they themselves see it—not in terms of frameworks imposed by the researcher. In this respect the analysis of the letters arguably produces more strongly valid results than that of the interviews, since parents are expressing themselves in their own words, with their own emphases, unprompted by anyone outside the family. In addition, the letters convey the parents' private, most deeply felt concerns to someone who is also the parent of a deaf child, with whom they are likely to be able to communicate most honestly and unreservedly. However, the letters tend to be short, providing a limited amount of information—they reveal key facts about the family's situation with regard to their deaf child and make clear the parents' main preoccupations, but they are silent about many details that a researcher might like to know. By contrast, interviews that systematically cover a broad range of topics produce more comprehensive information, thereby providing a fuller picture of parents' circumstances and their response to them. That fuller picture in itself contributes to validity, since it lessens the possibility that the researcher will draw false conclusions because relevant or possibly relevant factors were not considered; this argument is likely to be especially significant when the researcher is undertaking original research in a different cultural context.

The two studies taken together are significantly more informative than either study considered alone. This process, whereby different methodological approaches to a research topic allow cross-checking of the data as well as an increase in the level of insight, is sometimes referred to as "triangulation," a term borrowed from the field of land surveying; by looking at something from different angles, we obtain a better overall view (McNeill 1990). Triangulation effectively increases research validity and reliability.

When we evaluate the representativeness and generalizability of results of qualitative studies, it is useful to employ the idea of "fit"; that is, results and conclusions based on a study of one context can be generalized to another if the second context matches the first closely in key characteristics. Such an approach requires careful contextualization, which makes possible subsequent generalization (or qualified generalization) of the results to other similar populations and similar contexts (Schofield 1993). Using this reasoning, we can generalize from the conclusions reached in this research to other groups of parents with deaf children if key characteristics of the parents, their children, and their access to rehabilitation services all match. The parents interviewed in the first study and most of the parents who wrote the letters analyzed in the second study were living in urban areas rather than in the countryside; they were on the whole well-educated, middle-income families rather than poor and uneducated. Both groups of parents had children who were preschoolers at the time, although there was a significant difference in the children's ages—the average age of children whose parents were interviewed was 5.8 years (range 3.8 to 7.0 years); the average age of the children whose parents wrote letters was 2.6 years (range 0.7 to 7.0 years). Thus their attitudes and opinions reflect their different experiences: those interviewed had a child attending a rehabilitation center, while most parents writing letters were at an earlier stage, sooner after diagnosis and before any experience with rehabilitation services. Assuming that parents' socioeconomic circumstances, level of education, and place of residence (urban/rural) are key defining characteristics, and comparing the findings of my studies with the information presented in chapters 2 to 4, I believe that the findings from the interview data and from the analysis of letters are broadly representative of the views and attitudes of well-educated, urban Chinese parents with preschool-age deaf children.

A couple of final observations need to be made. I assume that many readers of this book, whether they are audiologists, teachers, researchers, or parents of deaf children, are familiar with deaf education in the West. They may perceive that many difficulties and shortcomings noted regarding the situation of young deaf children in China, often by Chinese professionals themselves, have still to be adequately addressed in Western countries: early diagnosis and intervention for *all* deaf children, for example, and optimal early development of language in profoundly deaf children of hearing parents. I do not intend this book as criticism of one society; the focus on China may draw attention away from circumstances in other countries, but many of the core issues and challenges faced by those involved in deaf education are universal.

CHAPTER TWO

THE CHINESE FAMILY AND THE DEAF CHILD

To understand how the presence of a deaf child affects the Chinese family, we need to understand the nature of Chinese families in general. The family system has been central to Chinese culture for thousands of years, and while certain key characteristics have persisted, significant social and political events in the last hundred years have had a tremendous impact on family life.

The traditional Chinese family was patriarchal, with power invested in the most senior male member of the family; paternalistic, in that individual responsibility was subsumed under the authority of the head of the family; and patrilocal, in that women after marriage left their own families to enter the household of their husbands. Direct descent was traced through the male, and the most important relationship was not between husband and wife but between parent and child — more specifically, between father and son (Jenner 1992). Although modern Chinese families, especially in urban areas, may seem to operate very differently, the influence of this pattern is still pervasive, particularly the principle of male dominance.

Traditionally, the ideal family was considered to consist of five generations under one roof, with many children, grandchildren, and great-grandchildren to testify to the wealth and prosperity of the family. In fact, only wealthier families could realize that ideal. The vast majority of Chinese families were poverty-stricken and were more likely to live in households consisting only of parents and children, perhaps with grandparents as well. Poverty severely limited family size, not only because of disease and malnutrition but also because parents were compelled to get rid of children they could not support; unwanted children were killed as infants, abandoned, sold, or given away for adoption (Baker 1979).

Male children were considered particularly valuable because they could be relied on to take care of their parents in old age, ensure the continuity of the family line with their own male children, and honor preceding generations through ancestor worship. The individual male was seen as a link in the chain of successive generations: he was responsible for looking after his parents, the preceding generation, as well as his own children, who would be the next generation. Thus there was a cycle of reciprocity and care within the family, since adults who cared for their children would in turn be cared for by them in their old age.

Female children, by contrast, could not carry out these crucial functions because they were lost to their natal family at marriage (it was assumed that all daughters would marry). Generally female children were regarded as a burden, since they had to be fed and raised until they were of marriageable age. Because female infants were seen as less valuable than male ones, female infanticide was widespread among the poor. The first daughter born into a poor peasant family might be saved, but subsequent daughters were usually drowned at birth. If a couple had more sons than they could support, however, the infant boy was more likely to be given away to be adopted, preferably by a close relative such as the father's brother. For childless couples the adoption of a son ensured the continuation of their family line.

The key cultural and philosophical influence on the Chinese family has been Confucianism; the "five relationships" (*wu lun*) of Confucian tradition came to govern the relationships within the extended family. The five relationships were, in order of importance,

1. ruler and minister
2. father and son
3. husband and wife
4. elder brother and younger brother
5. friend and friend

Mencius, the second great philosopher in the Confucian tradition, wrote in the fourth century B.C.E.: "There should be affection between father and son, righteous sense of duty between ruler and minister, division of function between man and wife, stratification between old and young, and good faith between friends" (qtd. in Baker 1979, 11). Mencius held that a man's moral character, as represented by the Confucian concept of "benevolence" (*ren*), was exemplified and demonstrated most fully in the parent-child relationship (Mencius 1970).

The five relationships were conceived as, and then developed into, a system that classified every human contact and determined the duties and obligations (and thus the behavior) of the individuals within a given relationship. Four of the *wu lun* are between dominant and subordinate partners; Confucian tradition legitimized the authority of the dominant partner. The fifth relationship, that between friends, was based on a relationship between equals but had considerably less importance than the others in daily life.

The traditional Chinese extended family thus had a prescribed hierarchy, with the eldest male at the head. Younger generations were subordinate to older generations; within generations younger siblings and their wives were subordinate to older siblings and their wives; and women were subordinate to their husbands. Lesser family members were expected to submit to the authority of more senior members, especially the head of the family, and if necessary sacrifice their own interests for the overall benefit of the family.

Twentieth-Century Changes in the Traditional Chinese Family

In twentieth-century mainland China, successive political movements have tended to reduce the size and power of the traditional extended family. The powers of government have increased, and the role of the individual has also become more prominent (Baker 1979). Family structure has been significantly affected by urbanization and modernization as well.

In the first decades of the twentieth century, political reformers saw that if China was to become a strong and unified nation, it was essential to reform the feudal system—including the family. A modern state could be built only if individuals were freed from the stranglehold of family allegiances and obligations and if they mobilized their efforts and abilities for the interests of the state. To achieve significant social reform, feudal practices perpetuated through the family—particularly those maintaining women's subjugation, such as arranged marriages, concubinage, and payment of bride-price — had to be eradicated. However, efforts at reform had little effect until the advent of the Chinese Communist Party.

Beginning in 1931 the Communist Party initiated key changes in the status of women in areas under its political control. Equality of men and women was promoted in legislation supporting free choice of partners in marriage as well as freedom to divorce; the beginnings of land reform, giving women the right to own land, also contributed to their independence and autonomy. There were urgent pragmatic reasons to support female emancipation and organize women's groups: Communist leaders regarded mobilization of women as crucial to support the war effort against the Nationalist forces that followed the end of Japanese occupation in 1945. For example, women were needed to carry out agricultural work while men were fighting (Davin 1976; Kane 1987).

After gaining control of the whole country in 1949, the new Communist government issued the 1950 Marriage Law of the People's Republic of China. This established principles on "the free choice of partners, on monogamy, on equal rights for both sexes, and on the protection of the lawful interests of women and children" (Baker 1979, 183). But not all tradition was abandoned: the law also confirmed parents' responsibility to rear and educate their children, and children's duty to care for their parents. As Baker points out, while eradicating many of the unjust patriarchal features of the feudal family system, the 1950 Marriage Law actually validated the importance of the nuclear family, composed of a couple and their children, and underlined the mutual responsibilities of family members.

Land reforms had an equally far-reaching and transformative impact on families. The 1950 Land Reform Law mandated confiscation of land from private landlords, effectively breaking up large feudal family units. Because land was reallocated on an individual basis, women and junior family members received the same amount as family heads, ensuring more equitable relationships within the family. The 1950s subsequently saw a process of transfer of land to public ownership: first in cooperatives, then farming collectives, and finally large-scale communes, which typically had populations of 20,000 to 50,000 people. In order to relieve women of child-care and food preparation tasks, communal nurseries and canteens were set up; Baker (1979) argues that this era of communal living posed a critical threat to the institution of the family.

A further assault on the traditional structures and values of family life came a decade later with the advent of the Cultural Revolution (1966–76). The first three years of this period were characterized by intense political upheaval and violent social disruption spearheaded by the activities of the Red Guards, young people who were themselves being manipulated by political factions in the leadership; the core institution of family life was greatly damaged. The overt aims of the Cultural Revolution were to radically transform education and culture in China; the country's leader, Mao Zedong, explicitly encouraged young people to challenge authority, including their teachers. Education was severely disrupted; between 1968 and 1975 ten million urban young people were sent to the countryside (Cleverley 1985). Families were torn apart as children criticized and attacked their parents. Those same children, now in their forties, have experienced the bitter effects of lost educational opportunities, and are especially motivated to ensure that their children receive a good education (Davin 1990a).

As part of extensive economic reforms undertaken in the early 1980s, the government phased out communal farming methods and initiated a system of household responsibility, whereby families sell their produce on the open market after contributing a set quota to the state. The welfare of elderly and disabled family members has now devolved solely on the family; the collective no longer offers any support. Croll (1983) describes how the status of women has been diminished in some respects—for example, it is now to families' economic advantage to stop daughters' education after only a few years of schooling so that they can work on the family plot or look after livestock. However, Greenhalgh (1992) argues that a decade of economic change in the countryside has also weakened authority relations in rural families and given younger family members and women more autonomy and opportunity to exercise their own initiative.

Urban and rural lifestyles differ greatly, and family structure, roles, and relationships are correspondingly different. Over a quarter of the Chinese population now live in urban areas, and this proportion will increase as the Chinese economy grows rapidly. Families living in large towns and cities tend to live in smaller family units—a couple with the one child they are currently permitted under the national birth control policy, with grandparents often living nearby. Sons are less important to guarantee security in old age because parents working in state enterprises are entitled to pensions; in cities many parents value daughters as highly as sons, will invest just as much in their education, and have as high aspirations for their future (Croll 1995; Davin 1995). Rural families, in contrast, operate as individual economic units that depend on the labor of family members for survival and on children for security in old age: children are still viewed largely in terms of their economic value to the family.[1] Rural families tend to have more children; they are also more likely to have grandparents living in the household. But whether in the city or the countryside, the Chinese family, although smaller than the traditional kinship unit of a century ago, is still very strong; family members give crucial support to one another, particularly through the obligations of the parent-child relationship.

Chinese Families with Disabled Family Members

In China, the welfare of individual citizens is the concern first and foremost of their families. The family is expected to look after all members that are elderly, sick, or disabled; any intervention by state services is secondary. The official view, expressed by Vice Minister Zhang, is that "socialist welfare services are seen as a supplement to family care and not a substitute for it" (qtd. in Sydenham 1993, 13). In some circumstances, local welfare services do step in: for example, elderly people without children are guaranteed food, clothing, shelter, medical care, and burial expenses (Chen Sheying 1996), and there are old people's homes provided by the community. Orphans and sick or disabled people without families are similarly protected. However, if elderly people do have children, those children are obligated by law to support them.

Influenced by centuries of Confucianism, the Chinese people respect conformity and value control of behavior, especially behavior directed at people outside the family; one's self-respect depends on the "face" presented to others. Family problems are kept within the family to avoid attracting idle comment and social contempt (Bond and Hwang 1986). According to one popular saying, "family ugliness should never be aired in public" (*jia chou bu ke wai yang*). The presence of a disabled child in the family is a serious threat to the family's face: family members contain this threat by refusing to discuss the child and by keeping him or her hidden away at home. Lucy Ching, for example, a blind woman who grew up in Hong Kong, writes of never being included in family outings as a child because her parents were ashamed of her; she describes other blind children being similarly treated (1980). Parents fear that the family will be regarded as tainted, harming the marriage prospects of siblings and other family members. Such efforts to conceal the existence of a child from outsiders may prevent remedial measures from being started early enough. A rural couple with a deaf six-year-old son whom I met during fieldwork in 1996 had wanted to buy a hearing aid and start speech training when he was three; but the paternal grandparents forbade this, saying they did not want other people to know their grandchild was deaf.

As in other countries, there appears to be a hierarchy of disabilities in China. A high degree of stigma is attached to mental illness (Phillips 1993); deafness, whether in children or adults, seems to be less stigmatized. Perhaps deaf people experience relatively less discrimination because they look like other people and are generally recognized as physically and intellectually capable despite the problems of communication. Nevertheless, a Chinese friend told me that some hard-of-hearing adults in China take care to remove their hearing aids in formal situations when they wish to present themselves well, in other words, when they wish to appear without "defect." During my fieldwork interviewing urban parents with deaf children in 1994, I found at least one family who removed their child's hearing aid when they went out in public because they did not want other people to notice and comment. Some parents I interviewed felt self-conscious about their children's voices and tried to keep them quiet when they were in public. I was told by a senior teacher at Nanjing Deaf School, who is herself deaf, that deaf signing adults are careful to suppress their facial expressions in the presence of hearing people "because they do not wish to attract attention." Such accounts indicate that deaf people themselves, and families with deaf children, are conscious of the stigmatizing features of deafness — hearing aids, the involuntary cries of deaf children, facial expressions accompanying signing — and may adapt their behavior in order to "pass" in certain public situations.[2]

In a detailed and very useful study of the impact of disabled family members on Chinese families, Phillips (1993) examines the coping strategies used to support them. He focuses on urban patients affected by schizophrenia, a condition that tends to start in adolescence or early adulthood. Phillips notes that the schizophrenic person has a severe impact on the family's economic circumstances: the patient's earning power is reduced; a family member, usually the mother, has to curtail work to care for him or her; and large amounts of money are spent seeking a cure for the illness. Most unmarried schizophrenic patients live with their parents, who exert a great deal of control over their lives. Since there are no social workers, parents are on their own in pleading that their child be allowed to stay in school or at work and in applying for medical and disability payments from their child's work unit if her or she is employed. Parents make every effort to arrange a marriage for their son or daughter, sometimes by concealing the illness from the potential spouse; typically a person of lower social status is chosen. Lin and Lin (1981) argue that parents of mentally ill sons hope that marriage will bring them male grandchildren, while parents of mentally ill daughters hope that marriage will rid them of an onerous responsibility; Phillips, however, finds that regardless of the child's sex, the parents are motivated primarily by the desire to relinquish responsibility. If grandchildren are born the grandparents may take over their care on the grounds that the mentally ill father or mother is not a fit parent.

In dealing with the severe social stigma of mental illness, families are torn between the need to obtain effective professional help and the wish to avoid publicly shaming the family (Phillips 1993). A typical response is to delay contact with psychiatric services until all possibilities suggested by the family's informal social network have been exhausted. And once the patient has begun receiving psychiatric treatment and medication, families may conceal the fact of mental illness even from close relatives or the individual's employer. In a discussion of the help-seeking behavior of Chinese families with psychiatrically ill members, Lin and Lin (1982) describe the reluctance with which the family consults outsiders; individuals with closer ties to the family are consulted first:

> Only when they find that their own material or knowledge resources and skills have not proved effective in solving the problem, will the family bring in outsiders. However, this process of seeking outside help is a cautious one and ex-

pands in concentric circles to include relatives, elders of the community[,] . . . school teachers and other trusted friends who the family regard as equal to their relatives. Their views on the etiology of mental illness are considered and their advice on treatment valued. The weight of such consultation increases with time in selecting treatment modalities, in inverted relationship to the failure of the efforts of intrafamilial coping. (392)

The family-oriented behaviors dictated by traditional Confucian standards and those encouraged by more modern patterns that place high value on individual effort and economic success are fundamentally in conflict (Phillips 1993). Families with a schizophrenic son or daughter feel compelled to revert to more traditional patterns, fulfilling the obligation to care for their children at the expense of their aspirations toward a better life and economic success. However, parents are caught in a trap: their children will not be able to complete the traditional cycle of reciprocal obligations by supporting them in their old age. In a society in which the state provides little help and the welfare of elderly people depends on their children, parents of children with mental illness or other major disabilities may face a bleak old age. The advent of the one-child-per-family policy has made it unusual for urban families to have more than one child (see below), so it is increasingly unlikely that there will be another child in the family who can support them.

The Family and Civil Society

The changes in China over the last century may have given greater emphasis to the individual and greater powers to state institutions, but there have been few alternative institutions to approach the importance of the family. Jenner (1992) argues that the marked distinction in China between the family or quasi-family structures, such as exist in schools or work units, and outsiders, or nonfamily, means that while individuals feel a strong sense of obligation to family members they have little commitment to anyone else, or to society in general: "in normal times there is only a weak sense of civic duty" (116).

Recent economic reforms have led to some significant changes in Chinese society, including the creation of new associations and institutions—for example, trade unions and business associations. However, their potential effectiveness is hampered by the tendency of the Chinese government to seek either to co-opt and control or to discourage and suppress independent nongovernmental organizations (White, Howell, and Shang 1996). These circumstances have important implications for the future of deaf children: in Britain and America, an enormous amount of constructive change has been brought about by the active campaigning of parents' organizations; in China, existing social structures do not favor such activity.[3]

Family Planning Policies and the Value of a Child

In the last twenty years family planning policies instituted by the Chinese government have transformed the size and nature of the Chinese family. Despite the official rhetoric of reform and equality, these policies explicitly incorporate traditional elements of social discrimination based on gender and disability.

Quantity Control: The One-Child Family Planning Policy

The Chinese government has encouraged limitation of family size since the 1950s. This policy was reversed in the early 1960s, when Mao Zedong declared that China could support a much larger population. However, by the end of the decade Chinese demographers realized that birth control was essential if China was to feed its own people and embark on planned development. Measures were introduced to encourage couples to have only one child, or at most two children. These included delaying marriage, spacing conception, and using birth control to limit the number of children born—the *wan xi shao* policy. As a result, the total fertility rate fell from 5.8 births per woman in 1970 to only 2.7 births in 1978 (Davin 1987). Yet planners saw China's development as still threatened by further population growth. Thus in 1979 the Chinese government introduced a more stringent family planning policy, still in effect, that permits each couple to have only one child. There is no national law; individual provinces and municipalities have issued their own regulations, which vary with local conditions. A number of incentives support couples who pledge to have only one child, and a range of fines and other penalties are levied on couples who have two or more children.

Most regional regulations specify exemptions to the one-child rule. For example, ethnic minority couples are permitted to have two or even three children, as one element of national policy favoring the ethnic minorities;[4] rural couples who are both single children are allowed a second child. "Special circumstances" can qualify parents for exemption from the one-child rule: thus couples may be permitted to have a second child when the first child suffers from a nonhereditary handicap that will prevent him or her from working normally as an adult (Greenhalgh 1986; Davin 1987; "Birth Planning" 1988). In such cases parents can request permission to have a second child, and the decision is determined by the birth quota allotted to the parents' work unit or village district. If permission is granted, parents have to wait at least four years before having the second child.

Compliance with the one-child policy has been high in urban areas, where women are more easily monitored through their workplace; in addition, having one child is more compatible with the urban than the rural lifestyle and aspirations (Davin 1990a; Gates 1993; Milwertz 1997). Workers in state enterprises receive retirement pensions, so parents do not feel that they must have more children to support them in their old age. A 1982 survey of 2,000 urban families in Anhui province showed that a couple's likelihood of taking the one-child pledge rose with their level of education and income; compliance was also greater if the couple had a son (Population Research Office, Anhui University 1982). However, data from the 1982 One-per-Thousand National Fertility Sample Survey showed no significant son preference in the pattern of compliance to the one-child policy in Beijing and Shanghai, China's two largest cities (Arnold and Liu 1986); in their analysis of national population statistics for that period Arnold and Liu also found son preference to be lower among more educated women and in urban areas.[5] Many urban families now feel that daughters are as good as sons and devote just as much attention to them (Croll 1995); indeed, girls are often perceived as easier to bring up than boys, and they are believed to be more likely to keep in close touch and care for their parents when they grow up (Chai 1992).

The one-child policy has proved much harder to implement in rural areas, where three-quarters of the population live. As already noted, the economic reforms of the early 1980s abolished communal farming and made households responsible for their own work. Thus each household now depends on a male labor force, with sons growing up to support and later replace the adults: rural families regard two or three children — at least one a son — as essential. Without a welfare system to provide pensions, elderly couples are dependent on their sons, since married daughters still follow the custom of living with their in-laws.

These intense pressures to have a son encourage rural families to evade family planning regulations. Some parents rely on age-old methods of getting rid of unwanted daughters: giving them away for adoption, failing to report their birth, abandoning them, or resorting to infanticide. Others take advantage of modern technology, using an ultrasound examination to discover the sex of their unborn child and then aborting a female fetus. In the early 1980s the Chinese government, faced in rural areas with pervasive noncompliance with the one-child policy and inflammatory reports in Chinese newspapers of widespread female infanticide, relaxed the regulations. Central Document Seven, issued in 1984, permitted rural couples to have a second child if the first was a girl, thereby acknowledging and accommodating the cultural preference for male children (Greenhalgh 1986; Davin 1990b).

The effects of this policy are to distort family composition (Davin 1990b). If we assume that all peasant couples will have a second child if the first is a girl and that couples will have no more than two children, then — leaving aside the effects of female infanticide or sex-selective abortion — we expect to find three kinds of families: roughly half the families will have one son, a quarter will have one daughter and a younger son, and a quarter will have two daughters. No daughter will ever be an only child receiving all her parents' attention. In a family with a girl and a boy, she will receive less attention than her younger brother. If she has a sister, whatever resources the parents have to give their children will be equally divided between the two children. So even though this policy may help prevent female infanticide, the resulting family structure continues to confirm the inferior status of daughters and to ensure that parents invest less in them than in sons.

In the 1980s and 1990s the one-child family policy has continued; and despite resistance, particularly in rural areas, it has dramatically curbed population growth. Its effectiveness can be attributed to the sustained political pressure, the resources devoted to family planning programs, and the great attention given to implementation at every level. In addition, increasing economic prosperity and improvements in maternal and child health have made the policy easier for many to accept. These changes have been accompanied by a growing consideration for the quality of family life—in particular, contemporary parents are more interested in investing in their children's education, including higher education (Greenhalgh, Zhu, and Li 1993). However, the costs of the one-child policy are also recognized: there is great concern that only children, spoiled by being the sole focus of their parents' and grandparents' attention, will grow up to be selfish and unwilling to contribute to society. It is also unclear how a generation of only children will be able to support parents and parents-in-law in their old age, as both law and custom still hold children responsible for their elderly parents' welfare.

Another effect of the one-child policy has been to exacerbate discrimination against female infants. The sex ratio at birth—in other words, the ratio of male babies to female ones—has increased steadily since the one-child policy came into force. There is a natural imbalance at birth of about 106:100, but in 1992 the ratio for the whole of China (disregarding regional variations) was 118:100: thus there were 1.7 million "missing girls" (Kristof 1993).[6] Sex ratios at birth are generally lower in the major cities, higher in towns, and highest in the countryside. Hull (1990) puts forward three explanations for the "missing girls": female infanticide, failure of parents to report female births (so that they can try again),[7] and sex-selective abortion following an ultrasound scan. Johansson and Nygren (1991), on the basis of 1987 population survey figures, argue that about half the missing girls can be accounted for by adoption by childless couples. Most adoptions are of infants, and most are unofficial and unregistered (Greenhalgh and Li 1993).

According to a team headed by Professor Zeng Yi of the Institute of Population Research at Beijing University, the main reasons for the increasing sex ratio are underreporting of female births and the practice of sex-selective abortion: they consider female infanticide a less significant factor now (Zeng Y. et al. 1993). Ultrasound machines have been used in China in hospitals and clinics for the last twenty years or so to monitor fetal growth and check for obvious abnormalities such as spina bifida. Since the early 1980s family planning authorities have been aware that they were being used to determine the sex of the unborn child, and this practice was outlawed. However, it is almost impossible to stop, as Zeng et al. explain: medical personnel are vulnerable to bribes or the demands of friends and relatives, and information on the sex of the fetus can easily be conveyed to parents without official knowledge. Given the widespread availability of ultrasound technology in China and the strength of son preference, they predict further increase in the use of ultrasound equipment for sex selection.

The marked rise in selective abortion of female fetuses, particularly in rural areas, has occurred despite government condemnation and opposition; it indicates not only that cultural discrimination against girls continues but also that abortion is widely accepted among the general population as a means of getting rid of an unwanted child. Abortion is readily available at government clinics, where it is a routine backup method of birth control when contraception has failed. One cross-cultural study of attitudes to euthanasia and abortion in the United States and China observes: "Though it may be considered to be morally wrong to have an abortion in the eyes of many people in the U.S., it appears that a majority of people in the PRC consider it morally right or at least acceptable to have an abortion" (Lee et al. 1996, 143). Drawing on data from students in both countries, Lee et al. found that the Chinese participants were more likely to favor infanticide of severely disabled babies and to believe that abortion was necessary to control population; the more educated they were, the more likely they were to favor abortion. The significantly different attitudes toward abortion in the two countries appear to be related to demographic as well as cultural factors.

Given the high level of discrimination against daughters in China, especially in rural areas, the widespread practice of sex-selective abortion may also be seen by couples as a lesser evil than the psychologically and morally repugnant act of killing a newborn baby; and in practical terms, infanticide—also a criminal act—is difficult to conceal (see Zeng Yi et al. 1993). This is not to say that individual women necessarily abort female babies willingly. They may be under intense pressure from their husband's family to have a son; if they give birth to a daughter they may be harshly criticized and treated badly (Davin 1987). In such circumstances they may have little choice in the matter.

Quality Control: Eugenic Family Planning Policies

Concomitant with family planning policies controlling population size, eugenic measures have emerged aimed at raising the quality of babies born; these are embodied in national law, the 1995 Maternal and Child Health Care Law. The preoccupation with "quality births" began in the late 1970s, when the one-child policy came into force (Banister 1984; Dikotter 1996). Government leaders emphasized the necessity for that one child to be healthy and intelligent; this coincided with parents' natural desire that their only child be a "quality" child. Officials also argued that the second births permitted to couples when their first child was disabled could be reduced if every first child was healthy (Banister 1984).

Policymakers were concerned with both *positive eugenics*—that is, measures to promote the birth of healthy infants, including good quality prenatal, obstetric, and infant health care—and *negative* or *preventive eugenics*—that is, the prevention or elimination of congenital defects, including genetically transmitted conditions. In the late 1970s and early 1980s the government focused on determining the number of "defective" people in China: surveys indicated there were between five and ten million mentally retarded people in the country ("Paying Great Attention" 1983; Banister 1984). The population of China was then one billion: thus about one percent were found to have mental handicaps, a relatively low figure.[8] However, these findings shocked Chinese scientists and leaders and persuaded them that preventive eugenic programs were essential. Their motivation was pragmatic: a healthy and productive population would best ensure a modern and prosperous China, and unproductive members of society burdened both their communities and the nation as a whole. Nevertheless, an editorial in the *People's Daily* affirmed, although every effort would be made to prevent the birth of congenitally defective babies, disabled adults such as mentally handicapped persons would be given proper care "out of humanitarian reasons" ("Chinese Population Policy" 1982). Efforts to eliminate defect from the population thus focus on the unborn child; official policies limit intervention to that which takes place before birth (Stone 1996).⁹ The 1990 Law for Disabled Persons states that children born alive with congenital defects should not be neglected or abandoned, and that disabled adults should be able to participate fully in their society.

In the 1980s several provinces implemented eugenic policies. In 1983 Jilin province introduced measures to prevent mentally retarded people from having children (Banister 1984). The 1987 Sichuan Family Planning Regulations state that couples with serious hereditary diseases, "such as psychosis, mental deficiency and malformation," must not be allowed to bear children; pregnancies that occur must be terminated ("Birth Planning" 1988, 372). Such policies have two aims: to avoid the transmission of hereditary defects and to prevent individuals deemed unfit to be parents from reproducing. These regulations also set up eugenic counseling centers at county level and above. In 1988 a wide-ranging policy was introduced in Gansu province forbidding individuals with severe mental illness, leprosy, AIDS, or sexually transmitted diseases as well as serious genetic conditions from having children; in Tibet similar legislation took effect in 1989. Given that both these provinces have large Tibetan populations, these measures can be viewed as deliberately discouraging the propagation of non-Han races. The association of poor genetic quality with ethnic minority groups was confirmed by the Chinese minister of health, Chen Minzhang: at the National People's Congress in 1993, he stated that the problem of "inferior births" was most severe among the "ethnic minorities, frontier peoples, and economically poor areas" (O'Brien 1995). In this statement three separate factors are conflated and all are linked with genetic defects. Thus ethnic minorities are often regarded as inherently, or genetically, inferior when in fact many of the observed problems probably result from economic disadvantage.

Consanguineous marriage—that is, marriage between second or first cousins—has been identified by Chinese experts as contributing significantly to the incidence of genetic defect. Marriages between first cousins were commonplace among the Han population before 1939 (Bittles 1994). There appears to be little systematic data available on the overall prevalence and patterns of consanguineous marriage in China since 1949; however, the relatively high incidence of congenital defect and mental retardation found in poor border regions and remote mountain areas, where minority groups live, has been linked with consanguinity and has revived concern at the prevalence of consanguineous marriage (Banister 1984; Bittles 1994). Since 1949, marriage legislation has prohibited marriage with close relatives; the 1981 Marriage Law confirmed the prohibition out to third cousins. Data from countries where consanguineous marriage is valued and practiced extensively—India, Saudi Arabia, and Turkey—indicate it is commonest in rural areas where people are poor and less well educated. The health of children of consanguineous marriages must be assessed in comparison with that of children from similar socioeconomic circumstances; otherwise, the genetic effects of intermarriage will be confused with the damage to maternal and child health caused by poverty, ignorance, and disease (Bittles 1994). In China, consanguinity has been identified as a cause of disability even though such studies have not been carried out.

The 1995 Law of the People's Republic of China on Maternal and Child Health Care, proposed to the Chinese National People's Congress in 1993 by Health Minister Chen as a "National Eugenics Program" to deal with the urgent problem of "births of inferior quality," went into effect on 1 June 1995.[10] Its official aims are "ensuring the health of mothers and infants and improving the quality of the newborn population." The first section of the law focuses on providing better health-care facilities for mothers and infants throughout the country. The second section deals with premarital health care, including compulsory medical examinations to be undergone by prospective marriage partners "to see whether they suffer from any disease that may have an adverse effect on marriage and childbearing." These are "genetic diseases of a serious nature, target infectious diseases, and relevant mental diseases."[11] "Genetic diseases of a serious nature" are defined as "diseases that are caused by genetic factors congenitally, that may totally or partially deprive the victim of the ability to live independently, that are highly possible to recur in generations to come, and that are medically considered inappropriate for reproduction." The last phrase in the definition is open to interpretation, which apparently is left ultimately to medical professionals. When an individual is found to have a genetic disease of a serious nature, as defined above, he or she may be permitted to marry only after agreeing to long-term contraception or sterilization.

Other articles mandate medical procedures. When genetic disease of a serious nature is detected or suspected in a married person of childbearing age, the couple concerned are required to follow the doctor's advice, which although not specified would presumably be to avoid conception or abort the fetus if the wife is pregnant. When fetal abnormality is suspected, a medical examination and diagnosis should be carried out; when an abnormality is detected during prenatal examination, "the physician shall explain to the married couple and give them medical advice for a termination of pregnancy if one of the following cases is suspected: (1) the fetus is suffering from genetic disease of a serious nature; (2) the fetus has a defect of a serious nature; and (3) continued pregnancy may threaten the life and safety of the pregnant woman or seriously impair her health due to the serious disease she suffers from." Although these measures underline the authority of the doctor in deciding whether to proceed with sterilization or termination of a pregnancy, the law stipulates that the person concerned should agree to the procedure, as demonstrated by a signature. A couple who have already had one child with a serious defect must avail themselves of genetic counseling.

Of the thirty-nine articles in the 1995 Law on Maternal and Child Health Care, six are concerned with preventing the transmission of genetic defects; the remainder are directed at improving maternal and infant health care, administrative measures, and so on. Thus it is a distortion to depict the new law as primarily concerned with negative eugenic policy, as some in the Western press seem to have done—for example, in coverage in the London *Times* (Hawkes 1995); Dikotter (1996, 1998) also takes an essentially hostile view. Others have pointed out that the law will greatly improve basic health care for mothers and children by mandating financial support for health centers at the local level (Hesketh 1996). The law also requires improved data collection regarding children born with congenital defects.

The argument for eugenic policies in China seems to have been fueled, particularly in its early stages, by a wish to prevent mentally retarded people from reproducing: proponents assume that mental handicaps are genetically transmitted. Since mental retardation in China is caused largely by poor nutrition, notably severe iodine deficiency, as well as by other environmental circumstances such as poor health care, their assumption does not hold. Inappropriate emphasis is placed on preventive eugenic strategies rather than on basic health-care measures to improve nutrition, upgrade obstetric and pediatric services, and provide rehabilitation for disabled children and adults. Similarly, children born with impairments such as deafness or blindness may have been affected by maternal infection during pregnancy, lack of oxygen or injury at birth, or other nongenetic factors; applying eugenic measures to these individuals as adults, or to their families, would clearly be inappropriate. It is often difficult or even impossible to identify the exact etiology of a disability, even in countries where the most advanced technology is available. Congenital deafness is a case in point—ascertaining its cause or causes can be very difficult.[12] Under these circumstances, efforts to fully implement China's eugenic legislation are bound to be fraught with ethical and practical problems. Lack of resources, especially the high level of medical expertise and sophisticated facilities required to support genetic investigation across the nation, will probably seriously hamper the law's implementation. Other difficulties are also likely: for example, individuals may hide relevant medical details in order to preserve their right to have children (Banister 1984).

Even applied to those conditions known to have a genetic basis, the rhetoric of engineering genetic purity through eugenic birth policies is at odds with the realities of genetic expression, which are very complex. The rationale invoked by the 1995 law is based on a model of straightforward transmission from parents to child by a dominant gene. However, many genetic conditions—for example, most types of hereditary deafness—are transmitted by recessive genes. There may be no family history of deafness and thus no suspicion that a particular couple carry these recessive genes; they are unlikely to be referred for genetic screening or counseling before having children. Some genetic conditions are determined by an array of genes whose expression is complicated and can be predicted only with sophisticated analysis, if at all. And because human genes slowly but spontaneously mutate, new and unpredictable defects continue to emerge.

The exact categories of genetic defect to be targeted have not been adequately identified or defined in the 1995 legislation, so local interpretations may vary somewhat, in accordance with particular social circumstances. Such variability makes inappropriate application of the preventive eugenic measures more likely, and points to the need for clear guidelines. However, while advances in knowledge about the genetic conditions and how they affect individuals are important, they also can be dangerous: if eugenic legislation contained strict definitions of the abnormalities or genetic conditions, leeway for making decisions in individual cases might be severely limited. In the United Kingdom, for example, a definitive list of targeted genetic abnormalities has not been drawn up precisely to avoid implying that certain abnormalities should automatically or probably lead to an abortion (Kent 1998).[13]

Some Western critics of the 1995 Maternal and Child Health Care Law are concerned that coercion may be used in its implementation. Although the law requires the patient's voluntary consent before a pregnancy is terminated on the grounds of fetal abnormality, critics question how much choice parents will in fact have. Dikotter is among them, arguing that "the coercive implementation of birth-control programmes indicates that eugenic legislation will be carried out without any respect for couples' wishes" (1996, 4). It may be parents will have little choice. But China's birth-control regulations demand a much greater level of sacrifice than does the eugenic policy: most Chinese families would like more than one child, but few mainland Chinese couples would wish to have a child with a disability if they could avoid it. Indeed, the one-child policy makes it more likely that parents would willingly take measures to ensure that their only child is perfect. Just as the birth-control policies have exacerbated discrimination against daughters, so they make giving birth to a disabled child seem even more undesirable. To be sure, in some cases the parents' wishes and the views of medical personnel may conflict—for example, couples with a family history of a genetic condition may avoid or resist medical advice not to have children. They may wish to take a chance, believing that a child with a disability would be better than no child at all.

Also highly controversial is the sterilization of mentally handicapped persons, the area on which eugenic policies in China were first focused. It seems likely that the rights of those with mental handicaps are being routinely ignored, as they have been in many Western countries. In Sweden, 60,000 people were sterilized over a period of fifty years because they were deemed to be genetically inferior; the program ended only in 1976. In Austria, it is still the practice to sterilize mentally handicapped men and women without their consent ("Scandal" 1997). In the United States, involuntary sterilization of mentally defective persons is explicitly authorized in fourteen states and when challenged the practice has been upheld in others; the grounds are usually the "best interests" of the person concerned, as determined by parents and professionals, but genetic reasons are invoked in nine states (Pfeiffer 1994). Pfeiffer also notes that in the United States strict laws regulate marriages of mentally handicapped people. Details on China's programs to sterilize mentally handicapped people are hard to obtain—for example, whether parental consent is involved, and what criteria are used to decide on sterilization. Much more information is necessary before we can fully understand the effects of this aspect of China's eugenic policy.

Western criticism of the preventive eugenic measures in the Maternal and Child Health Care Law has not gone unnoticed by the Chinese government (as the rewording of sensitive sections of the law indicates). Such criticism can have mixed effects, however. In 1995, international outcry followed revelations of the miserable conditions in Chinese orphanages filled with thousands of abandoned (mostly female) infants; the Western press claimed there was an official policy of allowing some babies in orphanages to die from neglect ("Orphanage Row" 1996). One immediate consequence of the adverse publicity was that some welfare organizations active in China found that relations with Chinese contacts became very strained, and work on their projects ground to a halt. Other major welfare organizations working in China, calling the criticism misplaced and counterproductive, stated that the root problem was severe underfunding of orphanages by the government. But the focus on conditions in orphanages also has led to some positive action: for example, UNICEF (the United Nations Children's Fund) has become involved in training staff and establishing procedural guidelines in orphanages. This incident suggests that perhaps more might be accomplished if informed sources such as nongovernmental Chinese organizations and foreign welfare organizations working in China are consulted before a major attack on government policy is considered.

The eugenic policy embodies the position of the Chinese state on disability, which is consonant with mainstream cultural attitudes. The policy also confirms the instrumental status of individuals in Chinese society: because citizens are valued by the state primarily for their productivity, disabled persons are worth less. A similarly instrumental view has traditionally been taken of children, whose benefits have been seen primarily in terms of their potential economic contribution to the family—not in terms of the emotional pleasure they may bring.

Families with Deaf Children and the Decision to Have a Second Child

Whether deafness is congenital or acquired, it is often not diagnosed in China before age two or three, when parents realize their child is slow to speak. Thus deaf children are less likely than those with visible disabilities to be abandoned or neglected in infancy. However, at least a small number of deaf children are rejected by their parents: a Swedish delegation visiting a Children's Welfare Institute in Shanghai noted several deaf children there (Liljestrom et al. 1982); an orphanage in Nanjing has one or two girls abandoned by their parents because of their deafness (Pan Le, conversation with author, 1994).

In most areas family planning regulations permit parents with a disabled child a second child, provided that the disability is not hereditary. In the case of deafness, if the parents are close relatives, or if there is a family history of deafness or other evidence that the deafness is genetic, *they cannot have a second child*. It is therefore crucial for parents to know the cause of deafness: but as we have seen, the cause is often impossible to determine, even with access to the best facilities. In their uncertainty, parents are apt to deny the possibility of genetic causation and have a second child, despite the risk that the second child may also be deaf. The China Rehabilitation Research Center for Deaf Children in Beijing (China's national center for developing model technological and educational approaches for the rehabilitation of preschool-age deaf children, hereafter called the CRR Center for Deaf Children) is actively investigating prenatal testing for genetic deafness that can be offered to parents who already have one genetically deaf child and would wish to abort an affected fetus. In light of recent advances in identifying the genes responsible for some forms of deafness, such testing will probably become available within a few years. It seems likely that Chinese parents themselves will demand it.

The urban lifestyle—parents working full-time, housing space at a premium, and grandparents often living far away—does not easily accommodate couples rearing two children. Furthermore, the cost, including education and health care, may be prohibitive. Thus there are strong incentives for couples who already have a disabled child not to take advantage of the exemption in the family planning regulations. In urban areas, deaf children are relatively well provided for: deaf schools provide education and welfare factories (which hire quotas of disabled workers) ensure paid employment. New rehabilitation centers, providing preschool aural/oral training for deaf children, are developing rapidly. Parents may prefer to invest in their deaf child rather than try for a second, particularly since the rehabilitation centers require heavy parental involvement as speech training teachers for their children; there may not seem to be enough time to devote to the needs of two children. Parents also must weigh their desire for a son, if their deaf child is a daughter — and as we have seen, for many urban parents the traditional preference for a son has lost much of its strength — as well as their attitude toward their child's deafness.

Almost no parents with deaf children attending the CRR Center for Deaf Children seek permission to have a second child, apparently at least in part because they have access to much better special education than is available elsewhere; the proportion of parents who have a second child is somewhat higher in the center's outlying rural center for deaf children — around 10 percent — and in the provincial rehabilitation centers, where it is more than 10 percent. An educational administrator at the center states that in his experience a higher level of education and a higher standard of living are key factors associated with the decision not to have a second child; younger parents are also more likely to have only one child, reflecting a generational shift away from the more instrumental view of children. Thus better-educated parents in favorable socioeconomic circumstances who know that their child can receive a good education are most likely to invest in one child, even if the child is deaf.

Parents of deaf children who decide not to have a second child, and who concentrate their resources on bringing up their deaf child, may come to be a force for constructive change. Just as urban parents of daughters will object to their being discriminated against in education or employment and will fight for their daughters' interests (Davin 1995), so we can expect parents of deaf children to expend a great deal of effort on improving opportunities for their children. In particular, they are likely to put pressure on school authorities to integrate their hearing-impaired children into local primary schools.

Rural families have retained an instrumental view of children and a strong preference for sons. Thus the decision of rural parents to have a second child if the first is deaf is likely to be strongly influenced by the gender of the first child, as well as by the family's economic circumstances. Both the birth of a daughter and the presence of handicap in a child provide strong practical reasons for desiring a second child: a daughter can contribute to her family economically for only a few years, until she marries; a disabled child may make only a limited contribution or may be a financial burden.

Severe or profound deafness is considered grounds for exemption from the one-child rule because it is seen as a handicap that prevents individuals from working normally as adults—yet deafness in itself is not incompatible with agricultural labor or a job in a welfare factory in the city. Behind this treatment are unstated assumptions that a deaf person is likely to be limited to menial, low-income jobs, thereby providing less for the family; and that the family will find it harder to educate a deaf child and arrange his or her marriage. The degree to which the exemption represents an accommodation to cultural prejudice against disabled and deaf people is hard to assess, but an analogy can be drawn with the state's accommodation to son preference. Here, too, the exemption is seen as a preventive against higher rates of infanticide (Liljestrom et al. 1982), or perhaps as a nod to the inevitable, since parents with a first deaf child might have a second regardless of the official prohibition, as would rural couples whose first child is a daughter. The dynamics of a family with a second child are also similar in both cases. A daughter who always has to share her parents' attention with a sibling who is favored if a boy is in the same position as a disabled child who has a younger sibling favored because he or she is whole. Furthermore, the younger child who perceives that he or she exists only because an older sibling is somehow devalued is always in an anomalous position.[14]

China's population policies have contributed to making the status of some children doubly undesirable—less valuable both because they are female and because they are disabled. Considerably higher numbers of handicapped girls than handicapped boys appear to be abandoned by their parents to be brought up in orphanages

(Dikotter 1996). The difference is likely to be most marked in rural areas where the economy is weak and the preference for sons is strong. Disabled girls may also have less access to education than do hearing girls, who are already educationally disadvantaged in comparison to boys: evidence from deaf schools in Jiangsu province, for example, indicates that enrollment figures are markedly higher for boys than girls: teachers say this is because rural parents often think that deaf daughters are not worth educating (Callaway 1999).

The complexities involved in implementing the population policies are highlighted by the treatment of deaf couples. Chinese authorities do not attempt to discourage marriage between deaf people as a means of eradicating genetic deafness—as did Alexander Graham Bell, for example, in the United States in the 1880s (Lane 1992). One reason for their reluctance may be that it is often difficult to distinguish genetically transmissible from adventitious deafness. If the 1995 Maternal and Child Health Care Law were implemented strictly, then deaf people whose deafness is genetic would not be allowed to reproduce; but deaf people apparently are permitted to have one child just as other couples are, even if the cause of their deafness is not clear. The right of every couple to have one child, one of the guiding principles in Chinese population policy (Greenhalgh 1986), seems in this instance to override eugenic policy directives. In practice, it is hard to see how the government could prevent deaf people from marrying and having children, given that deaf people themselves strongly desire to lead normal lives and their parents greatly desire grandchildren, who, according to the usual patterns of transmission of deafness in families, are very likely to have normal hearing.

Child Rearing and Socialization of the Chinese Child

The mainland Chinese government identifies three main arenas where child socialization occurs: the family, the preschool, and the primary school. Since this study is concerned primarily with preschool-age children, the following account focuses on the first two contexts.

Traditional Child-Rearing Values and Practices

In his comprehensive review of the literature, Ho (1986) finds that research on Chinese patterns of child socialization reflects a range of different perspectives. Much has been produced by Western anthropologists and political scientists; psychologists, both Chinese and foreign, have carried out a series of studies beginning in the 1960s on Chinese groups in America, and also in Taiwan; and more recently, psychiatrists in Hong Kong and Taiwan have contributed valuable qualitative analyses of family interactions and child socialization in Chinese families. Mainland Chinese academics have focused mainly on studies of the personality characteristics of the only child (Wu 1996). Data from these different sources relate to Chinese families living in a great variety of different geographical and socioeconomic circumstances; perhaps the most significant distinctions arise because of differences between rural and urban lifestyles. Yet the data show certain core values are characteristic of all Chinese families.

More than 2,500 years of Confucianism has established harmony as the most valuable ideal; attaining harmony in society requires orderliness and conformity in human relations. The "five relationships" (*wu lun*) outlined at the beginning of this chapter prescribe the role of an individual in their family and in society; the rules of propriety (*li*) set out the fitting behavior for each role. A person's morality and worth depend on obedience to the rules of conduct governing the social interactions of everyday life. Thus one core cultural value is self-restraint: spontaneous impulses must be strictly controlled since they threaten the mandate to conform and obey (King and Bond 1985). This "great tradition" of Confucian philosophy was essentially a set of abstract ideals formulated by the educated gentry. Its influence shaped the "little tradition," the values of millions of ordinary Chinese families, which are focused on attaining wealth and status, continuing the family line, and cultivating moral character. Traditionally, individuals worked hard to achieve merit or material success for the sake of their parents and family, not for themselves (Yu 1996). Educational achievement in particular has always been highly valued in Chinese society.

Underpinning the hierarchical family relationships of Confucian tradition is the crucial and pervasive concept of filial piety (*xiao*). Children must respect their parents and recognize their authority; they must also care for them in old age. In order for the family structure to remain intact and for the security of elderly parents to be guaranteed, children are encouraged to be relatively dependent, even as adults; independent behavior without reference to the wishes of family elders is viewed as selfish and inconsiderate. Parents expect to be consulted and involved in key decisions such as choice of marriage partner or job. Like independence, the qualities of assertiveness and creativity have relatively little value because they threaten the subordination of the individual to collective family interests.

Though particular circumstances lead to some variation, these traditional values emerge in family life in certain broad patterns. Many observers have noted how Chinese parents indulge their babies or young children, whose physical needs are anticipated and met with close attention. Affection toward children is very often expressed by giving them sweets or other tasty foods.[15] Traditionally, breastfeeding is relatively prolonged, continued for more than a year. Toilet training is relaxed, which according to Solomon (1971) delays a sense of personal autonomy. The heightened attention to children's physical needs promotes sensitivity to nonverbal interaction between parent and child; conversely, there is less verbal interaction than in Western families. As one psychologist reviewing studies of Chinese child socialization remarks: "The Chinese tend not to speak to their young children as much as Americans do, and treat them not as separate thinking beings but rather as physical extensions of themselves" (Bond 1991, 11).

The fear that children can be spoiled by parents (or grandparents) has been expressed in Chinese writings on child care for at least the last thousand years. They warn of *ni'ai*—"drowning in love": the child is simply swamped by overindulgence, frequently in the form of too many rich foods as well as too much of anything he or she asks for. The concern is that children treated in this way will be too willful and too pampered to fulfill their obligations to their family as they grow up. Even very young children in a traditional family are expected to respect their elders and follow the dictates of filial piety. Children as young as one or two are taught to address adults properly and to pay their respects every morning to their grandparents.

Somewhere between the ages of five and seven, there is an abrupt change in how children are treated by their parents: because they are regarded as capable of rational understanding (*dong shi*), they are ready to receive more formal moral training and education. As one would expect in a patriarchal culture, the most striking shift is in the behavior of father toward son: he becomes emotionally distant, strict, and demanding of respect. While the traditional father adopts a punitive approach to discipline, the mother remains a warm and affectionate figure.

According to the Confucian tradition, "a person by nature does not become an acceptable human being unless educated through deliberate efforts" (Wu 1996, 144). The primary responsibility of parents is to educate their children; that of children is to learn. Parents—and later teachers—teach by setting a moral standard for the child to follow: the principle of instruction through the power of exemplary models is deeply ingrained in Chinese concepts of education (and indeed such models have also been used extensively by the Chinese government for political purposes). Children who develop the ability to "listen" (*ting hua,* which, like "listen" in English, has the additional connotations of "heed" or "obey")—first to the instruction of their parents, then to other authority figures—are regarded as good and obedient. The right to speak depends on status in a rigid hierarchy; in traditional homes the older men speak most, while children are expected to say very little. As pupils in school, and later as employees at work, this pattern is reinforced. Conversational interaction, argument, confrontation, or feedback between participants of unequal status all run counter to traditional frameworks of communication (Gao G., Ting-Toomey, and Gudykunst 1996).

Contemporary Urban Child-Rearing Values and Practices

Chinese families in cities, particularly in thriving commercial centers, are in some ways living quite untraditionally. Cramped accommodations usually discourage grandparents from living with young couples—and even if grandparents live nearby, they tend to have less influence. Wives as well as husbands have full-time jobs, and the substantial economic contribution that they make to the household contributes to greater sexual equality.

Yang Kuo-shu has reviewed the research on the effects of societal modernization on Chinese families (1986, 1996). He outlines a number of methodological problems, notably the uncritical use of Western instruments with Chinese subjects and the reliance on unrepresentative sample populations; he also points to a lack of studies tracing the highly complex psychological processes involved in adaptations to modernization (Yang Kuo-shu 1986). Nevertheless, some conclusions can be drawn from the research to date. The motivation for achievement, traditionally oriented toward the group, is becoming individually oriented. There is also a trend toward greater independence and competitiveness, and more egalitarianism in relationships—including those between the sexes (Yang Kuo-shu 1996).

Yang Kuo-shu (1996) argues that societal modernization cannot be represented simply by a passage along a bipolar continuum with traditionality at one pole and modernity at the other. Instead, he makes the very useful suggestion that the two be treated as separate entities, each with several components and dimensions that can differ markedly across different cultures; for any individual within a given culture, levels of both traditionality and modernity may vary considerably in different social contexts. This model accommodates the coexistence of traditional values and modern ones. Yang Kuo-shu reports on a 1992 study he carried out with Taiwanese college students to test the correlations between selected factors of traditionality and modernity. The findings suggest that in the process of modernization, attitudes of submission to authority, conservatism, and male dominance are partially replaced by egalitarianism and open-mindedness. However, filial piety appears to be able to coexist with the independence and assertion that emerge with societal modernization. The view that filial piety comprises a particularly enduring set of values is supported by findings from a large-scale study of 1,123 young people in Hong Kong: while respondents thought love should be the basis for marriage and had fairly egalitarian attitudes about the husband-wife relationship, the majority were prepared to defer to their parents' wishes and many regarded the extended family household as ideal (Podmore and Chaney 1974). Ho (1996) argues that the practice of filial piety in Chinese families has changed: although the notion of obligations owed to parents persists, absolute obedience and submission to parents' wishes do not. He also points out that there may be a considerable gap between the values professed by the respondents and their actual behaviors.

A large-scale comparative study of child-rearing values carried out between 1991 and 1993 in Chinese communities in six different countries, including mainland China, has produced some interesting results (Wu 1996). In one part of the study, parents of five-year-old children were shown two videotapes of a child's daily routine (one local, one from outside the community), then asked to respond to three questions: What makes a child an ideal child? What are the traits of good parents? and What constitute good methods of family education for young children? The mainland Chinese group—a random sample of 600 households in Shanghai—most frequently answered the first question by emphasizing good moral character: a good child was respectful to elders, was mindful of others, had good manners, and so on. They also cited, in order of frequency, diligence in studying, obedience, good health, and good personality. They identified the most important trait of a good parent as being responsible for the child's receiving a good education, followed by setting a good example for the child. Parents felt that proper family education was first moral education, followed by encouragement to study. They thought it was important to support work done in school by making sure that children did their homework. Overall, the study demonstrated the parents' emphasis on moral training as well as formal education: traditionally, both have been highly valued in Chinese society. In another section of the same study, a survey of 500 Shanghai parents with children in kindergarten provided findings at variance with traditional child-rearing patterns: parents thought boys and girls should receive the same amount of education, and mothers took an active role in disciplining their children.

Parents in contemporary urban China want their child to be healthy, obtain a good education, get a good job, and be successful (Davin 1990a). Nowadays parents tend to define that success not by what their child can contribute to society but in terms of individual achievement. Yet few parents regard happiness per se as a desirable goal. There is a strong desire for children to succeed academically, and some parents also want their children to develop musical or other artistic talents. Because of the growth in their disposable income over the last few decades, many parents spend a quarter to a half of their income on toys, clothes, and other items for their only child (Davin 1990a). Although parents work full-time (recently reduced from six to five days a week), they spend their leisure time with their children, and weekends are often devoted to spending time in local parks, visiting grandparents, or going window-shopping. The only child is naturally the focus of their love and attention, although parents also worry about their child becoming spoiled; they often blame grandparents for inappropriate methods of child rearing, which they attribute to their parents' low level of education or old-fashioned ideas about bringing up children.

The traditional pattern persists, though perhaps to a lesser degree: relative parental indulgence in infancy and early childhood is followed by a stricter approach when children reach school age. Then parents become concerned about children's academic work; learning to read and write Chinese characters requires intensive memorizing and repeated reinforcement. Although corporal punishment is expressly discouraged by Chinese educators and childcare experts, many parents admit to smacking their child: in Davin's study (1990a) some parents said they hit their children on occasion, but regretted it afterward. Tobin, Wu, and Davidson (1989) report that most of the parents they interviewed in China managed their children's behavior not through disciplining or punishing them but through coaxing, humoring, and persuading them—actions covered by the word *hong* in Chinese.

Studies of Only Children

Parents, teachers, and child-care experts, as well as officials, show considerable anxiety about the numbers of only children in present-day China. They worry that an entire generation, after receiving all the attention of their parents as well as two sets of grandparents, will grow up selfish and irresponsible. Interested only in individual fulfillment, they will be unwilling to look after their elderly parents and to devote themselves to the interests of their country or fellow citizens. As we have seen already, such concerns over "spoiled children" are not new. They tend to reemerge whenever periods of social instability or transformation threaten, or appear to threaten, core cultural values; the most recent threats have been the effects of the one-child family planning policy and the impact of economic reforms (Press 1987; Davin 1990a; Wu 1996).

Since 1980 a number of research studies in China have focused on the physical, intellectual, and behavioral attributes of single children. When compared with children with one or more siblings, single children are on average healthier, enjoy better living conditions, and demonstrate superior intellectual ability (H. Yang, Kao, and Wang, cited in C. Ching 1982; Poston and Yu 1985). But studies of personality have produced conflicting results. For example, a 1980 study of 100 children in Shanghai found that 30 percent of only children were noncooperative at school compared with only 7 percent of children with siblings (cited in C. Ching 1982). A study involving 993 children in Beijing showed that only children were more egocentric, while children with siblings scored higher for persistence, cooperation, and peer prestige (Jiao S., Ji, and Jing 1986).[16] Yet Poston and Yu, in their study of 1,069 children in Changsha, found little difference in behavior: in fact, only children tended to be more cooperative than those with siblings. These studies tend to share a major flaw: their design, the methods of assessment chosen, and the interpretation of their results appear to be influenced by a powerful negative stereotype of only children. They are seen as self-centered and slow to share with other children, picky over their food, fussy about their clothes, and in general weak, delicate, and soft. Teachers complain that single children lag behind in practical skills such as brushing their teeth and dressing themselves. In the studies mentioned above, personality assessments were made by either teachers or peers who knew which subjects were only children—a procedure that Falbo (1982) singles out for criticism in research on only children.

Tao et al. (1995) carried out a six-year longitudinal study in Nanjing on 687 children who were preschoolers when the study started. Only children tended to show more neurotic traits while children with siblings tended to have externalized behavior problems (i.e., were more aggressive). While this pattern persisted throughout the study for boys, for girls it reversed in the first two years of primary school; the authors speculated that the change was related to their parents' expecting the girls to start doing housework at this age. The authors also investigated the relationship between stated parental preference for number and sex of children (most preferred one boy and one girl), actual number and sex of children, and children's behavior, and they found statistically significant effects for several groups. For example, when parents preferred only one child but had two, their boys showed marked immaturity; when parents wanted a boy, but had a girl first before a second child of either sex, the older girl scored very highly for neurotic traits. These results support the idea that children are strongly affected by parental attitudes.

Parents often attribute behavioral problems in only children to overindulgence by grandparents; teachers tend to blame both parents and grandparents for unwise child-rearing practices (Tobin,

Wu, and Davidson 1989). To prevent them from being spoiled, Chinese researchers strongly recommend that only children attend kindergarten rather than stay at home; they also stress the importance of educating parents and grandparents in proper child-rearing methods. That children learn to share and cooperate with others in the preschool is highly valued; parents are also encouraged to provide playmates for their child at home.

Socialization in the Preschool

Most children in urban areas attend kindergarten for at least one year when they are between the ages of three and seven; though day-care centers exist for younger children, parents generally prefer to leave their children with grandparents or other caregivers at home. Many kindergartens are attached to parents' workplaces — educational institutions, state enterprises, or administrative offices — and typically keep children for the whole day. Some kindergartens offer to board the children, who then go home to their parents on weekends, but these seem to have become less popular now that parents have only one child to look after. Urban kindergartens in China often have several hundred children, numbers that stretch thin their equipment and resources.

China has a long tradition of inculcating moral and social values in children, whether in the Confucian heritage or, after 1949, in socialist values. As the family has undergone tremendous change, the preschool has played a key role in maintaining continuity in the socialization of children. Today it is explicitly working to counteract the negative effects of excessive parental indulgence. Parents themselves, unable or unwilling to deny their only children, are often relieved to leave the task of disciplining children to the school. Thus children may experience a sharp contrast between discipline at school and relative indulgence at home (Tobin, Wu, and Davidson 1989); however, parents fully support teachers and their aims, and the underlying values in the two contexts are highly congruent.

Preschools aim at instilling the virtues of obedience, unselfishness, modesty, tidiness, and politeness. Children are taught to care for the environment, to help one another, and to know the difference between right and wrong behavior (Davin 1990a). On the one hand, individualistic behavior is seen as selfish and disruptive; on the other hand, conformity and obedience to the group are regarded in very positive terms. While competitiveness is encouraged, the children are made aware that achievement should be to benefit the collective and not to gratify the individual. Schools in some countries foster allegiance to the class or to the local community, but in China patriotism is emphasized most—children are acquiring their identity as citizens (Tobin, Wu, and Davidson 1989).

Kindergartens in China follow a national curriculum; adhering to the principle that children learn best through play, it outlines the knowledge and skills to be acquired by children in each preschool year. The subject areas are language development, simple arithmetic, general knowledge, arts and crafts, music and dance, physical education, hygiene, and moral education. Moral and social training are regarded as central elements: children are taught above all to think of others and to act for the common good.

Western observers often remark on how much more highly organized and regimented the daily schedule is compared with that of Western preschools (Kessen 1975; Breiner 1980; Liljestrom et al. 1982; Tobin, Wu, and Davidson 1989;[17] Davin 1990a). Lessons and other class activities are very structured. Kessen notes that "language learning . . . is highly formalized, places great stress on group recitation and memorization, and always serves as a vehicle for moral training"(87); Tobin, Wu, and Davidson comment that "the emphasis in language development is on enunciation, diction, memorization, and self-confidence in speaking and performing" (189). In drawing or coloring, children are asked to copy a picture precisely and to color it in neatly, rather than encouraged to exercise creativity; similarly, when children play with blocks they are asked to copy a model rather than build their own structure. Even during activities such as role play that are ideally suited to imaginative invention, Chinese children are expected to follow a set script in acting out the story. The emphasis is on skills acquired through structured activities rather than on cognitive development through problem-solving tasks.

Teachers create an orderly, highly structured environment in the kindergarten by maintaining firm authority over the children; their role is captured by the word *guan,* which incorporates the ideas of loving concern and care for the child as well as discipline (Tobin, Wu, and Davidson 1989). They frequently use positive reinforcements—praise of good behavior and skillful work—to ensure an atmosphere of warm approval. The slightest sign of fidgeting or antisocial behavior is picked up instantly by teachers, and reasoned admonitions follow; desired behavior is constantly and consistently reinforced. Prosocial behavior prevails because teachers project the expectation that children will behave well. The influence of example and the effect of a good teacher are regarded as crucial elements in the educational process (Liljestrom et al. 1982). In their demeanor toward children, teachers combine respect and affection, expressed not through physical contact but through frequent praise and encouragement; in this way, they persuade children to behave well. Kessen (1975) describes the effect of such a structured regime on Chinese children: they quickly learn to be compliant and obedient, yet display no signs of stress, tension, or flattening of emotion. The children show physical and emotional self-control, as well as the ability to concentrate on activities. They are skillful at dancing and art; they seem relaxed and confident, with very low levels of antisocial behavior.

Western critiques of Chinese kindergartens focus on the rigidity of the routine, arguing that its lack of choice for children encourages a passive approach to learning. As Kessen notes, "uniformly, children were being taught skills for performing preset tasks, rather than strategies for approaching new problems" (1975, 100). Indeed, some Chinese educators would welcome a more flexible and imaginative approach to kindergarten teaching, apparently on the grounds of pedagogical effectiveness rather than because they view freedom as valuable in itself (Tobin, Wu, and Davidson 1989). The overriding emphasis on the collective tends to obviate individualized teaching. One visiting group described a child with poor eyesight and cerebral palsy who was given only a little extra assistance: teachers on principle thought he should be treated as part of the group. They discussed him openly with the other children so they too understood his problems and could help him (Liljestrom et al. 1982). In the nursery for deaf children where I carried out my fieldwork, I observed that despite small classes of between four and seven children, and despite the different capabilities of individual children, teachers *always* taught their class as a unit; they took no advantage of opportunities to vary activities among the children or occasionally give them one-on-one attention. If a child was struggling with a particular aspect of class work, the teacher explained to parents what was required and asked them to deal with it as homework.

Socialization and the Deaf Child

Children in China are being socialized into a society with values and aims different in many respects from those of Western societies. Education of the deaf child both at home and at school will inevitably be shaped by those values and by the manner of socialization. The children experience great security in their early years. Infants and small children are treated with warmth and much physical affection, and parents are very responsive and attentive to their needs. Thus children's primary emotional needs are likely to be met. The concern with orderliness, routine, and control both at home and at preschool means that for a deaf child the world is relatively predictable, which helps ensure a sense of security and stability. However, unlike physical needs, emotional needs are not recognized or discussed as such, so insufficient weight may be given to the distress caused by an inability to communicate, especially as the child grows older. It is also likely that however secure a child's world is, he or she will be harmed by the emotional distress of parents once the deafness is discovered.

There is great emphasis on conformity, and on the appearance of conformity, in Chinese life. Parents will try to minimize their child's difference from hearing children in order to avoid being stigmatized. They will do everything possible to get their child into a mainstream school instead of a segregated school for the deaf. Small children are expected to be able to handle greetings in social situations and to fit in with everyday activities in the family and at preschool by understanding, and perhaps being able to say, common simple phrases. Such achievements may be more important for parents and for teachers than is the child's language acquisition in a deeper sense. Finally, the demands of conformity may make it more difficult to introduce approaches to education or child rearing that might be better suited to the deaf child but are in some way "different" from the conventional methods.

The attention paid to the physical needs of small children, who stay physically close to parents and other family members, suggests that they are able to communicate their basic desires by nonverbal means and are likely to have them readily satisfied. Parents are likely to feel that they "understand" their child and know what he or she wants—because the child's wants are fairly easy to identify at this stage. And even as the child becomes older, parents may consider conversations with their child to be relatively unimportant. Speech seems to serve a fairly instrumental function in Chinese households, and, as already noted, Chinese parents do not appear to talk as much with their children as Western parents do. More specifically, there seems to be little expectation that children should be full of prattle or self-initiated observations such as are encouraged and valued in many Western families, who tend to see such talk as stimulating children's minds and contributing to their knowledge and enjoyment of the world; nor is there a tradition of enjoying idle conversation with children. Perhaps such informal communication has little value because it lacks the status of speech in a formal teaching situation. Under these circumstances, parents of deaf children may feel relatively unconcerned about the poverty of verbal communication at home.

Chinese parents required to give their deaf child speech training at home are likely to find the role of teacher an extension of their traditional responsibilities to train and educate their children. Moreover, in this culture, where formal educational achievement is prized, parents are highly motivated to help their children, whom they hope will succeed academically and then obtain good nonmanual jobs. Difficulties may arise because of the conflict between a desire to indulge small children in the preschool years and the need to approach speech training early and methodically if any progress is to be made; however, early intervention is critical to a deaf child's ability to acquire language.

The approach to speech training currently advocated in Chinese preschools for deaf children is heavily influenced by the prevailing approach in mainstream education, which is formal, very structured, and teacher-directed. Children are expected to *ting hua* — listen to the teacher. These conditions support a systematic approach to inculcating language that relies on drilling in words and speech patterns rather than emphasizing interactional competence or child-centered learning. Because only stereotypical speech is demanded of children, a child's inadequate language acquisition may be masked until that time when language production is required in the form of written essays — usually at age nine in mainstream Chinese schools. This has enormous implications for the development of deaf education in China.

CHAPTER THREE

DEAFNESS IN CHINA

To understand the condition of deaf children in China, we must know something about the larger contexts both of China and of its deaf people. China is a vast country with marked variations by region in its geography, demography, and economy. Ninety-five percent of the population live in the fertile plains of the eastern half of the country, only 5 percent live in the mountainous and desert areas of western China. Government policies in the 1990s have promoted rapid economic development in "Special Economic Zones" on the east coast, so the already-pronounced wealth differential between eastern and western provinces is increasing. The disparity within provinces between urban and rural areas is also widening: in 1990 average rural incomes were a mere 31 percent of urban incomes ("Banknotes" 1998). The 72 percent of the Chinese population who live in rural areas earned on average less than $130 in 1998 (Thomas 1998).

In addition, adult illiteracy or semiliteracy is nearly three times higher in the countryside than in the cities (Gittings 1996). Urban dwellers enjoy a reasonably good standard of health care; workers in state-owned enterprises have part of their medical expenses reimbursed by their employers, although as China's economy is moving toward greater competition these entitlements are being eroded. Those who live in rural areas find access to health care more difficult, and recent agricultural reforms appear to be making their situation worse. A cooperative health-care system, which emphasized basic prevention and health education, has been replaced by state-subsidized hospitals and clinics where individuals must pay for treatment for which doctors can charge relatively high fees (Hillier and Zheng 1994; Oblau 1994; "When Illness Strikes" 1994; "Rural Health" 1997).

In any particular area, the prevalence of disease and disability is determined by local economic conditions and access to educational and medical services. We should therefore expect considerable variation in the prevalence and etiology of deafness.

The first systematic survey of disability in the Chinese population was carried out in 1987, providing the baseline information for planning appropriate medical and educational provision. The survey was based on data from 1.57 million people, selected as a representative sample according to specific socioeconomic and epidemiological criteria ("China Surveys" 1987; Wang H. 1988). In a smaller sample survey carried out at the same time and conducted with the assistance of UNICEF, more than 460,000 people in eight provinces were interviewed, 26 percent of them under the age of fourteen: this study focused on childhood disability (*Children and Women of China* 1989).

According to the 1987 national survey, 17.7 million people in China (about 1.7 percent of the population) had a hearing or speech impairment ("China Surveys" 1987; Wang H. 1988).[1] In the United States, by comparison, 8.6 percent of the population have hearing impairments (Holt and Hotto 1994); the figure for the United Kingdom is 7 percent (Palmer 1990, 13). Wang Hua believes that the Chinese figures are a considerable underestimate; he interviewed doctors involved in the 1987 survey who suggested that milder degrees of hearing loss were not picked up; in addition, poor equipment and errors limited accuracy of screening, and some respondents were reluctant to admit to a handicap. The UNICEF investigation produced a more realistic estimate of 120 million people in China with hearing loss, both mild and more severe — 10 percent of the population.

Hearing loss was also investigated in a large-scale genetic-epidemiological survey carried out during 1986–87 in Sichuan province, with a representative sample population of 127,000 (Liu Xuezhong et al. 1993, 1994). This survey is particularly useful because those found to have hearing loss underwent further detailed medical examination and a careful investigation of their family history. *Profound* deafness in the general population was found to be 0.186 percent. Ninety-six percent of subjects identified as profoundly deaf had lost their hearing before the age of ten; in 44 percent of cases the hearing loss was congenital.

TABLE 1: CHILDREN AGE 0 TO 6 WITH HEARING
IMPAIRMENT, 1987

Age (years)	Number	Percentage
0–1	33,300	0.12
1–2	34,200	0.17
2–3	51,900	0.34
3–4	65,400	0.28
4–5	87,000	0.44
5–6	94,300	0.43

SOURCE: Li S., Zhou, and Guo 1993, p.17, citing statistics from the 1987 National Survey of the Disabled.

According to the 1987 survey, there were 1.71 million hearing-impaired children under the age of fourteen in China: 740,000 of these children were under seven. Table 1 shows the numbers of children ages 6 or younger found to be deaf, along with their proportion of the total population of children. The incidence of hearing impairment rises with age both because some deafness is acquired and because some congenital cases are diagnosed late. The UNICEF-assisted survey's figure for the incidence of hearing and speech impairment in children under the age of 14 is comparable: 0.34 percent of the children surveyed (*Children and Women in China* 1989). These are broadly similar to U.S. statistics: 1 child in every 1,000 in the United States is born with profound deafness and an additional 2 children per 1,000 acquire deafness in early childhood (Northern and Downs 1991), a childhood prevalence rate of 0.3 percent. However, the Chinese figures may well be underestimates: in a country where the standard of living for much of the population is lower and medical services in many areas are not so well-developed as in the United States, one would expect the rates to be higher.

The 1987 survey statistics show an overall ratio between male and female hearing-speech disabled children up to age fourteen of 60:40; this gender bias was found to be about the same for urban and rural areas. The gender discrepancy is not easy to explain. As we saw in chapter 2, discrimination against girls means that more boys are born and survive infancy, and also that many girls become officially "invisible" because their births are not reported. Thus there is already an imbalance in the recorded numbers of male and female children. But statistics from other countries also indicate a higher prevalence of deafness in boys; for example, in the United States there are 54 boys with hearing impairment for every 44 girls in the three-to-seventeen age group (Holt and Hotto 1994). In rural China the higher incidence may have other causes: parents spend more money on their sons' health than their daughters' (Burgess and Zhuang 1996), so it is possible that more boys are exposed to the harmful effects of ototoxic antibiotics (discussed below).

Another possibility is that some deaf girls are abandoned or neglected once their deafness is discovered, but evidence that might support or disprove this conjecture is hard to obtain. According to an educational administrator at the CRR Center for Deaf Children in Beijing, it is not uncommon for couples in rural areas to divorce following the diagnosis of deafness or to consign the deaf child to the care of grandparents; but outright rejection of the child is rare. As mentioned in chapter 2, welfare institutions sometimes have a few deaf children, usually girls, among their inmates: presumably their parents could not accept their deafness.[2] As already suggested, the relatively late diagnosis of deafness in China may protect the child; it may be much harder for parents to abandon a deaf child at two or three than to reject a child with an obvious defect at birth.

In the 1987 survey the distribution of hearing-speech disabled children between cities, towns, and countryside was found to be 5.6 percent, 11.2 percent, and 83.2 percent respectively, although the distribution of the total population of children was 9 percent, 16 percent, and 75 percent: children in the countryside were more likely to be hearing impaired.[3] This is what one would expect, given that they suffer lower standards of living and receive less adequate medical care. Untreated chronic ear infections and illnesses such as meningitis and measles are both commoner in rural areas and contribute to the higher prevalence of childhood deafness. Liu Xuezhong et al. (1993, 1994) found no significant difference between the incidence of congenital deafness in rural populations in Sichuan and that in urban populations, supporting the view that the higher incidence of deafness among children in the countryside is due primarily to environmental factors such as infection and disease.

TABLE 2: DEGREE OF HEARING LOSS BY CATEGORY, 1987

Category	Subcategory	Hearing Loss	Percentage of All Children with Hearing Loss
Deaf	grade one	> 91 dB	39
	grade two	71–90 dB	17
Partially hearing	grade one	56–70 dB	18
	grade two	41–55 dB	26

SOURCE: *Canji ertong ziliao* 1991, citing the 1987 Survey of the Disabled.

The deaf children identified in the survey were classified as "deaf" or "partially hearing," with further subdivisions according to the degree of hearing loss (see table 2). These figures indicate that well over half the children with impaired hearing identified in the 1987 survey were either profoundly or severely deaf: however, we must remember that a substantial number of children with milder losses probably were not identified.

According to data in the 1987 National Survey of the Disabled, shown in table 3, the most common cause of deafness in children is middle ear disease, which is responsible for 17.5 percent of cases. Febrile illness and ototoxic drugs account for 13 percent and 12 percent respectively. Hereditary deafness, so identified when another family member is congenitally deaf or when the parents are related, accounts for only 9 percent of cases. Over a quarter (27.8 percent) are of unknown causation. Ototoxic drugs appear to be a more important cause of deafness in cities (23 percent) than in the countryside (11 percent). Conversely, middle ear disease and febrile illness are more prominent causes in the countryside—20 percent versus 4 percent in the cities, and 14 percent versus 8 percent, respectively. Maternal illness in pregnancy, which includes rubella infection, appears to account for only 2.8 percent of cases of deafness in children.

It is useful to compare statistics for childhood deafness in the United States with the Chinese figures. Genetic factors are responsible for more than 50 percent of cases of childhood hearing loss in the United States ("Statistics on Deafness" 1998). The 1992–93 Annual Survey of Hearing Impaired Children and Youth carried out

TABLE 3: CAUSES OF DISABILITY IN HEARING-SPEECH DISABLED CHILDREN, INCLUDING THOSE WITH MULTIPLE HANDICAPS

Cause of Disability	Residence of Child			Total	Percentage of All Auditory Disability
	City	Town	Country		
Middle ear disease	6	32	412	450	17.5
Febrile illness	14	33	287	334	13.0
Ototoxic drugs	39	46	222	307	11.9
Hereditary/ consanguineous marriage	11	31	192	234	9.1
Developmental malformation	29	24	126	179	6.9
Maternal illness in pregnancy	9	7	56	72	2.8
Trauma	2	5	18	25	1.0
Endemic disease (Keting disease, etc.)	0	2	15	17	0.6
Birth trauma	3	0	7	10	0.4
Noise	0	1	1	2	0.1
Other causes	18	26	186	230	8.9
Cause not known	36	106	574	716	27.8
Total	167	313	2,096	2,576	100.0

SOURCE: *Canji ertong ziliao* 1991; percentage column added.

by the Center for Assessment and Demographic Studies at Gallaudet University indicated that pregnancy and birth complications, including Rh incompatibility, prematurity, and birth trauma, were the second most common cause at 8.7 percent (Holt and Hotto 1994). As neonatal technology and expertise improve, so does the survival rate in Western countries of very premature babies, who are at greater risk for deafness and accompanying disabilities; up to 7 percent of babies who have been in neonatal intensive care units are found to have a hearing impairment (Balkany and Luntz 1998). But maternal rubella, which caused around 20 percent of cases of deafness fifteen years ago, now accounts for only 2.1 percent (Holt and Hotto 1994) thanks to extensive immunization programs. Bacterial meningitis is now the most common cause of acquired childhood deafness, identified as responsible in 8.1 percent of cases. Middle ear infection and other infections and fever, in contrast to the Chinese figures, account for less than 5 percent each (Holt and Hotto 1994). Ototoxic antibiotics such as gentamycin are not a significant cause of deafness for children in the United States. As in China, however, a substantial proportion of cases of deafness — about a quarter — are of unknown cause.

Data from China's 1987 national survey show that 9 percent of deafness in children has a hereditary basis, but this figure far understates the prevalence of genetic causes. The Sichuan study, which focused on people with profound deafness in the general population, found a genetic cause in 43 percent of cases; furthermore, some of the 20 percent of unknown cause may also have been genetic (Liu Xuezhong et al. 1993). Of those cases ascribed to genetic causes, 92 percent were due to autosomal recessive genes and 5.4 percent to autosomal dominant genes. The Sichuan researchers attribute the very high levels of autosomal recessive forms (which are usually considered to account for about 80 percent of cases of genetic hearing impairment; Parving 1996) in part to the high incidence of consanguinity in some of the populations included in the study. In light of this explanation, it is clear that in China as elsewhere, genetic factors are very significant causes of hearing impairment, though easily overlooked or underestimated because the genes responsible are predominantly recessive and therefore difficult to detect.

Families are often very unwilling to accept that deafness in children or adult relatives is genetic.[4] There is a great reluctance to admit to "deafness in the family," which parents may hide from doctors and deaf school teachers (Dr. Fei Zhao, conversation with author, 25 July 1995; Dr. Liu Xuezhong, conversation with author, 8 September 1995; Liu F. 1995). I found that in several families living in the countryside near Nanjing, each with two children with congenital deafness, the parents were still anxious to blame the deafness on birth trauma or other nongenetic causes. There seems to be little understanding that recessive genes can cause deafness even though no relative in an earlier generation was deaf; indeed, the lack of a family history of deafness is presented as evidence that the deafness is not inherited (letters to Zhou Hong, nos. 63 and 113).[5] In contrast, interbreeding between close relatives is widely recognized as causing abnormalities and defects in children: this information has been extensively publicized by the government in marriage and family planning regulations.

Mothers appear more often to be held culpable, by themselves as well as by others, on the grounds that something ingested during pregnancy, some illness at this time, or some lack of care on their part is responsible for the child's deafness (Lu Hui, conversation with author 1994; Zhang Manhua, conversation with author, 1994).[6] The unborn child is traditionally believed to be affected by the mother's physical and moral qualities, as well as by external factors that influence her during the pregnancy (Dikotter 1992). Recent research on cultural practices associated with pregnancy and maternity among women in Hong Kong has revealed the widespread persistence of traditional restrictions on food and behavior that pregnant women are expected to observe to ensure the well-being of their child (D. Martin 1997).

Most Chinese do not recognize the possible role of the rubella virus as a causative agent, although historically it has been responsible for a large proportion of childhood deafness in Western countries (especially following epidemics).[7] In China as elsewhere, rubella is endemic; a high incidence of infection in children leaves about 95 percent of the population over ten years of age with natural immunity (M. Young and Prost 1985). However, as Young and Prost point out, 5 percent of women between the ages of twenty-one and thirty-five thus have no immunity against rubella: should they become infected in the early stages of pregnancy, their infant may be born with congenital defects that include deafness. Currently women in this group are not immunized against rubella. Serological testing for rubella is not routinely carried out; it is likely that some cases of deafness of unknown causation are due to the virus (Liu Xuezhong et al. 1993).

Ototoxic drugs cause a significant—and, over the past forty years, growing—proportion of the cases of deafness in children (Callaway 1986). The 1987 survey indicated that the incidence of ototoxicity in children in urban areas was over twice that of children in rural areas, suggesting that it is becoming a more prominent cause of deafness as measles and other infectious diseases are being treated more effectively. According to surveys of special populations such as deaf schools and ear, nose, and throat (ENT) outpatients, between 50 and 70 percent of cases are caused by ototoxicity. Perhaps doctors attribute deafness to ototoxic drugs if there is a history of their use and no other obvious cause can be identified: many cases that are in fact genetic may be put into this category. For these special populations in cities, a more realistic figure for ototoxicity may be 30 percent, which is still quite high (Dr. Liu Xuezhong, conversation with author, 8 September 1995). Liu Chan, referring to the Beijing area, also estimates 30 percent (conversation with author, 7 July 1995).

Drugs most often implicated in causing deafness in children are the aminoglycoside antibiotics (gentamycin, streptomycin, kanamycin, and neomycin), which are all relatively cheap and in widespread use, though they are often prescribed inappropriately. An infant or small child with a cold, fever, or diarrhea rarely should be given an antibiotic injection. Yet a detailed survey carried out in Henan province involving 437 children deafened by gentamycin found that 284 (65 percent) had been given the drug to treat a feverish cold, and 66 (15 percent) had been given it for diarrhea (Yang Jianmin 1995). This study also showed that children under two years of age were more susceptible to the ototoxic effects of the drug and that the dosage was a crucial factor, especially in younger children. Many parents seem to believe that injections are the best form of treatment for childhood illnesses. Furthermore, doctors have a financial incentive to give injections: they can charge a specific fee for this service. There appear to be no structural disincentives to the unrestrained use of gentamycin and related antibiotics, as doctors are not held professionally accountable for any adverse side effects.

Hereditary susceptibility to the ototoxic effects of the aminoglycosides, which appears to be relatively common in Asian populations, may be present in as many as a third of the individuals with aminoglycoside toxicity in China (Snow 1995). That several generations in a family may suffer deafness due to ototoxic drugs (Yan 1979) demonstrates the lack of awareness of risk and the failure to take precautionary measures. In the Henan study 47 children had relatives already deafened by ototoxic antibiotics, and Yang Jianmin (1995) uses these findings to emphasize that doctors must check the child's family history before administering gentamycin. Recent development of an inexpensive blood test that can detect hereditary susceptibility to the aminoglycosides could be crucial in preventing further harm; to ready the test for widespread use, Dr. Xiaomei Ke at Beijing Medical University has been screening families of children attending a deaf school in Beijing to identify patterns of inheritance of this characteristic.

Government directives in recent years have warned doctors to use ototoxic drugs with caution, especially in children. Increased awareness concerning this issue may be beginning to have some effect in major urban areas: thus at the CRR Center for Deaf Children in Beijing, the proportion of children enrolled who were thought to be deaf because of ototoxic drugs fell from 70 percent in 1994 to 60 percent in 1995.[8] However, for various reasons, including the dearth of inexpensive alternative drugs and the lack of systematic enforcement, the directives seem to have been relatively ineffective so far, especially in rural areas. The Ninth Five-Year Plan (1996–2000) includes the goal of reducing deafness due to ototoxicity by one-third; the China Disabled People's Federation (CDPF, China's national organization for disabled people; see below) undertook a major public awareness campaign on ototoxic drugs in 1997. If such campaigns, combined with parental education on how to deal more appropriately with minor childhood illnesses, can be conducted effectively, then cases of childhood deafness in China should decrease significantly.

Medical Services and the Provision of Technology

Since a substantial number of cases of deafness in children in China are acquired, through disease or the effects of ototoxic medicines, certain intervention approaches are likely to be favored. For children with moderate or severe hearing losses who have become deaf in the first or second year of life, early audiological assessment followed by early intervention with the fitting of hearing aids and stimulation of speech for communication and language development will be regarded as appropriate measures. Where resources are scarce, they will probably be focused selectively on this population rather than on children with congenital profound deafness.

There is no comprehensive program in China to screen for hearing loss in children. Children are usually tested only after parents, or sometimes teachers, notice a lack of reaction to sound or a delay in speech. The CRR Center for Deaf Children puts the average age for diagnosis of deafness in China's cities currently between one and two; in the countryside it tends to be later. Early diagnosis is clearly a problem in China, but it is also difficult to achieve in more developed nations: in the United States, a sizable number of children still have their hearing loss, including profound hearing loss, identified only after the age of two (Northern and Downs 1991; "Recommendations" 1997; "Statistics on Deafness" 1998).

There are very few trained audiologists in China; until quite recently there were no postgraduate audiological training courses available.[9] However, audiological services are provided in large city hospitals, usually by ENT doctors and by some medical technicians as well. Audiometry can be carried out in most ENT departments, and brain stem evoked response (BSER) testing is available in hospitals in the major cities. Parents living in remote areas may travel long distances to bring their child for testing.

Diagnostic Services

In the diagnostic interview, the doctor simply informs parents of their child's hearing loss as shown by testing. Doctors have no professional responsibility to counsel parents and little appreciation of the underlying psychology of the diagnostic process—the force of parents' emotional reactions, the difficulty they have absorbing information when in a state of shock, and their need to deal with overwhelming emotions so that they can plan for the future and start to take constructive action (e.g., see Luterman 1990). By contrast, audiologists in the United States and Britain now generally take such measures as putting parents in touch with other families with deaf children and making arrangements for follow-up sessions for counseling and discussion of educational options. Some Chinese doctors do, however, provide helpful information; parents usually ask about the possibility of a cure, and doctors will explain that there is no treatment for sensorineural deafness. They may advise parents to purchase a hearing aid and may refer them to the nearest rehabilitation center for preschool deaf children for further information, particularly advice on speech training.

Chinese parents show a striking disinclination to accept one medical opinion. They tend to consult a series of doctors in different major hospitals, especially those in Shanghai and Beijing that have a high reputation. The same tests are repeated; parents have to pay for the consultation and the tests each time. One of the parents who wrote to Zhou Hong had BSER tests carried out five times, at different hospitals, to confirm his son's deafness (LZH, no. 56). When the initiative for testing lies with parents, there is clearly considerable scope for inappropriate use of expensive specialized services.

Treatments for Deafness

Certain diseases that can lead to deafness in children are amenable to standard medical treatment. Ear infections, for example, can be treated with antibiotics. Appropriate treatment depends on access to good medical care; while this is available in urban areas in China, families in rural areas may not be so fortunate.

However, many deaf children with severe or profound hearing loss in both ears have sensorineural deafness, which cannot be cured — as the Chinese ENT doctors tell parents at the time of diagnosis. This convinces parents that Western medicine has nothing to offer. Typically, after going from doctor to doctor to confirm the diagnosis, they then turn to Chinese traditional medicine, which has an array of treatments reputed to cure deafness. Many preschool deaf education professionals have observed this behavior (Zhang Mingliang 1991; Liu F. 1995; Wang Youguo 1995a, 1995b; Chen Suzhen 1995); in one of the few studies that provide actual figures, parents of 90 out of the 98 deaf children surveyed in Henan province sought traditional medical treatments for their children (Xu X. et al. 1995). Rehabilitation professionals regard parents' search for a cure as one of the major obstacles to successful rehabilitation of deaf children.

Although Western medicine became established in China in the first half of this century, it never supplanted traditional medical care: treatment has been, and remains, markedly pluralistic. Traditional medicine was indispensable in establishing and maintaining a comprehensive health-care system in China, since Chinese herbal medicines were much cheaper and more readily available than most Western drugs. Its prestige and popularity derive from its strong roots in traditional Chinese culture (Hillier and Jewell 1983). Chinese people generally look to Chinese medical treatments if Western approaches are not available or are ineffective, and they often use both at the same time. As Phillips remarks, "Chinese families are very pragmatic in their utilization of health-care providers: they often try a variety of modalities (either sequentially or concurrently) to find the method that generates the most desirable outcome" (1993, 290). Phillips also notes that even well-educated people and high-ranking officials will consult dubious shamanistic practitioners if other courses fail.

Treatments resorted to by parents of deaf children include acupuncture, *qigong* (a traditional therapy described below), and herbal medicines. In deciding on a particular treatment, parents are strongly influenced by the practitioner's reputation. They may read about certain traditional practitioners and their particular skills in newspaper articles as well as in specialist magazines such as *Qigong and Science,* which carries information about individual *qigong* masters, some of whom specialize in treating sensorineural deafness (LZH, no. 82). The journal of the CDPF, *Disability in China,* publishes accounts of "cures" effected by traditional Chinese medicine—the January 1995 issue, for example, contains the personal account of a deaf teenager who regained his hearing through the practice of *qigong* exercises (Wang K. 1995). With this kind of official endorsement and publicity, traditional Chinese therapies achieve a credibility that must impress parents seeking cures. It is perhaps unfortunate that Zhou Hong, who taught his deaf daughter to speak, advocates acupuncture and other treatments to the hundreds of parents who consult him about their deaf children. Out of a sample of 135 letters written to Zhou Hong by parents of deaf children, 65, or 48 percent, contained specific requests for information about treatments for deafness; 53 parents (39 percent) mentioned in their letters that they had already tried various cures (see chapter 6).

Acupuncture is widely regarded in China as an appropriate treatment for deafness. The acupuncturist inserts fine needles into the patient at particular points, which are situated along special channels known as meridians, in order to stimulate and redistribute the flow of *qi,* the body's vital essence, thus restoring the harmony necessary for wholeness and health (Kaptchuk 1983). Its apparent success in treating children at a deaf school in Liaoyang in Manchuria in 1968 was widely publicized at the time and has since become part of popular mythology.[10] Acupuncture subsequently became

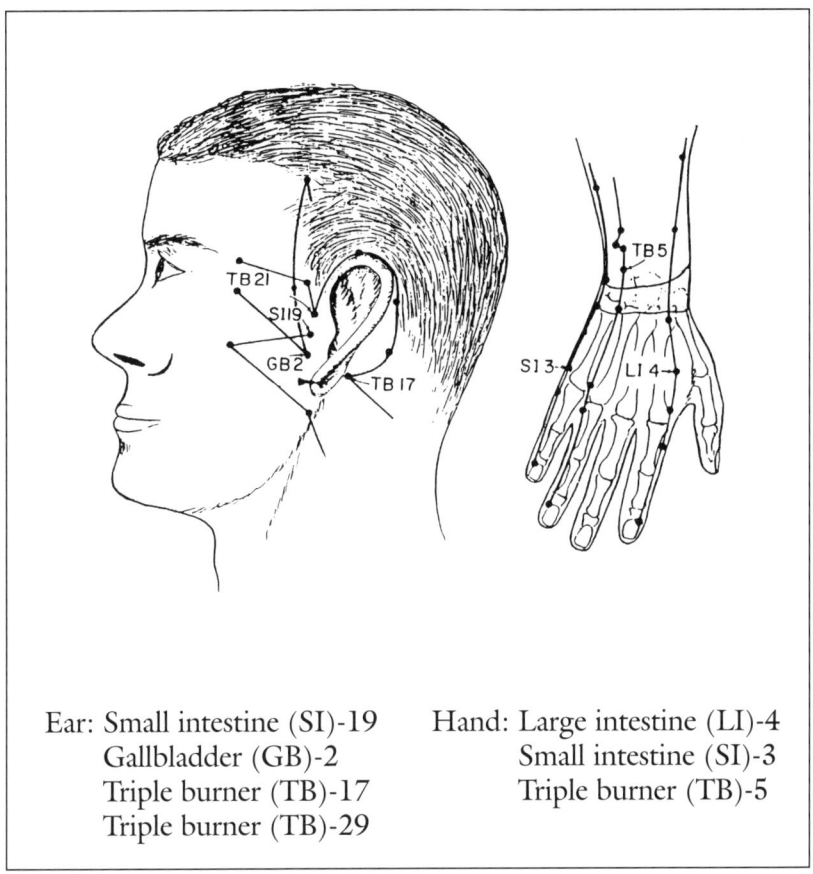

Ear: Small intestine (SI)-19
    Gallbladder (GB)-2
    Triple burner (TB)-17
    Triple burner (TB)-29

Hand: Large intestine (LI)-4
    Small intestine (SI)-3
    Triple burner (TB)-5

FIGURE 1. Location of acupuncture points used in the treatment of deafness. From Eisenberg, Taub, and Dicarlo 1974, 1944.

widely used in teaching hospitals and schools for the deaf as a treatment for sensorineural deafness (Rosen 1974).

There are specific acupuncture points for the treatment of deafness on the head near the ear, as well as on the hand (see figure 1). However, there may be considerable variation in how the needling is done—for example, whether it is "deep" or "shallow." A course of one to four years of treatment is often recommended (Rosen 1974). Acupuncture practitioners regard deafness of relatively recent onset and milder hearing losses as more amenable to treatment; a favorable outcome is also held to be more likely if the patient is in good general health (Dr. J. H. Chen, conversation with author, December 1997). Children are considered to be particularly sensitive and responsive to acupuncture treatment, yet many practitioners prefer not to treat very young children, presumably because of the discomfort involved and the difficulty of making young children lie still; parents may also be reluctant to place their children in such an uncomfortable situation. In variations on traditional acupuncture methods, acupoints may be stimulated using low-voltage alternating current or by means of lasers, pressure, massage, or even injection at the site. Moxibustion—carried out by slowly burning moxa-wool, the shredded dry leaves of the Chinese wormwood, near the diseased area or at the acupuncture points (Fu 1975)—is sometimes combined with acupuncture. Individual practitioners freely develop their own approaches after long experience and experimentation.

Much research has been carried out in China and elsewhere on the efficacy of acupuncture in treating deafness. As Liu Qian et al. comment in their study of acupuncture treatment for sensorineural deafness involving 1,001 subjects, "many acupuncturists as well as patients have always hoped that scientific evidence could be procured consistent with the subjective improvement in hearing following the treatment" (1982, 21). Eisenburg, Taub, and Dicarlo's evaluation (1974) included a control group given acupuncture using acupoints not associated with hearing or deafness; other careful studies include those by Fairbanks, Wallenburg, and Webb (1974); Roeser, Campbell, and Glorig (1975); and Rosen (1974). Both Chinese and Western researchers have found that although in some cases transient improvements are demonstrated, both subjectively and on hearing tests, no such changes can be conclusively shown to be independent of psychogenic effects or of practice in taking the test. Fairbanks, Wallenburg, and Webb conclude: "We concede that a certain number of patients or, more particularly, parents of deaf patients will feel compelled to 'leave no stone unturned' even in the face of data such as that presented. They should be made aware that at the present time acupuncture is uncontrolled human experimentation" (1974, 401).

Herbal treatments for deafness are widely regarded as working more gradually than acupuncture but with a particularly lasting effect. There are a range of herbs that may be used, and the medicine typically consists of a combination of several herbs prescribed according to the characteristics of the patient. They are usually taken as a bitter-tasting infusion once or twice a day. Herbal medicines are very often used in combination with other treatments, including acupuncture.

Qigong, another traditional form of therapy, is currently enjoying a massive increase in popularity (Phillips 1993). As in acupuncture, the aim is to regulate the flow of *qi*, or vital spirit, along the meridians until a harmonious balance is attained: however, this is achieved not through needling but by employing the power of the mind and movements of the body. There are many different forms of *qigong*, some of which are still being developed by current *qigong* masters, but essentially all forms fall into two groups — passive, in which the body is motionless, and active, which involve specific physical movements. Hospitals specializing in traditional Chinese medicine have *qigong* doctors who treat patients by making a series of hand movements over them to affect the patient's *qi* (McNamara 1995): this would seem especially appropriate for small children, who might not be able to perform complicated breathing exercises or the more active forms of *qigong*.

Besides these widely used traditional approaches, various other treatments have been adopted in China to cure sensorineural deafness. These include injections of adenosine triphosphate (ATP) and injections of vitamin B. In their letters, several parents mention to Zhou Hong a "desensitization" treatment for sensorineural deafness caused by ototoxic drugs, but it is not clear how the desensitization is carried out or what drugs are involved.

Doctors offer a great number of different treatments for deafness. One designed specifically for sensorineural deafness caused by ototoxic drugs that was reported in *British Deaf News* (Dimmock 1995, 19) is typical in its eclectic combination of methods: a Dr. Gao Lihua developed a treatment consisting of acupuncture, electrical stimulation, physiotherapy, and Chinese herbs. According to the report, his first patient was an eight-year-old girl who had lost her hearing two years before, after being given streptomycin injections for glandular fever. Apparently after a few weeks' treatment "she started to hear sounds when people spoke." Zhou Hong advises parents to go to the Railway Hospital in Lianyungang in northern Jiangsu province, where children receive a course of intravenous infusions whose content is not divulged to patients. He also recommends electrical acupuncture treatment at a traditional Chinese medicine clinic in Nanjing. These approaches all have in common their development by individual doctors, or teams of doctors, and a lack of proper testing or control over their use. Parents may also seek treatment from traveling doctors, who journey from town to town offering their unique "cures" for various illnesses; typically, the ingredients of the medicines are a closely guarded secret, handed down from father to son. Many of these traveling doctors are charlatans who take advantage of desperate parents.

Despite the claims made by the practitioners, there is no firm evidence that any of the treatments described above result in a sustained improvement in hearing in cases of sensorineural loss. In the Henan survey, "some effect" was seen in 21 out of the 90 children who had treatment; in 69 there was no effect at all (Xu X. et al. 1995). The report provides no details as to the nature of this "effect" or its persistence—and in circumstances such as these, when both practitioners and parents are highly motivated to perceive an improvement, very careful and accurate pre- and posttreatment testing would have to be carried out to rule out a placebo effect. Children who do show definite improvement after treatment may have had a conductive component to their hearing loss, caused by a middle ear effusion that has cleared up. In a few cases of childhood deafness due to ototoxic drugs the damage is reversible, and hearing may show some recovery over time (Wright, Forge, and Kotecha 1997): improvement attributed to a treatment may in fact be spontaneous. Thus claims that some traditional medical treatments can mitigate hearing loss need to be treated with great circumspection.

Parents characteristically refer to speech training as a form of treatment no different in kind from the medical treatments described above. Just as mutism until recently was regarded as inseparable from deafness in children, with the reason for the inability to speak not clearly understood, so parents often appear not to separate the effect of the improvement in hearing promised by the medical treatments from the remedial effect of speech training, as if both work in the same fashion. In classifying speech training with medical cures for deafness, parents also reveal how thoroughly they perceive, or wish to perceive, its value as a process of eliminating the deafness and returning the child to normal—not as a means of enabling communication despite their child's hearing deficit.

Hearing Aids

Only a small percentage of the Chinese population who could benefit from hearing aids obtain them. Tyler and He (1990) point out that in China in 1988, 155,000 hearing aids were expected to be sold to a population of one billion, whereas in the United States in 1989, 1,500,000 were sold to a population of about 260 million—thirty-seven times as many per capita. America has an older population than China, with a higher proportion of elderly people requiring aids: nevertheless, the difference is enormous.

Chinese-made hearing aids have been produced by a factory in Tianjin since 1960. These are relatively inexpensive; a behind-the-ear (BTE) aid costs between 300 to 400 yuan (about $50). Chinese hearing aids accounted for 90 percent of sales in 1990 (Tyler and He 1990). Imported hearing aids are also available, and are typically much more expensive—up to 3,000 yuan or more, according to the make. This would be equivalent to at least six months' wages for most workers. Most hearing aids sold in China are body-worn aids, which are worn with foam ear plugs (Tyler and He 1990). However, the preschool rehabilitation centers ask parents to purchase BTE aids for their children, and good-quality soft ear molds can now be made, at least in large cities.

The majority of hearing aids are sold over the counter in medical shops, pharmacies, and department stores; in such sales, little or no advice is given to the customer (Tyler and He 1990). Hearing aids can also be obtained through hospitals and hospital commercial units, who mainly provide good-quality BTE aids and can refer families to doctors who provide comprehensive advice and follow-up. But there is considerable variation both among hospitals and among doctors, for whom this is often a profit-making service (Steen Teisen, letter to author, 15 April 1996). Because demand is low, and mainly for the cheaper aids, there are few hearing aid services in the countryside and remote areas in China. Those who wish to buy a hearing aid must travel to large towns or cities; for repairs, they have to make another journey or use the postal system. Hearing aid companies have little financial incentive to extend their services to rural areas (Steen Teisen, letter to author, 15 April 1996).

Hearing aid use in deaf children is still far from prevalent. In the 1987 survey, 28 out of 2,576 hearing-speech disabled children under the age of fourteen (1.1 percent) were found to have hearing aids.

However, they appear to be becoming more common, at least in some areas: in a recent survey in Henan province, 44 of 98 preschool deaf children (45 percent) had hearing aids (Xu X. et al. 1995). As we might expect, children living in urban areas are more likely to have hearing aids than children in rural areas.

The time between diagnosis of deafness and obtaining a hearing aid is frequently considerable: Xu Xiaoming et al. (1995) note that although 90 percent of the children in their survey were diagnosed before the age of three, all those children with hearing aids received them after the age of three. Parents have difficulty getting their children to use them, especially without professional support: in the same study, 21 out of 44 children with aids, or 48 percent, "did not like" their aids. Typically, after parents purchase an aid they are disappointed that no significant change can be observed in the child's hearing. I found that some parents believe that use of a hearing aid will damage or atrophy a child's residual hearing. Furthermore, wearing a hearing aid makes a deaf child conspicuous; some parents may feel uncomfortable with the hearing aid as a visible sign of their child's disability.

The establishment of the rehabilitation centers for deaf children has been the key to getting preschool-age deaf children properly fitted with appropriate hearing aids and ear molds. Teachers keep a check on maintenance, and they reinforce the wearing of the hearing aid at the rehabilitation center as a daily habit. At home, behaviors vary: some children remove their aids after school, some wear them for homework only, some keep the aids in until bedtime. Because the aids are expensive, parents may ask children to keep them safe by removing them before they go out to play. Indeed, expense is a significant issue: while children at the CRR Center for Deaf Children in Beijing are nearly all binaurally aided, most children at the rehabilitation center in Nanjing where my fieldwork was carried out could afford only one hearing aid.

Cochlear Implants

Cochlear implants have been developed in China since 1979. In the 1980s several institutions in China carried out implantations with single-channel devices (Peter Alberti, letter to author, 26 September 1995); by 1993 about 1,000 deaf people in China, including 50 under the age of 12, had received single-electrode devices in a relatively inexpensive procedure (F. Zeng 1995).[11] Alberti noted the lack at that time of proper selection procedures and habilitation and rehabilitation support for patients. According to Tyler and He (1990), many of these patients did not benefit from their implant because of problems with infection as well as technical malfunctions; many patients lived far away from the hospitals, making follow-up difficult. After evaluating the single-electrode devices, Chinese doctors concluded that they were not effective enough; attention therefore turned to multi-electrode implants.

Although there is interest in developing indigenous cochlear implantation programs in China, they face a number of barriers. The production of Chinese-made multichannel devices has been hindered because local manufacturers do not possess the necessary hermetic sealing technology (F. Zeng 1995). Fangang Zeng also points out that although surgical implantation may be successful, the device may not be properly calibrated because of lack of biotechnological expertise; also, postoperative rehabilitation services are not available. Thus attention has shifted recently to obtaining implants from Australian companies and to learning methods of rehabilitation from colleagues in Australia and America.

Until recently there has been a reluctance to implant devices in children. In late 1994 officials at the CRR Center for Deaf Children told me that they were not developing cochlear implant programs in preschool-age children because parents would be reluctant to submit their children to such an operation. In May 1996, however, I was told that several major hospitals in Beijing intended to start such programs for children. A delegation was going to Australia to acquire further expertise in cochlear implantation, with the aim of establishing a post-implantation rehabilitation program. Apparently the parents of the children concerned will have to bear the high cost of the device, which suggests that only children from relatively well-off families will receive the implants.

Some have suggested that cochlear implants may be particularly effective for enhancing aural reception of spoken Chinese, since essential linguistic information is conveyed through changes in tones marked by variations in pitch that the cochlear device can pick up and emphasize. Tests carried out with a bilingual patient with an Australian Nucleus device showed recognition rates of 65 percent for Chinese words and 44 percent for English words; these may have been skewed, however, because the subject's native language was Chinese (Xu S., Dowell, and Clark 1987).

Government Policy and Special Education

The first school for deaf children in China was started in Tengchow (now Dengzhou), Shandong province, in 1887 by Mrs. Annetta Mills, wife of a Presbyterian missionary. In 1898 the school was relocated to Chefoo (now Yantai), also in Shandong province, and came to be known as the Chefoo School.

Mills had previously taught at the Rochester School for the Deaf in New York and she used methods she had learned there — notably Bell's Visible Speech and fingerspelling based on the Lyon phonetic manual — in her Chinese school. A contemporary pamphlet describes her approach: "The school is conducted on what the Americans call the combined system. Finger-spelling is freely used, aided by pantomime, gesture, and picture cards; while all who can are taught to speak and lipread" (Entrican [1905?], 28–29). We should note that sign language was not used in the classroom at the Chefoo School.

The Chefoo School greatly influenced the first stages of development of deaf education in China, introducing educational methods that were subsequently replicated elsewhere. For example, the fingerspelling system for Chinese developed by Mills formed the basis for the finger alphabet used in Chinese schools (Zhou Y. 1980), and the graded primers that she translated and adapted from American works were the first course materials used in deaf education in China (Entrican [1905?]). Deaf graduates of the school, and in some cases their hearing relatives, founded or taught in a number of deaf schools set up in China in the first half of the twentieth century.

According to the educator Liu Zhenxing, who is himself deaf, twenty-five deaf schools had been established in China by 1937. Between 1937 and 1949, when China withstood not only Japanese invasion but also the civil war between the Nationalist government and Communist forces, many educational institutions including schools for the deaf were temporarily shut down or relocated. But where refugees fled, some new schools were also set up — many by deaf people (Liu Z. 1992).

In October 1949 the People's Republic of China was founded. Two years later, the policy document "Decision on Reforming the Education System" stipulated that "governments of every level shall establish schools of special education for the deaf and blind and offer education to handicapped children, youth and adults" (182). By this means deaf education became a responsibility of the state, and government at all levels — provincial, municipal, and below — was obligated to provide education for deaf children in their area. Steps were taken to implement the policy in six main areas:

1. The government took over control of existing deaf schools and certain textbooks were designated as standard.

2. A Bureau of the Deaf and Blind was set up in the Central Education Ministry.

3. The government developed a curriculum for deaf schools that set standards in academic, physical, and moral education. Deaf schools were to complete the curricular material specified for mainstream primary schools and also to provide vocational training. Teaching plans were designed.

4. The government conducted research to improve oral teaching and promoted the use of better methods.

5. Budgets were set for deaf schools that were more generous than those for ordinary schools. Staffing requirements were fixed, and to encourage recruitment the principals, deans, and teachers at deaf schools were to be paid 15 percent more. Class sizes were to be limited to no more than fifteen students.

6. The government issued special textbooks in Chinese language and mathematics for use in deaf schools. (Piao 1987)

The number of deaf schools in existence in 1948 is uncertain. According to Piao (1987) there were 23 schools for the deaf and 9 for deaf and blind children, making 32 in all; H. T. Li, who is cited in Tyler and He (1990), put the number at 42, with about 2,000 students; a Russian source, S. A. Zykov, cited in Gryffed-Williams (1962) counted 27 schools with 1,415 children. The discrepancies may be due either to incomplete gathering of information, since most of the schools were private, or to differences in definition. At any rate, by 1957, when all schools were under government administration, there were altogether 66 schools for deaf, blind and deaf, and blind children (*China Statistical Yearbook* 1991, 623). Astonishingly, over the next five years the number of schools quadrupled, to 261; after a slight drop during the Cultural Revolution, when schools were closed down and staff sent to the countryside, there has been a steady increase to the present day. In 1992 there were 642 schools for the deaf, with 57,281 pupils and 12,559 teachers ("Work for the Deaf" 1994); in 1996 there were 980 schools for deaf and blind children, with 90,149 pupils and 19,060 teachers (*China Statistical Yearbook* 1997, 668). The number of deaf children in school has expanded accordingly. By government estimates, in 1987 30 percent of deaf children attended school and only 23 percent completed six years' basic education; now 60 percent of deaf children have access to education ("Eastern Red" 1998). The Ninth Five-Year Plan sets a goal of 80 percent for the year 2000 (*Development* 1997). Generally speaking, deaf children in urban areas have good access to education in deaf schools, but some children in rural areas have no deaf school in the immediate area and have little chance of education unless they are admitted into a local school: there they find no specialized support and may have great difficulty learning in such circumstances.

Children are enrolled in urban schools for the deaf at the usual age for starting primary school—seven, or a year or two older (e.g., Nanjing Deaf School enrolls children only between the ages of seven and nine); deaf schools in the countryside admit children considerably older than this, in some cases even in their teens. Most will not have attended preschool; in urban areas, a few children may have gone to mainstream kindergartens or one of the new rehabilitation centers for deaf children before starting deaf school. The first year at deaf school appears to be a difficult stage: according to the head teacher of Nanjing Deaf School, teachers regard first-year pupils as very undisciplined, and there are communication problems — "they can't understand anything." By the second year, however, most seem to have settled down. Teachers believe that deaf children should have access to preschool education so they can be properly socialized through the experience of being with other children in a disciplined environment.

The population of children in deaf schools includes, as one would expect, many severely and profoundly deaf children; but there are also children with lesser degrees of hearing loss who have been refused entry to mainstream schools.[12] In the future, as services for preschool-age deaf children improve and official directives supporting the integration of disabled children in mainstream schools take effect, such refusals are likely to be less common. Children admitted to deaf school must be of normal intelligence and have no other disabilities; indeed, there is little provision for deaf children with multiple disabilities, other than state welfare institutions.

Large urban deaf schools generally provide a ten-year course based on a national curriculum — six years of primary education followed by four years of middle school. Subjects include Chinese language, math, science, history, geography, art, sports, and rhythm dance. Moral training is an important element in the curriculum. In the middle school years vocational training is strongly emphasized, with classes in sewing, carpentry, and arts and crafts providing pupils with practical skills to use in their employment (Callaway 1986). Many urban deaf schools now have a computer room and teach word processing.

The majority of deaf schools in China rely primarily on sign-supported Chinese in the classroom. Although a comprehensive aural/oral approach has always been held up as optimal (Piao 1987; "Work for the Deaf" 1994), few schools have been able to implement such an approach because of the lack of hearing aids and speech trainers as well as appropriately qualified staff.[13] That deaf pupils often have a relatively late start in education also poses a serious obstacle to acquiring speech and language. Most of the teachers learn signs on the job: during the first few months of their assignment to a deaf school, they sit in on more experienced teachers' classes (Zhu Juling, conversation with author, June 1996). Therefore some inexperienced teachers probably have quite limited ability to communicate with their students and to teach effectively through signing.

Outside the classroom, students use a more natural form of sign language, dropping the word order and the redundant elements of signed Chinese and employing more colloquial and local signs. Teachers constantly deplore this "irregular" use of sign language, noting the difficulties that pupils have with reading comprehension and in writing characters in the correct grammatical order of the spoken language. Teachers believe that earlier teaching of sign-supported Chinese to deaf children, and its vigorous repetition and reinforcement, will prevent these problems: this is one reason why teachers would welcome the use of sign in preschools for profoundly deaf children. Thus the sign language used by deaf children and deaf people is regarded as inferior, while sign-supported Chinese is fully legitimized through its use by teachers, the vast majority of whom are hearing, in formal education in the deaf schools.

Older generations of deaf school teachers were trained on the job, but the trend in the last decade has been for teachers to attend special education teacher-training institutions such as the Normal School for Special Education in Nanjing, which opened in 1985. The new emphasis on formal certification has resulted in deaf people being squeezed out of the profession: whereas in the 1950s deaf schools had a significant number of deaf people on the teaching staff, now only those deaf young people who obtain specialist qualifications are able to get a teaching post in a deaf school (e.g., Nanjing School for the Deaf has two young deaf art teachers who graduated from a special college in Changchun that runs art courses for deaf students). According to one deaf man who was admitted to the Normal School in Nanjing, it is extremely rare for deaf people to be accepted into a teacher-training course at one of the provincial normal schools (Liu Zhenxing, conversation with author, November 1994). Administrators are reluctant to admit students who may have difficulty accessing the curriculum or finding employment later; there are as yet few, if any, initiatives to support deaf students in such courses.

Government Policies for the Disabled

In the 1980s the combination of a number of factors led to a powerful new set of initiatives for disabled people in China. In 1978 China started its "open-door" policy toward the outside world, and Chinese educators began to have better access to information on programs of special education in developed countries. The UN Decade of Disabled Persons, from 1983 to 1992, focused international attention on disability issues and lent support to those concerned for the welfare of disabled people and promoting new policy initiatives on their behalf. The individual in China most closely connected with these new policies is Deng Pufang, son of the former premier Deng

Xiaoping — he himself is disabled and in a wheelchair. In 1983 he established the China Welfare Fund for the Handicapped, which in 1988 became the China Disabled People's Federation (CDPF). Deng Pufang has played a crucial role in bringing disability issues to prominence nationally and in promoting programs to benefit disabled children and disabled people (Shapiro 1989; China Association of the Deaf 1990).

The CDPF is a "semigovernmental" organization that protects the rights of disabled people and works with the government in formulating policies, laws, and development programs. The level of representation by disabled individuals in the CDPF is high — the federation's regulations mandate that more than half the members of the National Congress and Presidium of the CDPF, which formulates policy, and more than two-thirds of the CDPF's Advisory Committee must themselves be disabled people — strengthening the CDPF's claim to represent their interests (China Association of the Deaf 1990). The federation has branches in every province, in all major cities, and in large county towns, enabling systematic implementation of centrally formulated policy throughout the country. CDPF-sponsored institutions in the capital are set up as models for similar institutions nationwide.

Work plans are set in Beijing, and the numbers of disabled children to be rehabilitated in each area are fixed; feedback from the CDPF branches to the central administration influences the next round of policies. One drawback of this top-down control of policy and planning is that no official connections are maintained between branches of the CDPF at grassroots level and local education bureaus; this lack of coordination can lead to practical difficulties — for example, when deaf children from the preschool rehabilitation centers organized by the CDPF enter local primary schools or are admitted to deaf schools, both of which are administered by the local education authorities.

The 1987 National Survey of the Disabled established the size of the population of disabled people and the nature of the services required; the data obtained for deaf children and deaf people were summarized at the beginning of this chapter. A year later, the Chinese government introduced a "Five-Year Plan for Disabled People" (1988–93). Three main areas, named the "three rehabilitations," were given priority: operations for people with cataracts, orthopedic operations to correct disabilities caused by polio, and hearing and speech training for deaf children. Target quotas were set for each province. In its provisions for disabled people, China's Eighth Five-Year Plan (1991–95) outlined additional quotas for 1994 and 1995; the Ninth Five-Year Plan (1996–2000), contains new policies affecting families with deaf children. How the implementation of these policies is affecting the rehabilitation of preschool-age deaf children is described in greater detail below.

One result of work done in the 1980s to raise the profile of disabled people in China was the 1990 Law on the Protection of Disabled Persons, which both confirms the new status and rights of disabled people and outlines future policy in specific areas such as providing employment, education, and social welfare. Its core intention is to ensure the "equal and full participation in social life [of disabled people] and their share of the material and cultural wealth of society" (Article 1).[14] Not only are disabled people to be treated without prejudice as full citizens, but they should enjoy equal access to economic opportunity. Article 8 specifically designates the CDPF as the organization responsible for implementing government policy for the disabled by representing disabled people, safeguarding their interests, uniting them, and providing essential services (including education).

The 1990 Law for the Protection of Disabled Persons describes society's responsibility for rehabilitating disabled people as follows:

> The state and society shall adopt measures of rehabilitation to help disabled persons regain normal functions or compensate for lost functions, thus enhancing their ability to participate in social life (Article 13).

Rehabilitation is assumed to be a process of normalizing abnormal or deficient functioning so that the disabled individual can join the mainstream of "normal," able-bodied people. However, the law confirms the government's determination to leave the primary responsibility for the care of disabled children and disabled adults with their families, who are expressly forbidden to mistreat or abandon them. Yet disabled individuals should not be dependent on their families: "family members and guardians of disabled persons should encourage and assist disabled persons to enhance their capability of [*sic*] self-reliance" (Article 9). The emphasis on self-sufficiency makes clear the government's belief that disabled individuals should become economically independent and self-supporting.

The rights of disabled people to education are confirmed in the 1990 law. In each administrative area, provision should be made to ensure that disabled children have access to education, including preschool education. Crucially, Article 22 forbids mainstream educational institutions at any level from excluding disabled pupils who are capable of participating: "Ordinary primary schools and junior middle schools must admit disabled children or juveniles who are able to adapt themselves to life and study there; ordinary senior middle schools, secondary polytechnic schools, technical schools and institutions of higher learning must admit disabled students who meet the state admission requirements and shall not deny their admission because of their disabilities." A procedure is outlined whereby disabled students denied admission or their parents can appeal to "the relevant authorities," who will require the schools concerned to accept the students. Ordinary preschool institutions are also required to admit disabled children according to the same guidelines. Moreover, disabled children can be exempted from some or all school fees, and grants should be made available for poor disabled students.

To date, the implementation of the 1990 legislation for disabled people has been only partial. One serious problem is lack of resources when so many other priorities are compelling: for example, in remote rural areas where it has proved difficult to provide able-bodied children with basic education, disabled children find it even more difficult to obtain the education to which they are legally entitled. Nevertheless, this unequivocal statement of the Chinese government's current stance is a landmark in the development of rights for disabled people in China.

1988 Onward: New Initiatives for Preschool-Age Deaf Children

As has already been noted, developing programs for hearing and speech training for deaf children was one of the three priority areas designated in the Five-Year Plan for Disabled People for 1988 to 1993. A target was set: 30,000 children were to receive rehabilitation training during this period. Although this number seems large, it was still only 4 percent of the deaf children in this age group. China's Eighth Five-Year Plan for 1994 and 1995 added another 20,000 children (Tang 1992).

The program for deaf children consists of hearing and speech training of preschool-age deaf children—in other words, children between the ages of three and six—in special rehabilitation centers set up by the CDPF nationwide. The aim is to enable deaf children, especially those with residual hearing, to acquire sufficient speech and knowledge of language so they can enter a mainstream kindergarten or a mainstream primary school at age seven. To this end, the importance of the "three earlies" is underlined: early diagnosis, early fitting of hearing aids, and early hearing and speech training. The percentage of children from rehabilitation centers being integrated into the mainstream is 11 percent nationally (from the CRR Center for Deaf Children, at least 15 percent enter mainstream schooling); the goal in the Ninth Five-Year Plan (1996–2000) is to raise this to 12 percent. The remaining children go on to segregated education in deaf schools.

The rehabilitation centers provide a full-time curriculum based on that of the mainstream kindergarten, but emphasizing activities that train hearing and practice speech. The approach to speech training is very structured and systematic: the first drills are based on children reading *pinyin* syllables and learning to recognize them by sound;[15] to these is added practice in everyday phrases such as greetings, then gradually longer phrases and sentences. In line with mainstream kindergarten policy, few Chinese characters are taught at this stage. The rehabilitation centers also play a crucial role in providing education to parents and in fitting hearing aids and ear molds. By ensuring that children have good-quality functioning aids and get in the habit of wearing them and using them properly, the rehabilitation centers help counteract the parents' difficulties in making their children wear hearing aids.

The CRR Center for Deaf Children in Beijing, with its rich resources in diagnostic, educational, and research sections, is the model for rehabilitation centers for preschool-age deaf children throughout China. In the educational section, children between the ages of three and six—there were eighty-four in 1995–96—receive rehabilitation training. The classrooms are colorfully decorated, well-equipped, and attractive; teaching standards are excellent, with young, enthusiastic, and qualified teachers. The atmosphere is cheerful and purposeful.

Rehabilitation centers all over the country are currently suffering a severe shortage of suitably trained staff. In 1993 the Early Childhood Education Department of Nanjing Normal University, in cooperation with the CCR Center for Deaf Children, started a two-year intensive program to produce the specialists needed: the first class of forty-five teachers graduated in 1995 (Jiao Zhimin 1995).[16] Otherwise, typical training for staff at the rehabilitation centers, many of whom have no previous teaching experience, consists of short courses in auditory and speech training techniques, which are sponsored by the local branch of the CDPF. The rehabilitation centers have been hampered by a severe shortage of funds to build, equip, and staff them (Tang 1992). The logistical problems in identifying families with deaf children of preschool age and encouraging attendance at the rehabilitation centers are discussed in more detail in the next chapter.

In its provisions concerning the rehabilitation of deaf children, China's Ninth Five-Year Plan (1996–2000) marked important new developments in policy, particularly regarding the role of parents. It recognizes the basic problem of demand far outrunning capacity: "Deaf children's rehabilitation in China is still in process, the number of deaf children is great, rehabilitation institutions are few in number, and very far from being adequate for the demand" (*Zhongguo canji ren* 1996, 56). To rehabilitate thousands of preschool-age deaf children with some residual hearing through auditory and speech training, existing facilities and training of specialized staff must be expanded:

> China now has 800,000 deaf children under the age of seven, and each year 30,000 more deaf children appear. The vast majority of deaf children have residual hearing, by means of which auditory and language training can be enough to promote aural-oral communication. During the period 1996 to 2000, 58,000 deaf children should enter auditory and language training, 1,765 deaf children's rehabilitation setups should be established at different levels, and 3,540 deaf children's rehabilitation teachers and various other specialized personnel should be trained. (*Zhongguo canji ren* 1996, 56)

The plan lays out five objectives:

- Sixty thousand deaf children should enter auditory and language training, *among whom 20,000 should receive training at home;* after receiving training the number of deaf children entering ordinary nursery schools and primary schools should be at least 12 percent.
- The national system for deaf children's auditory and language training should be established and completed, so that by the year 2000 there is the capacity to train 20,000 children.
- Two hundred language training units should be established.
- *Twenty thousand parents of deaf children should be trained,* as well as 2,000 personnel.
- Early intervention work should be developed in the thirty provincial deaf children's rehabilitation centers. (*Zhongguo canji ren* 1996, 56–57; emphasis added)

The provincial rehabilitation centers, as well as language departments "with suitable conditions," have the responsibility of running training courses for parents, whether or not their children are enrolled in rehabilitation classes. The teachers are required to help parents, carry out home visits, and so on; some of the support is provided through correspondence.

The Ninth Five-Year Plan also outlines the responsibilities and functions of the different levels of administration; overall direction of programs for deaf children is by the CRR Center for Deaf Children in Beijing. This institution is responsible for heading research into preventing deafness, developing screening tests, fitting good-quality hearing aids and ear molds, and developing teaching methods and materials; it also trains teachers and other specialized personnel and collects statistics on childhood hearing impairment.

Deaf People in China: Language, Culture, and Community

The preceding discussion has focused on medical and educational aspects of deafness. Societal attitudes toward deafness, and the status of deaf people and their language in China, affect the lives of deaf children and deaf adults and their families at least as deeply. What follows is a brief introduction to these complex and relatively unexplored issues.

Deaf Children and Deaf People

Traditional attitudes toward deaf children and deaf people in China were very negative. In nineteenth-century China they were feared and avoided because they were believed to be inhabited by evil spirits. Annetta Mills's successor as principal of the Chefoo School for deaf children, Anita Carter, observed that "in China the deaf are more truly outcasts than even the blind; these are sometimes looked on as wise men, but the deaf are, according to current belief, being punished for previous sins, and are possessed of a devil" (Carter 1938, 51).

One contemporary observer described the situation of deaf people in China at the turn of the century:

> Their condition is supposed to be entirely hopeless. They are not treated with any special unkindness, but they are considered as little better than dumb animals. They are clothed and fed, but have to learn to do whatever they can by watching others. If it is a son the parents offer a double marriage dowry to get a hearing wife, and if it is a daughter, a small dowry is claimed, and she is married into some poor family, where she is practically a slave. Both blind and deaf girls are frequently sold into slavery, and driven into every kind of sin and vice. (Entrican [1905?], 9–10)

Carter's description (1911) of the backgrounds of the girl pupils who entered the Chefoo School provides much evidence to substantiate this account of the fate of deaf girls, considered worthless both because of their sex and because of their disability. There were apparently far fewer deaf women than deaf men in China at the time: even healthy female babies had little value, and those who were found to be deaf were often killed; but deaf boys were more likely to be saved because they could still continue the family line (Entrican [1905?]).

The education of deaf children, whether boys or girls, was generally regarded as a waste of time. Before 1949 education was available to relatively few children at all. Chinese parents evidently found it strange that teachers at the Chefoo School went to so much effort for deaf children when many hearing children had no chance to attend school: "If it is difficult to persuade parents to meet the expenses of their hearing sons in mission schools, it is far more so to get them to expend anything on the deaf. 'What can a deaf boy do?' 'Can a deaf boy learn letters,' &c., are the contemptuous remarks often heard, while to gather them into a school and try to teach them is considered quixotic indeed" (Entrican [1905?], 10). Christian missionaries in China in the early years of the twentieth century judged the indigenous religions of China—Buddhism, Confucianism, and Taoism—to be lacking in sympathy or pity for the less fortunate and unwilling to make provision for them, and they contrasted these attitudes unfavorably with Christian compassion for the poor and afflicted that leads to philanthropy (Mills 1910).

In describing her experiences growing up in Hong Kong in the 1940s and 1950s, Lucy Ching, who is blind herself, also attributes lack of sympathy in Chinese society toward disabled people to the influences of Confucianism and Buddhism (1980). Confucianism is centered on a system of graded social obligations and prescribed social behavior toward others: personal merit is gained through fulfilling these obligations correctly, especially within the family. Buddhism teaches that being born into a lowly station in life is a sign that a person committed bad deeds in a previous existence; suffering, which is an unavoidable part of life, can be transcended only by cultivating abnegation of worldly desires and following a virtuous way of life. Although in theory individuals gain merit by doing good deeds and demonstrating charity and compassion to others, the practice of Buddhism in China did not seem to lead to any systematic effort to provide for the deaf, blind, or mentally ill. Thus the indigenous moral belief systems in China in the first part of the twentieth century did little to counteract societal prejudice against disabled people or to establish institutions to help them.

We should not generalize from evidence of prejudice against deaf people in the China of fifty or more years ago to contemporary views, particularly among well-educated people living in urban areas. Nevertheless, the grandparents of today's generation of children were brought up with such beliefs, which may still color their attitudes and behavior; and Lucy Ching (1980) observes that traditional prejudices against disabled people do still persist. In chapter 2, we examined how a disabled child is stigmatized: he or she is not only an emotional and economic burden for their family, but a source of shame for the family in their relations with others. Sydenham (1993, 29) notes that official materials acknowledge and perpetuate negative images of disability and points to a statement from a circular sent to households in Jiamusi, in northeast China: "a disabled child is a misfortune of human society, it not only causes the parents suffering and shame, but is also a great burden on society."

The great progress made in highlighting disability issues that has taken place in the last ten years under the aegis of Deng Pufang and the CDPF has been accompanied by official rhetoric intended to change attitudes and behavior toward disabled people. This publicity campaign portrays disabled people as willing and able to work hard, to contribute to national development, and to play a positive role in society; individual disabled people who have achieved success are held up as exemplars and their stories are published widely in the media.[17] The normative construction of desirable attitudes through official propaganda not only creates a positive public image of disabled people but also makes it clear that the appropriate response of able-bodied people is to support them and help them solve their problems (Sydenham 1993).

To be sure, there can be a considerable gap between rhetoric and reality. When Chinese parents are told that their child is deaf they are shocked, as they immediately conjure up images of their child's future as a deaf-mute person isolated from the family. Parents coping with their own grief also become sensitive to the reactions of others in daily life: many are upset when other children or even adults point out their child as "little mute." Parents worry deeply about their child's chances for education and a good job. Their anxieties are well founded: huge practical barriers hinder their children from gaining access to mainstream education or employment, and parents must deal with an enormous amount of ingrained social prejudice, not only from outsiders but also from other family members and even from within themselves (Sydenham 1993).[18]

The Status of Sign Language

In the 1950s, when the curriculum and structure of deaf schools were being set, regional variations in sign language were perceived as an obstacle to the uniform and regulated development of deaf education, as well as to communication between sign language users from different parts of China. In response, in 1958 a Sign Language Reform Committee was established (Piao 1984). Signs were collected from all over China; they were then sorted, printed, and redistributed to regional committee members for their comments and suggestions. Deaf people were consulted both at the collection and discussion stages, and hearing teachers in deaf schools apparently also played a major role in this process. New signs were also invented to cover various occupations, family relationships, topics in politics, and other areas (Yau 1987). Because these signs were based on the spoken language, many two-syllable words were represented by two signs rather than one to express the concept in question. The "standard" sign language devised in this process consisted of 2,000 signs, which were then popularized in study classes. The work on standardizing Chinese sign language was halted during the Cultural Revolution, but in 1979 a sign language forum was held and a two-volume book published containing 1,000 signs; the 1992 edition contains over 3,000 signs. This has been designated "Chinese Sign Language"; in other words, Chinese Sign Language officially comprises the standardized signs in the most recent dictionary.

In late-nineteenth-century America, the desirability of imposing some sort of uniformity on the many variations of different signs used in different educational programs was also discussed — but never carried out. Nor has recent concern over the increasing number of different sign systems used to manually encode English in schools led to standardization (Stedt and Moores 1990). Nevertheless, as Stedt and Moores point out, American Sign Language has not splintered into a number of debased regional versions but has proved resilient and survived. A recent television debate in the United Kingdom considered the standardization of British Sign Language, or BSL (*See Hear on Saturday*, BBC 2, 26 September 1998). One of the participants, Susan Gregory, emphasized the importance of developing conceptually rational sign vocabulary for teaching math and science in schools. Panelists also noted an emerging nationally used BSL vocabulary, which may be gaining dominance over distinct regional variants; this trend seems to be reinforced by the greater use of sign language on television.

The standardized Chinese Sign Language achieved by the Sign Language Reform Committee is perceived and defined by hearing Chinese educators as a tool for communication and education: its signs and fingerspelling follow the word order of spoken Chinese. Forms of sign language developed by deaf people themselves are called "gesture language"; characteristically they do not employ fingerspelling, and they "follow the grammatical rules of spoken language incompletely, without a fixed order of expression" (Piao 1992, 3). Thus the natural language of Chinese deaf people is not officially defined as a "sign language": that phrase has been adopted by the sign language reformists to refer to their artificial system, which they call "deaf people's sign language." Not surprisingly, this terminology leads to some confusion. China accepted sign language as an official language in 1990 ("Eastern Red" 1998), but it is not clear in what terms "sign language" has been defined. In an official context, however, it most likely means signs used in the order of spoken Chinese, rather than indigenous Chinese sign language.

Piao Yongxin, one of China's most authoritative figures in special education, declares in his recent book on sign language that "because of its innate limitations, sign language is ultimately somewhat inferior to spoken language" (Piao 1992, 5). He lists its weaknesses: its use is limited to deaf people and a few others, it has a limited vocabulary and a limited range of expression, it cannot convey abstract concepts, and it is imprecise in the meaning of some of its signs. Piao goes on to claim that the use of sign language harms cognition and language development in deaf children:

> Sign language is often related to concrete objects, so the development of abstract thought in deaf students is hindered. They become accustomed to using gestures and consequently give up using speech, or use it only seldom. They avoid using difficult expressions and choose easy ones, with the result that some of their signing becomes separated from the spoken language. This leads to mistakes in their written language, which affects their ability to learn. (5)

At the same time that Piao deplores the use of sign language, he suggests that it is much more important for deaf children to master written Chinese, the measure of formal academic achievement, than it is to communicate easily using sign language.

In discussing whether "gesture language" has its own grammar, Piao shows some appreciation of particular syntactic patterns used by deaf people: for example, topic-comment constructions, negative and interrogative constructions in sign, and directionality with certain verbs. But he otherwise does not mention the unique grammatical features of sign language, particularly the use of space and the inflections of signs to produce a range of meanings; nor does he mention the crucial role played by facial expression and other nonmanual features. It is perhaps significant that the Chinese phrase for "sign language" (*shouyu*) literally means "hand language," a term that deflects attention from the other essential components of communication in sign. Piao concludes that the observed differences in deaf people's ordering of signs is a matter of habit, which can be corrected (i.e., made to approximate the word order used by hearing people) with formal education:

> As the level of deaf people's education increases, deaf people will have a better understanding of signs used according to the rules of spoken or written language. As deaf education becomes more widespread, deaf people will become more proficient in spoken and written language. . . . Deaf people's sign language will become more closely related to spoken and written language, and the situation whereby deaf people put words in the wrong order will gradually improve. (1992, 6)

Ironically, hearing educators still call the reformed sign system "deaf people's sign language," as though under such circumstances it could still belong to them.

The standardization of Chinese signs and publication of the dictionary of Chinese Sign Language should have made it easier, at least in theory, for hearing teachers to learn signs in a systematic way and to teach the national curriculum in deaf schools. However, in practice it appears that teachers use many local signs rather than following the standardized lexicon. Frances Parsons, an American deaf woman who traveled around China in 1986, observed marked differences in the different deaf schools she visited; she notes that "each school said that its signs were right and the others wrong"

(1988, 131). Indeed, it may not be possible to impose a standard set of signs throughout the educational system, let alone among the Chinese deaf community.

Educators and teachers in deaf schools believe that the use of signs in the order of spoken Chinese, without the unique syntactic features of indigenous sign language, benefits the academic development of deaf children by remaining close to the forms of the spoken language. They seem not to appreciate the cognitive and intellectual advantages for deaf children of communicating with each other in indigenous sign language or to recognize the importance for a deaf child's sense of identity and self-esteem of such communication with other deaf people. In practice, however, many teachers, whether experienced or just starting to teach, may not stick rigidly to the word order of spoken Chinese when they sign; instead they express themselves more economically in a manner more accessible to their students. Teachers are required to speak and sign at the same time, but this mandate is difficult to sustain; according to a senior teacher at Nanjing Deaf School, sometimes teachers drop the speech and just use signs with their classes.

Although teachers rely on sign to communicate with deaf students and teach, official descriptions of the approach used in the deaf school system do not reflect this key practice. The method of teaching is described as "oral," with "sign assisting"; together the two components constitute a "combined system" (Callaway, 1999). When a third modality—the written language—is added, it is called a "comprehensive approach." In such descriptions, sign plays a subordinate role in assisting communication, and it is aligned and synthesized with spoken and written forms of the Chinese language.

The insistence on using signs in the order of spoken Chinese also shapes discussion of bilingual education for deaf children. The term "bilingual" and its application to deaf education appear to be very recent imports from Western countries. In the 1996 *Dictionary of Special Education,* edited by Piao, the entry for "bilingual environment in schools for the deaf" assumes that there are two languages in the classroom: sign language and Chinese (oral and written). In fact, the sign language used simply encodes spoken Chinese—it is not the separate, living language of deaf people. Here again the argument is made that because the two forms of communication cannot be precisely aligned, they interfere with one another. The entry recommends that deaf children should master both the rules of grammar (of the Chinese language) and everyday (spoken) language, so that the two languages, sign and Chinese, can become "even more combined and unified."

Many of the concerns and arguments of Chinese deaf educators who support the use of a Chinese-based sign system in schools for the deaf are very similar to those employed by U.S. supporters of "methodical" signs in the late nineteenth century (see Stedt and Moores 1990). But a key difference is that the American educators were engaged in a long and complex debate with a significant number of American deaf school teachers who preferred the use of "natural" signs in the classroom as more accessible to students and argued publicly for their use. No such substantial group of people in China appears to be advocating the use of indigenous sign language in education. In a paper titled "The Place of Sign Language in Deaf People's Education and Culture" (1998), a retired deaf Chinese teacher, Mei Fusheng, does provide a clear analysis of the language issues in deaf education that both recognizes the distinct and different grammatical features of indigenous sign language and presents a strong argument for its use in the education of deaf children — but this position is a striking exception. According to Shen Yulin, deputy editor of China's principal special education journal as well as a qualified teacher of the deaf, many teachers in Chinese deaf schools do not know that sign language has its own grammar (letter to author, 28 August 1998). The centralized bureaucracy in China, which issues guidelines on all aspects of education, including the deaf schools, undoubtedly makes it more difficult for individual schools or teachers who might have new ideas to try out different methods of teaching.

The efforts to adapt indigenous Chinese sign language (or sign languages) for use in education as well as other social contexts, especially the undertaking to produce a standardized vocabulary, parallel the state's manipulation of spoken and written forms of Chinese for various purposes. Mandarin Chinese (*putonghua*) has been adopted as the official spoken language of China; its use in the media and educational institutions provides a unifying, common language for all Chinese, although many speak home dialects far removed from the standard Beijing dialect on which *putonghua* is based.[19] Its systematic nationwide introduction began in 1956; in 1958 the Foreign Minister Zhou Enlai stated that "our promotion of Putonghua aims at the removal of the barriers among the dialects but not at the suppression or destruction of the dialects" (qtd. in Freeman and Habermann 1996, 91). The position taken by the Chinese government was that because it was impractical to attempt to eradicate regional dialects, a policy of bilingualism in the spoken language should be implemented. Even as a national spoken language was introduced, *putonghua*-speaking government officials were required to learn the local dialects of the regions where they were working: thus there was some effort to make the language policy work in both directions (Freeman and Habermann 1996). This stance on bilingualism resonates with the goal of the Chinese Sign Language Reform Committee: "to provide the deaf population with a full-scale standard lexicon while continuing to tolerate dialectal signs" (Yau 1987, 65). However, the extent to which a standardized sign vocabulary can be imposed on deaf people is questionable.

Jenner (1992) describes the "centralizing, authoritarian tradition" of Chinese civilization that permits only one culture and one set of values—as well as only one written language. He notes that "while a huge variety of local low cultures, mainly Han but also non-Han, could continue to exist, *they were not 'civilisation'*" (225; emphasis added). The appropriation and adaptation of natural forms of sign language by hearing educators clearly follow exactly this pattern: setting up one language as official, legitimate, and proper while at the same time designating all other forms as uncivilized and inferior. But there is also an important difference between adopting an extant and widely used version of Chinese, *putonghua*, as the official spoken language and officially designating an artificial language—a collection of standardized approved signs used in the order of spoken Chinese—as "Chinese Sign Language."

Just as many other cultures, languages, and regional dialects flourish in China alongside the main, official spoken language, so we might expect there to be many forms of indigenous Chinese sign language used by different communities of deaf people in China: these have still to be fully investigated (apparently the Shanghai dialect is the most influential; see Yau 1987). Probably the richest languages will be found among communities of deaf school graduates; and it would not be surprising if the sign language that deaf people use among themselves shows some influence from the sign-supported Chinese taught in deaf schools, just as the English-based system of signs first used in American deaf education in the last century has influenced the development of American Sign Language (Stedt and Moores 1990).

The ideographic written language is of overriding importance to Chinese culture and civilization; its "primacy is felt to belong to the character, which has an existence and meaning independent of mere speech" (Jenner 1992, 212). Moreover, despite its disadvantages it provides a unified communication system. The attainment of literacy is highly valued, and this helps to explain why Chinese educators attach much more importance to sign communication that matches the written language than a natural form of signing that departs from it (it also explains the efforts to modernize the written script in the 1950s and early 1960s by simplifying it systematically). For communication between deaf and hearing people, including among family members at home, the use of written Chinese is customary and essential: "At present, sign language has not been very popular in China, so they [deaf people] can not communicate freely with their family members, colleagues or the communities. Conversation by writing is still the chief means between people with hearing impairment and hearing people who don't know sign language" ("Work for the Deaf" 1994, 3). Under these circumstances, parents of deaf children and teachers in deaf schools have an additional reason to place special emphasis on deaf children's achieving literacy.

Deaf Culture and Deaf Community

Drawing on information concerning the families of the 1,548 deaf children identified in the 1987 National Survey of the Disabled, we can estimate that between 3.5 to 5 percent of Chinese children with hearing impairments have at least one deaf parent (*Canji ertong ziliao* 1991). A survey of twenty-two deaf schools in Jiangsu province showed that 5 percent of children had deaf parents, although this figure may not be representative of the general population as some deaf parents may not be able to afford to send their children to deaf school (Callaway 1999). These numbers are of the same order as those for the United States and the United Kingdom, which are generally placed at between 5 and 10 percent,[20] although one might expect a somewhat lower figure for China because of the greater incidence of acquired deafness. There appear to be relatively few families in which sign language, the core element of deaf culture,[21] is the language of the deaf child's parents and therefore the language of communication at home. Furthermore, in families in which parents are deaf, the intergenerational transmission of sign language is likely to be weakened if hearing grandparents take responsibility for care of their deaf grandchild and decide to use speech at home rather than sign.[22]

Strong and lasting bonds among deaf individuals in China begin to develop in the deaf schools, which are found mainly in urban areas. They are fostered in the welfare factories, which are state enterprises that employ fixed quotas of disabled people: welfare factory managers maintain close connections with deaf schools in their area, and visit them each year to select new employees from the graduating class. This process ensures that deaf people who attended the same deaf school often work together as well. Continuity between school and work is also strengthened in smaller ways; for example, the deaf school teachers may inform prospective employers of the new employee's name sign (Yau and He 1989).[23] Thus in the cities, at any rate, there are groups of ex-schoolmates who remain in close contact throughout their working lives. Deaf community life follows patterns that are characteristic to China; in particular, there are no fixed public meeting places equivalent to the deaf clubs that exist in the United States and other Western countries. The branches of the Chinese Deaf Association in different Chinese cities provide a focus for some social activities, but these tend to be officially organized functions or celebrations that occur only a few times a year. Deaf informants have told me that they usually meet deaf friends in their own or their parents' homes, sometimes in quite large groups; they may also arrange to assemble in a restaurant, park, or other public venue. Gatherings and celebrations are also organized at deaf people's workplaces. Personal connections are crucial in every aspect of Chinese life, from obtaining scarce goods and services to finding a marriage partner or establishing business networks, and the network of relationships within the Chinese deaf community in a particular locality presumably affords the same essential benefits: smoothing deaf people's passage through life as well as providing a sense of identity and companionship. Such networks appear to underlie business activity by Chinese deaf entrepreneurs.

A key issue in the lives of Chinese deaf people is the balance between the influence of their (hearing) families and that of deaf peers; given the centrality of the family in Chinese life, these different allegiances may be a source of tension and conflict in some cases, especially over the question of whether a deaf son or daughter marries a deaf or a hearing spouse. In rural areas where deaf children do not go to deaf school, their only ties may be with their families; they have no contact with other deaf children or adults. This was my impression on a visit to a poor area in northern Jiangsu province in 1994: the deaf children I met were attending local mainstream primary schools (though most were unable to fully participate in the classroom because they had little support) and had no contact with other deaf children (Callaway 1998a). Yau Shun-chiu, a linguistics researcher based in France, met many deaf people in the Chinese countryside in the 1980s, and he noted their isolation from other deaf people (1996).

Fangang Zeng, who works at the House Ear Institute in Los Angeles, expresses a typical mainstream Chinese attitude in claiming that "the sense of deaf culture does not seem to be strong, if existing at all, in China" (1995, 62). More accurately, although a strong sense of shared identity and a shared language exist in urban areas among deaf school graduates and among deaf people working together (often in the welfare factories), the features of a deaf way of life are neither visible to nor valued by hearing society. Zeng gives three reasons for his statement: most deaf Chinese people live among hearing people; signs used by deaf people in China are not as developed as American Sign Language and are not recognized as a language; and deaf people, who are economically disadvantaged, must rely on family and government for financial support. Because "the general public opinion in China is that deafness is a handicap and should be treated if possible" (62–63), the government has recently emphasized rehabilitation; moreover, Zeng argues, the absence of deaf culture makes the low-cost cochlear implant an appropriate technology for China.

While such views may predominate in China, others exist. Teachers in deaf schools spend their daily working life with deaf children and remain in contact with them when they leave school; they are likely to be well-informed about deaf people's lives and their patterns of association. When I was talking to a senior teacher at the deaf school in Chongqing in Sichuan province about the way deaf young people continue to associate after leaving school, the teacher observed, "The way they always want to be together, they're like an ethnic minority" (*gen minzhu yiyang*). We had not been discussing concepts of deaf culture—the remark was completely spontaneous. Other hearing people in China who work closely with deaf people may similarly perceive them as a linguistically and culturally distinct group.

It would be very valuable to know more about the views and opinions of deaf people themselves on their identity as a cultural group: no one has done much research into Chinese deaf communities. Chinese deaf people have written about their experiences for various magazines in articles that tend to confirm the stereotype of deaf people being defined by their disability—hardly surprisingly, given that this is the official and publicly promulgated image of deafness. It may be that now in China, as for deaf people a generation ago in America and Europe, the concept of deaf culture has little meaning—or perhaps some deaf people in China do have a strong and conscious sense of their identity as a group distinct from hearing people, possessing specific, shared characteristics.

Following the introduction of an experimental bilingual sign class for preschool-age deaf children in Nanjing, after contact and cooperation between myself and my colleagues at the Center for Deaf Studies in Bristol and our counterparts in China—a class described in greater detail in chapter 7—I learned much about Chinese deaf professionals' views on their roles in deaf education. While Chinese policymakers may not be concerned by the drop in the numbers of deaf staff in deaf schools, deaf teachers themselves have very different views on the value for deaf children of having a deaf teacher. Liu Zhenxing, who managed to overcome many difficulties to qualify as a teacher of the deaf, states emphatically that the example of having a deaf teacher like himself helps deaf children understand that they too can have a normal life and participate in their society. In his statement in a newsletter for parents of deaf children, Liu emphasizes how powerful the example of a successful deaf person can be; he thus draws on the Chinese tradition of exemplary models. In addition, he stresses that contact with, and learning from, a deaf teacher will help prevent deaf children from becoming isolated and lonely, and will help them develop self-confidence and self-esteem: their deaf teacher will give them a better understanding of their society and a more constructive outlook on life (Liu Z.

1996). Deaf adults are important as positive role models because they and deaf children share a common identity that can be beneficial for the children concerned. For similar reasons, deaf professionals involved in bilingual programs in Western countries value deaf adults' involvement in the education, socialization, and language development of deaf children (see, e.g., A. Young 1995). Such views conflict with a medical model of deafness, which requires that teachers and role models should be hearing people, or deaf people whose ability to speak makes them equivalent to hearing people. Liu's statements and other evidence from Chinese deaf people themselves challenge the assumption that the official and mainstream views concerning deafness and deaf people are necessarily all-pervasive or indeed especially relevant in real-life situations.

China has one official organization for deaf people—the China Association of the Deaf (CAD), which falls under the administration of the CDPF. According to information put out by the association, any individual with a hearing loss greater than 40 dB is automatically a member ("Work for the Deaf" 1994).[24] The CAD has branches in every province as well as in the larger cities, and it is currently expanding to the county level. Leading officials in the CAD are all deaf people: the president, Dai Mu, became deaf when he was six years old. Fu Zhiwei, chief executive of the CAD became deaf in adulthood, but he is married to a deaf woman, uses sign language, and interacts frequently with other deaf people. The CAD, which both raises its own funds and receives funding from the government, has contributed greatly to creating the national (standardized) sign language; to a large extent, its activities reflect government interests and policies. That the CAD makes a point of working closely with the Chinese government was confirmed by Fu Zhiwei when I interviewed him (Callaway 1998b). It is clearly of practical importance as well as symbolically significant that many CAD officials are deaf. Nevertheless, we may well question how responsive to and how truly representative of the views of deaf people in China the CAD and its branches are; they appear to be primarily an instrument of government policy for the disabled.

CHAPTER FOUR

The Role of Professionals and Parents in the Education of Deaf Children

During the last decade of rapid development in preschool rehabilitation for deaf children, Chinese professionals working in this field have increasingly recognized that parental involvement is essential for success. To implement the key objectives of early childhood intervention—early diagnosis, early fitting of a hearing aid, and early speech training—parents must be motivated and take initiative. Although most parents whose children are in deaf schools do not themselves learn sign language and thus leave the main responsibility for educating their children to the school, those whose children are enrolled in rehabilitation centers need to reinforce work done in class and to keep up speech practice at home. Many articles on rehabilitating deaf children published in the early 1990s emphasize this pivotal role of parents (Wang Yarong 1992; Zhang S. 1992; Ge 1993; Xu T. 1993; Chen G. 1993; Hua 1995; Wang Youguo 1995a, 1995b; Gao Chenbo 1996). Indeed, the main theme of the first national conference for hearing and language specialists in deaf children's rehabilitation in 1993 was family rehabilitation (Tang 1993). Researchers have sought to demonstrate that children with conscientious parents make better progress (e.g., Wang Youguo 1995b).

Parental involvement is perceived as valuable for a number of reasons:

1. Parents are strongly motivated to invest time and trouble in their own child.
2. They know their child best, and can therefore teach their child in a way that is most likely to be effective for him or her.
3. They are with their child for much of the time, especially at the preschool age, and can make use of any time available to teach him or her.
4. Grandparents and other relatives living with or near the family can also act as teachers.
5. The family provides a rich linguistic environment, in which the child is exposed to a variety of everyday language. (Tang 1993; Ge 1993)

Overall, professional discussions strongly emphasize the importance of parental closeness to and sense of responsibility toward their child.

Moreover, there are too few specialized personnel and too few rehabilitation centers for the speech training of all preschool-age deaf children. So many children require these services that the centers cannot meet the goals on their own. Thus many parents are being forced not simply into partnership with their child's teacher but into becoming their child's only teacher. Assessing early progress in the Eighth Five-Year Plan (1991–95), Tang stated the problem quite bluntly:

> In order to accomplish the objectives of the Eighth Five-Year Plan, the key solution is to establish deaf children's family rehabilitation. . . . The 30 provincial centers train 50 children a year each on average; the 400 language training units train 12 children a year on average; altogether 6,300 children a year can be accommodated. Bearing in mind that deaf children spend over a year in training, the number that can actually be trained each year is 5,000 plus. This leaves a shortfall of 3,000 children still requiring training each year. The initiation of family rehabilitation models for deaf children in provinces such as Zhejiang and Hubei is an extremely important step forward. (1992, 5)

He also specified why the "family model"—that is, parents' taking responsibility for giving their children speech training at home—is necessary:

1. Only in this way can deaf children in remote areas receive training.
2. It is 38 times cheaper for a child to be rehabilitated at home.
3. The rehabilitation centers can accept only limited numbers of children.
4. Family training is particularly suitable because there are more opportunities for language and speech interaction in the home.

These arguments reveal the logistical and economic pressures shaping policy on preschool rehabilitation, which is ambitious in its aims of setting up nationwide services despite lack of resources and trained personnel. In stressing parents' involvement the government not only acknowledges the particular benefits the family can provide, but also follows the established pattern of meeting social and political objectives by mobilizing the efforts of ordinary people.

Other arguments have been advanced for parental involvement. Parents can provide continuity in education and speech training, by starting speech training before their child is old enough to attend a rehabilitation center, then acting as partners to the teachers at the center, and finally providing essential follow-up education if their child is placed in a mainstream nursery or primary school (Wang Yarong 1992; Wang Youguo 1995a). In addition, Wang Yarong (1992) stresses that parents are crucial because the optimum time for speech training is before the age of six. He points out that 91 percent of deaf children are deafened before the age of three; most of these children do not attend an ordinary preschool but stay at home, "so the family has a great influence on the child's speech development" (26).

Chinese researchers tend to stress the period between three and six years of age, as this is when deaf children and their parents are in contact with rehabilitation teachers; the focus also reflects their emphasis on speech training (the result of a formal and systematic educative process) rather than on language acquisition (the result of interactive communication from infancy). Yet Western audiologists and education professionals believe that intervention needs to begin very early—auditory stimulation before eighteen months of age is critically important to development. Language deprivation during this period diminishes the child's chances of achieving a good command of language later (Northern and Epstein 1998). Some urban Chinese parents are able to obtain advice from rehabilitation facilities when their children are younger than three; nevertheless, scarce government resources and state provision in China currently concentrate on the older children, between three and six.

Concepts of Rehabilitation in the Family

In the first issue of the professional journal for preschool hearing and language rehabilitation professionals in China, *Rehabilitation of Deaf Children in China,* the director of the CRR Center for Deaf Children in Beijing presents the following definition: "The rehabilitation of deaf children is aimed at making full use of residual hearing, employing medical, educational, and social means to bring about their full rehabilitation in all aspects of hearing, language, psychology, etc., so as to prepare them to start school and return to mainstream society" (Gao Chenghua 1991, 5). In other words, the deaf child with residual hearing is to be normalized as far as possible, enabling him or her to attend an ordinary school and to become integrated with the rest of society. By casting the desired outcome as a "return to mainstream society," Gao Chenghua suggests that the child originally belonged to mainstream society and was removed from it by deafness—even if this may have been congenital. Rehabilitation is thus a kind of restoration to the norm.

The director also warns against understanding the "rehabilitation of deaf children" simply as "speech training of deaf children"; he says that if insufficient attention is paid to other aspects of their rehabilitation—particularly auditory training and psychological counseling—these children will have to be withdrawn from mainstream primary schools when they reach the third or fourth year. That this point is made in so prominent an article suggests there has in fact been considerable overemphasis on speech training in the rehabilitation of deaf children and that some professionals are aware of the inadequacies of such an approach.

Family Education and Rehabilitation for Deaf Children

Prospective rehabilitation teachers at Nanjing Normal University find the following definition of "family education" in their textbook:

> Family education refers to the social activity by means of which parents (mainly the father, mother, and other adult members of the family) exert educational influence on children in the family. This activity is carried out in accordance with social norms and takes into account characteristics of the child's physical and mental development, by parents' consciously and conscientiously using personal example and verbal instruction, and practicing the routines of family life. This activity is extremely important since the family is the fundamental unit of society. Children spend most of their time with their families, so the family is the ideal environment for early education to be carried out. Evidence shows that children's success in education can be attributed in large measure to good family education. For this reason, more and more importance has been attached to family education nowadays. (Li S., Zhou, and Guo 1993, 287)

The idea that the family environment has a crucial influence on children's early development has long been accepted by Western educators; the Chinese definition, however, has several striking features. The process of teaching is characterized as a conscious, deliberate, and relatively formal activity. It is the sole responsibility of adult members of the family—not siblings or cousins, for example—so an age-based relationship of authority is maintained between teachers and pupil. Only the teachers, whether parents or other adults in the family, are active in this process: there is no mention of response from the child or interaction between parent and child. Also, this definition points to "good family education" as leading to future academic success rather than to gains in the child's confidence, happiness, or emotional health.

Family education has assumed a new importance in recent years in China with the implementation of the one-child family policy, as chapter 2 described. Government propaganda has linked limiting family size to the importance of raising children who are looked after very well and are well-educated (expressed in the slogan *you sheng you yu,* meaning "quality birth, quality upbringing"). In addition, parents whose own education was disrupted in the Cultural Revolution are particularly eager to ensure that their children will have every advantage. Many urban parents therefore devote much time and a substantial part of their income to their one child's education (Croll 1995). In Chinese cities, the competition to get into good schools and later to obtain good jobs is fierce; from early on, parents feel the pressure to invest in education and to push their child to achieve academic success.

Parents of deaf children face the same pressures and more. They have the additional responsibility of providing a good environment for the development of speech and language in their child,[1] turning "family education" into "family rehabilitation." The textbook outlines the full extent of parents' responsibilities:

1. Parents should help and encourage their child to adapt to their new circumstances when they start attending the rehabilitation center.

2. Parents should encourage children's intellectual development by buying them books, telling them stories, giving them craft work, and taking them on outings. They should use the opportunity to stimulate and satisfy their child's desire for knowledge by talking about the new surroundings.

3. Attention should be paid to children's health. Parents should ensure that their children eat nutritious food at mealtimes and avoid indulgence in snacks, have sufficient rest, and have enough time to play. In addition, parents should pay attention to children's psychological health by refraining from too much impatient criticism.

4. It is very important for parents to cooperate with the teachers at the rehabilitation center. Cooperation is necessary so that the educational aims of the center can be incorporated into family education.

5. Children should be taught good habits in their daily routine that apply to studying, mealtimes, sleeping, personal hygiene, and so on. They should be taught to respect their teachers and older people, to be polite, and to show good manners in simple sentences. In order to instill good habits in their children, it is sug-

gested that parents explain the reasons for good behavior to their children, set a good example, be firm and consistent, and use positive encouragement rather than punishment as an incentive. (Li S., Zhou, and Guo 1993, 290–94)

Much of this is simply current advice for good parenting, with some additional reminders of parents' responsibility to cooperate with rehabilitation center personnel. Discipline is emphasized because the spoiling of only children is felt to be a matter of great concern nowadays in China. However, there is little practical advice given to parents of a deaf child: how, for example, can they explain that something is wrong? Because the difficulties that result when parents and children cannot effectively communicate are hardly acknowledged in current professional discussions, they are barely addressed or analyzed here.

Social Rehabilitation and Community Rehabilitation

The phrase "social rehabilitation" most often is applied when the deaf child enters the mainstream of society, that is, starts ordinary primary school. Thus discussions in the professional literature about the "social rehabilitation" of deaf children generally focus on their integration in the mainstream school setting. Sometimes it refers more generally to the situations in which the deaf child or adult has the opportunity to meet hearing people—when shopping, for example, or in the local park. Less often, "social rehabilitation" is applied broadly to the socializing of the deaf child, including that which occurs in the family in the early years.

The term "community rehabilitation" appears infrequently in the Chinese literature concerned with preschool deaf children. International definitions of community-based rehabilitation (CBR) differ (see, e.g., Lang 1998), but generally it refers to grassroots, low-cost initiatives generated in the local community to help its disabled members, and it is contrasted with high-cost, institution-based solutions involving expensive equipment and the importation of professionals to manage rehabilitation. It presumes that disabled people should be encouraged to participate fully in the life of their community, including making contributions through their work, and that they should not be labeled as different or segregated in any way. Instead of taking a narrow, medical focus, CBR emphasizes a holistic approach to rehabilitation in the community setting; it has been promoted by nongovernmental organizations and aid agencies as particularly appropriate for rural areas in developing countries.

In practice, the rehabilitation of preschool deaf children in China (and elsewhere) cuts across these definitions. The centralized top-down network of rehabilitation facilities takes precedence over community initiative; the introduction of professional expertise and relatively expensive equipment in the form of hearing aids is not a grassroots approach. Nevertheless, the emphasis on the role of parents does to some degree move responsibility for the rehabilitation process outside the professional network and institutions.

In addition, there are a few clear examples of community rehabilitation for deaf children; for example, the outreach work carried out in China's remote countryside. Jiao Zhimin et al., (1995), who discuss different models for rehabilitation, contrast correspondence school courses, which require parents to travel to a central location to make contact with the teachers, with the work of professionals based in "family rehabilitation guidance stations" in rural areas: as part of community rehabilitation, they make regular home visits to parents with deaf children (see also Yang Rongxian 1995, who uses the term in discussing similar services in the rural northeastern province of Jilin).

The Impact of Diagnosis on Parents

Professional publications tend to deal briefly with parents' attitudes and emotions at the time of diagnosis, regarding them of interest only insofar as they influence parents' contact with medical or educational services. However, a few researchers have examined parents' emotions in greater detail.

Li Shaozhu, Zhou, and Guo (1993) describe the enormous stress experienced by parents when their child is diagnosed as hearing-impaired, identifying six main patterns of emotional response: a sense of loss because their dreams for their child's future are shattered; feelings of inferiority, because they think that other people will look down on them and their child; feelings of guilt, because they feel responsible for their child's deafness; feelings of helplessness, because they do not know what action to take; a sense of determination to educate their child so that he or she can achieve as much as possible; and, finally, feelings of impatience when their child appears to be making slow progress. This list is followed by, though not explicitly linked with, a description of the different types of upbringing deaf children receive because of the different personalities, backgrounds, and circumstances of their parents. Four types of parents are identified:

1. Parents who work hard to educate their child in cooperation with the rehabilitation system.
2. Parents whose sense of loss and feelings of helplessness prevent them from taking active steps to rehabilitate their child: they limit their care of the child to looking after his or her physical needs only.
3. Parents who depend on the rehabilitation institution to educate their child: "once their children are admitted to a rehabilitation center, they cease to care about their children's education at all" (290).
4. Parents who are unrealistic and impatient for quick results in training their child to speak and in other areas: they may punish the child repeatedly, with the result that the child becomes resistant to rehabilitation education.

In a detailed analysis titled "Notes on the Psychology of Parents with Deaf Children" (1995), Liu Fudian of the CRR Center for Deaf Children approaches the question of parents' response to the diagnosis of deafness somewhat differently. He specifically relates parents' sense of shock and grief to the increased expectations caused by the implementation of the one-child policy:

> As society's level of civilization rises, every young couple hopes they will have a healthy, intelligent child. As birth planning work is strengthened, and implementation of the one-child policy is broadened and deepened, parents' expectations of their children are becoming correspondingly higher — they hope their sons will be dragons, their daughters phoenixes: nowadays this way of thinking on the part

of parents is universal. However, when the reason for their child's impediment to language development is diagnosed as sensorineural deafness, it is undoubtedly an enormous blow for parents, and produces a significant effect on their emotions and behavior. (12)

He goes on to explicitly connect parents' emotional responses to the diagnosis and their subsequent behavior toward their child. Parents are divided into two groups. On the one hand, those with "reasonable attitudes"—representing, Liu estimates, 30 percent of the total—accept the diagnosis and spend only a relatively short time searching for a medical cure before they get their child fitted with a hearing aid and start on a program of speech training. Parents perceive the reward for their sacrifice and persistence is that their children will become "like, or nearly like, normal children," and about 25 percent will be able to enter mainstream schools. These parents are described very positively: they are characterized by "stable emotions, strong willpower, broad-mindedness, and a warm personality, so that they have a relatively rational approach toward setbacks, do not slacken from the hard work, and can change unfavorable circumstances and overcome setbacks." By their exemplary behavior, they "have caused their child, though deaf, not however to be mute; they can feel proud of what they have done, and become the model that very many parents with deaf children can study" (12–13).

On the other hand, parents with "unreasonable attitudes"—the remaining 70 percent—react to the diagnosis with negative or hostile emotions. Liu identifies seven different emotional states, each linked with harmful behavior toward the child. Although these are depicted as common and even to be expected, there is nevertheless a strong tone of moral condemnation in Liu's descriptions. First, some parents take out their anger on others. A small number of parents respond to the diagnosis by turning on the doctor; others blame their spouses. These couples may divorce, or they may leave the child to be looked after by the grandparents. Second, some exhibit regressive behavior and refuse to deal with their difficulties maturely. They hurry to have another child without obtaining medical advice first, with potentially disastrous consequences—"another deaf child, creating enormous misery for the family, and another burden for society" (13). Liu warns that such behavior is socially irresponsible and tells a cautionary story:

A couple in the Beijing area had four children, three of whom were deaf. The eldest was a girl, and when she was two or three years old and couldn't speak, her parents discovered she was deaf; they very quickly had another child, a daughter. This daughter was speaking at a little over a year old, and the parents thought that with two daughters, one of whom was deaf-mute, they must certainly have a son. So two years later they had a son; when he was two or three years old he still wasn't speaking, and when examined was found to be deaf. Having already suffered severe punishment, they had a fourth child, another boy, but this child reached four years of age and was still unable to speak—examination showed him to be severely deaf. Of the four children, the eldest, who is twelve, is at deaf school. The youngest is four years old. Because there are so many mouths to feed, the family's financial situation is very straitened, and the parents haven't been able to afford hearing aids for their three deaf children. (13)

Two elements in this story are worth noting. One is that the desire to have a son played an important role in the parents' decision to have their third child. The other is the observation that having many children results in poverty, which in turn greatly reduces the deaf children's chances of education and rehabilitation.

A third category of parents blame themselves and are overcome with remorse and guilt. These feelings make them much too indulgent with their child, who becomes spoiled and dependent, making it more difficult to carry out rehabilitation. Fourth are the stubborn parents who refuse to listen to professional advice and persist in searching for a cure for their child's deafness instead of starting speech training. Examples of two families are given: one family wasted two years in this way, and spent 40,000 yuan; another persisted until their daughter was six, and only then—after she had missed the optimum period for rehabilitation training—was she fitted with a hearing aid. Asked the reason for this long delay, the mother of this girl replied, "We kept on thinking some medical treatment would cure our daughter's condition."

The fifth emotion is denial, which Liu describes as a defense mechanism against painful feelings. Parents who deny their child's deafness may make excuses, perhaps saying that their child is just slow in learning to speak. Or they insist that their child cannot be deaf because there are no deaf people in the family. In some cases one or the other parent may refuse to admit to a family history of deafness out of a wish to avoid blame or divisiveness. Other parents refuse to accept the difficulty of the task ahead of them. Those with the sixth attitude, "compensation," think that they have discharged their responsibilities when they buy a hearing aid for their child. Finally, some parents expect to see immediate results after their child gets a hearing aid and starts speech training—their impatience is counterproductive and hinders effective rehabilitation.

Liu emphasizes that rehabilitation professionals must understand these psychological reactions because they profoundly affect parents' subsequent behavior. Although he advises that they act positively "to guide [parents] as quickly as possible through these wrong areas, and get them to face up to the reality of their deaf child in a correct way, so that the implementation of deaf children's rehabilitation work can be smooth and effective" (14), he offers no suggestions for how this emotional transformation is to be effected. Liu seems to be aiming primarily at creating a typology of parents' emotional states and their behavioral manifestations.

The markedly judgmental tone of Chinese descriptions of parental behavior contrasts strongly with the accepting and nonjudgmental attitude advocated by, for example, David Luterman in counseling Western parents with deaf children (1987, 1990); the Chinese approach appears to emphasize establishing norms of desirable behavior so that rehabilitation work can be carried out more effectively. Moreover, the Chinese models are relatively static: there is no sense of moving from one stage to another over time, as most Western models posit. Perhaps this simply reflects practical realities: Chinese professionals who diagnose deafness in children typically do not see the families again, because there are no systematic follow-up arrangements, and thus their impression of parents' emotions are usually based on one meeting. It is also possible that many Chinese parents do in fact remain stuck in a stage of denial and rejection of their child's deafness, unable to resolve their original emotions.

The practice in China of consulting a series of doctors seems to be widespread: even Liu Fudian's "reasonable" parents spend some time searching for a cure before they accept rehabilitation training for their child. Western explanations for this behavior cite not just denial but also the inadequacy of the explanations and counseling that parents initially receive. The "doctor shopping" that takes place in China occurs in a sociocultural context in which alternative treatments, mostly derived from traditional Chinese medicine, are extensively advertised and have considerable credibility. However, when parents persist in seeking a cure for their child's deafness, Chinese professionals blame the parents for not accepting their advice rationally and for being "stubborn" as well as denying the reality of the situation; they fail to consider that handling the diagnostic interview differently might alter parents' subsequent behavior. This tendency to blame parents leads more generally to their being characterized as problematic when they somehow interfere with the goals of rehabilitation workers.

Parents as a "Problem"

Parents' Material Circumstances

Professionals see parents' low income, low educational level, and residence in a remote area far from rehabilitation facilities as hindering the rehabilitation of deaf children. All three problems are far more pressing in the countryside, where most deaf children live.[2] Another problem that affects both urban and rural families is that when both parents work they have little time to teach their child.

The Anhui Province Disabled People's Rehabilitation and Research Center provides evidence of how parents' financial circumstances affect their children's opportunities for rehabilitation (Lian 1992). Of over 300 children found to be deaf at the hospital, only 109 came to the center for speech training. Of these, 72 lived in the city and 37 in the countryside. According to this study, relatively few children from the countryside attend the speech training center primarily because their parents find the cost of transportation to or accommodation in the provincial capital too high. Many parents do not enroll their children in a rehabilitation center because they cannot afford the fees. Fees range between 30 and 100 yuan a month (roughly $5 to $17),[3] which are often prohibitive for rural parents, whose monthly income may be 100 to 200 yuan a month (Ge 1993). Hearing aids, together with the needed ear molds and batteries, can amount to the equivalent of several months' income.

Parents' level of education is perceived to be an important determinant of successful rehabilitation (Tang 1992; Wang Youguo 1995a, 1995b; Chen Suzhen 1995; Yin and Liu 1995). In his study of families with deaf children in Anhui, Lian (1992) finds that parents who are well-educated are able to cooperate closely with the teachers in the rehabilitation center and carry out training effectively at home. In contrast, those with a low level of education (especially from the countryside) are unable to carry out family education effectively and do not know how to give their children speech training, as their children's slow progress demonstrates. Of the 217 parents whose children were enrolled at the center and who took training classes there, 23 (11 percent) had technical college education; they were mostly urban. One hundred and four parents (48 percent) had received junior middle school education: these parents were also mostly from the city. Ninety parents (41 percent) had primary school education only, or were illiterate; they were mostly farmers from the countryside. To judge the success of rehabilitation, Lian analyzed the number of children going on to a mainstream nursery or primary school. Out of 50 urban children, 18 (36 percent) were mainstreamed, but of the 33 children from the countryside, only 6 (15 percent) went on to ordinary nursery or primary schools. He concludes that the relatively poor achievement of rural children is related to their parents' low level of education.

However, a group from the CRR Center for Deaf Children in Beijing assert firmly that there is no direct relationship between children's learning to speak and their parents' level of education (Jiao Z. et al. 1995), pointing to a couple living in rural Shandong who were able to give their son effective speech training even though they were both illiterate. They provide no other evidence for their claim; their main argument appears to be that rehabilitation professionals and parents should not assume that, or behave as if, parents' low level of education is necessarily an obstacle to the successful rehabilitation of their children.

Researchers have also focused attention on the link between parents' occupations and their children's progress: Pan Longsheng, from the Hubei Province Rehabilitation Center for Deaf Children, investigated the academic progress of deaf children who had left the Center and entered mainstream primary schools (1993). He found that the children of cadres (government officials) were most successful, making up 22 of the 27 children gaining the highest marks even though overall fewer than half the parents (48 percent) were cadres. The children of factory workers (also 48 percent of the parents) did less well, though most achieved passing marks.

Access to rehabilitation programs is difficult for those living in remote areas. Providing medical and educational services to remote and mountainous areas has always been a problem in China. Even deaf schools set up in rural areas have been found to serve wealthier families who live in or near rural townships rather than the more isolated poorer families. Liu Zhenxing, a deaf man who succeeded in qualifying as a teacher of the deaf, investigated the family backgrounds of students attending a deaf school in Ruyang county in Henan province; he found that although two-thirds of the county is made up of seven mountainous rural areas, all of the twenty-four students in the school came from the remaining third (1993). He explains that families in the isolated mountain villages of this region are often very poor (in 1990, some had average annual incomes of less than 220 yuan), travel is difficult, and towns are too far away. Liu concludes that in rural communities, special education facilities should be attached to mainstream schools.

Professionals engaged in developing rehabilitation services for preschool deaf children in rural areas report the same difficulties: families living in remote villages find it difficult to travel to urban areas, and cannot afford the expense of travel or the cost of rehabilitation (Lian 1992; Ge 1993; Chen Suzhen 1995; Jiao Z. et al. 1995). Additional complications may face rehabilitation workers trying to contact families who live outside cities. For example, some families with deaf children in Jinghu county in Jiangsu province live on boats, and their location is always changing; they are thus very difficult to reach (Yin and Liu 1995).

Finally, parents may have little time to devote to their child when both are working (Ge 1993; Guo Z. 1995; Wang Youguo 1995a). Perhaps because educators generally assume that this problem can be resolved only by the individual families concerned according to their individual circumstances rather than by changes in rehabilitation policies, it has been little discussed in the professional literature. Parents — usually mothers — who change their job or give up their work are praised for their sacrifice, as in the article by Liu Fudian (1995). Conversely, parents who through apathy or irresponsibility do not become involved in their child's education are viewed as creating problems (Wang Youguo 1995a, 1995b). In

China, both parents have to work in order for the family to survive financially. Some families manage to educate their deaf children under these circumstances, but the professionals expect that all parents should do so.

Parental responsibility is central to the Chinese government's policies on disability; however, policymakers have also put forward solutions to alleviate some of the practical difficulties, including financial subsidies and outreach programs. The cost of each deaf child at a rehabilitation center is an estimated 1,000 yuan a year, which pays for teachers' wages, equipment for the center, and so on; most of this expense is covered by the government (Tang 1993). However, deaf children's families have to bear the costs of medical consultation and the fitting of hearing aids, as well as fees for education in the rehabilitation center. Although in general parents cannot expect financial assistance, some rehabilitation facilities do subsidize certain costs, such as the purchase of hearing aids or their own fees. Such funding is at the discretion of individual centers, and it often depends on their financial health. In addition, some allowances may be made for a parent who stops working to devote more time to educating his or her child. Thirty percent of mothers with children enrolled at the CRR Center for Deaf Children in Beijing have given up their jobs so that they can educate their children (an unusually high proportion that is far from norm throughout the country). These families are charged fees of only 50 yuan per month—half the normal cost.

In addressing the question of parents' educational level, the professional response is to stress the importance of educating parents about rehabilitation and to support them through regular meetings. Teachers are instructed to discuss the program the parents should follow with their child at home to make both their efforts consistent and systematic. When parents are not well-educated, teachers are asked to compensate for this disadvantage by increasing their efforts to educate and support them.

For the many hundreds of thousands of parents with deaf children living in remote areas, the Ninth Five-Year Plan proposes setting up family rehabilitation guidance stations in rural areas. These outposts are to be staffed by one or two rehabilitation workers who will make contact with and support parents with deaf children in their area; personnel from nearby rehabilitation centers in urban areas will visit the stations regularly (Shu 1995). Correspondence schools can also help families living in remote areas (Chen Suzhen 1995).

Parents' Attitudes

Many articles by rehabilitation professionals describe parents' persistence in seeking a medical cure for their child's deafness, behavior that may go on for years and delay the start of speech training until after the critical preschool period has passed (Zhang Mingliang 1991; Liu Fudian 1995; Wang Youguo 1995a, 1995b; Chen Suzhen 1995). The professionals also note that many parents do not believe that their child can be rehabilitated through a program of auditory and language training (Lian 1992; Wang Youguo 1995a, 1995b). If they do enroll their child at a rehabilitation center, they may think it is the responsibility of the center to educate their child, and do not take any active part in their child's rehabilitation (Wang Youguo 1995a, 1995b; Chen Suzhen 1995).

As we might expect, given the number of "unreasonable attitudes" toward a diagnosis of deafness that Liu Fudian (1995) identified, other attitudes toward rehabilitation are also seen as problematic. Some professionals complain that many families are thinking only of having a "normal" child instead of devoting themselves to the rehabilitation of their deaf child (Ge 1993; Liu F. 1995; Chen Suzhen 1995). Out of shame and concern for what other people might say, some parents keep their deaf child at home; as a result, the child both loses the benefit of seeing new people and places and becomes very dependent on his or her parents (Li C. and Guo 1995). Some parents are impatient to see results (Li S., Zhou, and Guo 1993; Wang Youguo 1995b); others are inconsistent and educate their child unsystematically (Ge 1993).

The professional literature emphasizes that the solutions for these problems are essentially educational. Professionals are given the responsibility of explaining the aims of rehabilitation to parents and teaching them how to educate their child at home. A wide range of media are used to reach and inform parents: television programs (many people in China, even in rural areas, now have access to television), newspaper and magazine articles, videos, and specially prepared booklets and materials (Lian 1992).

Parents' Responsibility for Children's Behavior

The focus on parents as "problems" has another aspect. Rehabilitation professionals often hold them responsible for bad behavior in their deaf children, without acknowledging the role played by failures of communication. According to Liu Yanxia (1995), the main cause of willful behavior in preschool-age deaf children is spoiling by parents, who are acting out of a sense of guilt:

> The development of a willful disposition in deaf children is due mainly to spoiling, pampering, and accommodation on the part of their parents. Although the deaf child's physiological disability may be due to a number of causes, the adult members of the family feel a sense of guilt, and blame themselves for the deafness. Because of this, they give their deaf child whatever the child wants without any limits. In time deaf children become completely self-centered. On occasions when they do not get what they want, there is a tearful scene. Once willful behavior becomes part of their disposition, deaf children use it as a means to force their parents, teachers, or other members of the family to give them what they want. (11)

Nowhere does Liu mention the frustration experienced by parents or child when they cannot adequately communicate. He suggests simply that parents can prevent undesirable behavior by adopting an encouraging but firm approach toward their children.

Liu Xin and Meng (1992) also stress the importance of being firm with deaf children. They attribute bad behavior to the same cause—overindulgence by parents who blame themselves for their child's deafness and are compensating for their feelings of guilt—and they advocate the same solution. Again, no connection is made between the behavior of deaf children and problems with communication. The professional literature thus makes no distinction between behavioral problems in deaf and in hearing children. The current anxiety over spoiled only children seems to overshadow and prevent a more specific analysis of how impoverished communication affects deaf children.

To be sure, some attention is paid to the emotional problems of deaf children, who are characterized as typically low in self-esteem and self-confidence (Li C. and Guo Zaixiang 1995; Li L. 1995), although the reasons for their condition are not addressed in the literature. However, it is considered important to raise children's level of confidence so they can be educated more effectively, and parents are given advice to that end:

> Deaf children readily develop emotional barriers. They lack self-confidence—they have low self-esteem. Their low self-esteem is an archenemy; it causes deaf children to lose many educational opportunities, and seriously hinders normal mental and language development. For this reason one of the first conditions for speech training is to help deaf children build up their self-confidence.
>
> In order to develop deaf children's self-confidence, the first thing is to let them enjoy the taste of success: the more they experience success, the more self-confident they will become. Parents can let deaf children do some activity where application will lead to success—such as practicing pronunciation, reading characters, sweeping the floor, and so on—and when they have completed the task, praise them, so their achievement makes them feel pleased and take pride in themselves, and their self-confidence is raised. (Li C. and Guo 1995, 193)

Just as with deaf children's misbehavior, a problem here is recognized but not analyzed. Practical child-care advice is given to parents without further investigation into the underlying cause of these emotional difficulties.

Research in the United States and other Western countries in the last twenty years has revealed that in their early interactions, hearing mothers and deaf children often fail to connect; by contrast, deaf mothers are able to use a range of strategies to establish effective, synchronized interaction with their deaf children. Furthermore, the language provided to deaf children from the speech of hearing mothers is generally less easily understood, poorer in quality, and simpler in form than that provided to hearing children from their hearing mothers or to deaf children from their deaf mothers if sign language is used. Ineffective and impoverished communication makes it harder for a child to establish secure attachment to others and to learn what is considered appropriate behavior in his or her community (Meadow and Trybus 1979; Stokoe and Battison 1981; Greenberg 1994). The ability of a child to handle feelings and behavior depends on being able to identify and name emotional experiences (Meadow and Trybus 1979), and without language and communication this understanding cannot develop. Hearing parents of preschool-age deaf children have difficulty handling misbehavior in their child because they cannot explain that a particular behavior is undesirable, or why—and they have to resort to physical means to stop it, since verbal means are ineffective. Western researchers cite the damage caused by impaired communication in early childhood, together with negative parental attitudes toward their child's deafness, in explaining the high rates of emotional and behavioral disorders in school-age deaf children in the United States and Britain (Meadow and Trybus 1979; Gregory 1994; Hindley 1994). Significantly, deaf children of deaf parents appear to show relatively less emotional and behavioral disorder (Stokoe and Battison 1981). According to Stokoe and Battison, the feeling of acceptance and belonging conveyed to the deaf child by his or her deaf parents establishes a foundation of emotional health. Communication and understanding develop at home because there are effective, shared systems of communication instead of the frustrating and destructive barrier experienced by hearing parents wishing to communicate with their deaf children.

Disturbed behavior in the deaf child is the outward manifestation of a dysfunctional parent-child relationship resulting from poor communication: inwardly, the child is likely to have suffered some degree of damage to his or her sense of identity and self-esteem. In a study based on interviews with deaf young people and their parents, Susan Gregory, Juliet Bishop, and Lesley Sheldon found that about one in nine of the deaf interviewees showed strong feelings of low self-worth. These young people attributed this to rejection of their own deafness, and in some cases this rejection could be linked with their parents' negative attitudes toward deafness—for example, in forbidding their children to use sign or to watch television programs with subtitles (Gregory, Bishop, and Sheldon 1995).

In the United States and Britain, where the crucial importance of effective parent-child communication for a child's psychological and emotional health has been recognized, special programs have been developed to improve interaction in the home. These initiatives for families with deaf children include introducing parents to better communication strategies, offering sign language courses to parents, devising programs aimed at fathers, and facilitating meetings with other deaf children as well as deaf adults (see, e.g., Greenberg 1994). Mark Greenberg and his colleagues at the University of Washington initiated the PATHS (Providing Alternative Thinking Strategies) project: their curriculum seeks to develop self-control, emotional awareness, and interpersonal problem-solving skills in hearing-impaired children of primary school age, and it has been shown to be effective in increasing the children's social understanding, problem-solving skills, and reading achievement (Greenberg et al. 1984). In Britain, the NDCS Deaf Children in Mind project, based on the PATHS curriculum, was begun in 1995 for deaf children ages eight to ten; it includes a family intervention package that aims at fostering more positive parental attitudes and expectations regarding their deaf children, as well as improving communication at home (Reed 1995).

Such research studies and practical programs focusing on communication between hearing parents and deaf children have not yet been undertaken in China. Though limited resources obviously constrain researchers, they are also influenced by their own perceptions: at the moment, they do not see much need for these programs. As we have seen, professionals in China have paid little attention to the long-term adverse effects of poor communication on deaf children's social and emotional development, both in their literature and in the information they give to parents. There is certainly plentiful evidence of poor relationships between parents and their preschool-age deaf children: teachers in deaf schools consistently find pupils in the first-year class, at age seven or eight, badly behaved and difficult to discipline. Their tendency to attribute this unruliness to the children's spoiling by guilty parents rather than to communication problems in the early years also appears to be related to a larger cultural bias toward placing little value on informal communication in the home environment but great value on conformity (e.g., deaf children acquiring speech so they can be like "normal" children) and formal academic achievement. There seems little appreciation that age-appropriate linguistic, cognitive, and intellectual development in preschool children, which depends on access to plentiful informal communication at home, is essential for later educational achievement. The deprivation of deaf children is exacerbated by the widespread perception that speech is the only legitimate form of language. Parents see no obvious benefits to using sign language with preschool children—indeed, it is perceived as detracting from the all-important efforts at training their child to speak.

Parents' Responsibilities in the Education of Their Deaf Children

Early diagnosis, early fitting of hearing aids, and early intervention with hearing and speech training, the main objectives of the current drive for the rehabilitation of preschool-age deaf children in China, can only be achieved if parents actively cooperate with rehabilitation professionals. A more detailed outline of parents' role in family rehabilitation, derived from correspondence course material for parents in Zhejiang province, is provided by Tang (1993). They must do three things: get their child fitted with a hearing aid, use scientific methods to train their child, and show persistence and strong willpower. In Tang's account, parents play a leading part in family rehabilitation: their first responsibility is to seek medical advice to obtain effective hearing aids; then, guided by rehabilitation center teachers, they must learn effective methods of rehabilitation training to bring out the children's ability to communicate using hearing and speech, so that they may develop physical, mental, and moral health. Parents have specific tasks—to get a hearing aid for their child and to start giving their child speech training at home—as well as a specific relationship to the professionals concerned, who are to guide them. The goals of family rehabilitation are also made clear: hearing and speech training are only part of the whole rehabilitation of the child, which should also include physical, intellectual, and moral development. "Scientific method"—a systematic, formal approach to the training—is emphasized. The requirement that parents "must show persistence and strong willpower" reflects a strong element of moral exhortation. The literature normally refers simply to "parents" or "family," but researchers and educators understand that mothers are more likely to take the main role in educating their preschool-age children, for they are closest to the young child. The point is occasionally made that fathers as well as mothers should be responsible for their child's rehabilitation training, but the father's role generally receives little discussion.

This responsibility to teach their own children may seem very heavy to some parents. Because many who now have preschool children had their own educations disrupted by the Cultural Revolution, they may feel less than competent. Parents may have to learn *pinyin* in order to carry out speech training with their children. In today's primary schools, unlike the schools of their day, this romanized form is taught in the first year as an aid to learning to read. For some, a much more taxing requirement is that they teach their deaf children to speak standard Chinese (*putonghua*), even if they ordinarily speak a completely different dialect of Chinese at home. Hua (1995) has observed that after children have stayed for several months at residential rehabilitation centers where they are taught standard Chinese return to their parents in the countryside where a completely different dialect is spoken, they cannot understand what people are saying; such linguistic variation obviously makes it very difficult for parents to support the work carried out in the center (deaf children from ethnic minority families in Western countries can have analogous problems). Hua's not very realistic solution is that parents should learn to speak standard Chinese and use it to communicate with their child. However, some professionals are advocating the opposite approach, insisting that especially if rehabilitation work in the countryside with peasant families is to be effective, speech training will need to be in the local dialect. In the journal *Modern Special Education,* Guo Xi, an associate professor in the linguistics department at Nanjing University, argues strongly for relaxing the policy specifying that the language for education in the rehabilitation centers be standard Chinese; he stresses that peasants speak regional dialects, and their deaf children have to be able to communicate with their families and those around them (Guo X. 1993).

Parents as Exemplars

Those parents who are successful in rehabilitating their children may be given wide local or even national publicity: they are treated as exemplars to inspire other parents to increase their efforts. Through newspaper and magazine articles and television programs, large numbers of people in rural as well as urban areas can learn of their experience. The practice of publicizing certain people whose actions or achievements are regarded as ideal has been common in China since 1949: one of the best-known exemplars is Lei Feng (1940–62), a soldier in the People's Liberation Army whose example of patriotism and self-sacrifice is held up to thousands of schoolchildren and young people in China.

Among people with disabilities, one of the most prominently publicized was Zhang Haidi, a young woman in a wheelchair whose story received broad media coverage — particularly in 1984–85, during a massive government initiative to bring disability issues to the fore. In the journal *Disability in China,* Xu Qianren, Gu Baofeng, and Chen Xiaoping (1995) relate how a young deaf boy, Qi Zhaolong, read about Zhang Haidi in a magazine and, inspired by her example, became an excellent student and later a teacher at the deaf school he had attended; he also began a career as a writer. The exemplar need not be Chinese: Helen Keller's story has appeared in China in book and magazine versions as well as on film and is widely known.

Such examples of triumph in the face of adversity seem to be effective in raising the hopes of disabled people and their families and encouraging them to take positive action. There are two widely cited examples of successful rehabilitation of deaf children. One is Wan Xuanrong, an actress who taught her severely deaf son to speak: he attended an ordinary school and is now at college. The other is Zhou Hong, originally a factory technician, who taught his severely deaf daughter, Zhou Tingting, to speak: she has just finished high school through home study. They appear in the professional literature: for example, Wang Yarong (1992) uses the story of Zhou Tingting and her father to illustrate the importance of the family environment for the development of deaf children's speech. Zhou Tingting's father himself has ensured that her achievements have become well-known — together they wrote a book called *From Mute Girl to Child Prodigy* (Zhou H. and Zhou 1990); in it, he points to his own use of exemplars, crediting Helen Keller for inspiring him not only to believe that his daughter could be educated but also to try particular methods of teaching deaf children. Both Wan Xuanrong and Zhou Hong, although untrained and unqualified, now have influential posts in preschool deaf education because of their experience in educating their deaf children. Both of them have received hundreds of letters from parents of deaf children asking for advice (see chapter 6). Many who have written to Zhou Hong mention that reading about his success in teaching his daughter to speak gave them renewed hope.

While only a few individuals have received widespread attention in the national media, other parents of deaf children who have made significant progress are also publicized, if on a more humble scale. They are mentioned by name in professional articles, praised most often for their persistence and selflessness. Parents or other family members who have been able to teach their children effectively may themselves publish articles about their experiences in professional journals: for example, Huang Kaicheng (1994) describes how he taught his deaf granddaughter to speak and recognize characters—she is now coping well in a mainstream primary school. Zhang Meijuan (1996) relates how he taught his daughter to speak, giving details of the language learning strategies he employed as well as the importance he attached to her developing a healthy, confident personality. Because they have achieved success in the rehabilitation of deaf children, they can encourage other parents by their example: they are not simply sharing their personal experiences. Here, as in other areas of life in China, exemplars are used extensively to inspire others to emulate socially desirable behavior.

Parents Who Become Professionals

The family rehabilitation model requires Chinese parents to become informed about the effects of deafness in children, to learn "rehabilitation knowledge," and also to acquire intensive practical experience, for they must train their deaf child to speak as well as attend to other aspects of his or her rehabilitation. Some parents of deaf children become deaf education professionals. A number of Western parents have made the same transition: for example, Kathy Robinson and Lorraine Fletcher, both mothers of deaf children who wrote books about their experiences, became respectively a teacher's assistant in a deaf school and a fully qualified teacher of the deaf (see Robinson 1991; Fletcher 1987).

These parents, who are forced by the unwelcome responsibility of caring for a deaf child to gain training and experience in a previously unfamiliar body of theoretical and practical knowledge, find their lives given a completely new direction. One mother wrote to Zhou Hong that she is at a special education college training to become a teacher of the deaf: she chose to leave her previous job as a math teacher and start a new career because she felt in this way she could help her deaf son more effectively (LZH, no. 36). Li Yingui (1993) tells of a poor farmer who taught his deaf daughter to speak at home, as he could not afford to live in the city while she attended a rehabilitation center. His persistence was rewarded: his daughter progressed, and when she was admitted to a mainstream nursery class, he was appointed teacher at the auditory- and language-training facility for deaf children in Xuchang city. In this case the father won his position on the strength of his practical experience in teaching his own daughter rather than on the basis of relevant professional qualifications: clearly his demonstrated expertise was felt to be particularly valuable.

Parents of deaf children who become rehabilitation workers themselves are seen by other parents as able to offer especially useful advice: many of those writing letters to Zhou Hong tell him that he knows how they feel and can understand their suffering, because he has experienced it himself. Therefore they are more likely to listen to and have faith in what such a person has to say: such parent-professionals are perceived as being particularly effective teachers.

Relationships between Professionals, Parents, and Children

At the time of diagnosis the professional's job is to examine the child and then advise parents about rehabilitation. As we have already seen, parents' reaction to the diagnosis and subsequent actions are often judged harshly. That there is little discussion of how the professional involved could ameliorate the situation—no mention, for example, of any kind of "counseling"—is perhaps not surprising. There is no tradition of psychological analysis in Chinese professional practice, and the Chinese people are deeply reluctant to engage in discussions of their feelings or emotions with anyone outside their own family: such exposure could leave them open to ridicule and loss of face. Chinese parents have to cope with the emotional impact of diagnosis on their own, aided only by their families;

there is no professional responsibility to support parents emotionally when they are under such stress.

In contrast, practitioners in the United Kingdom and the United States have consciously developed a procedure for dealing sensitively with parents. Luterman (1990) argues that the most effective relationships are "client-centered": concentrating on the parents' needs at any given stage and being more responsive to these needs results in more fruitful cooperation between professional and parents, which ultimately benefits the child concerned. He emphasizes that one of the most useful things the professional can do at the time of diagnosis is to listen attentively and nonjudgmentally to parents:

> Careful responsive listening allows the release of the pent-up emotions that most parents hold within themselves and that can be quite destructive. When the clinician is caring, responsive, and, above all, nonjudgmental; when the clinician's attitude acknowledges that feelings just *are,* not right or wrong, but just the way parents feel; then the parents can more readily take constructive action, free of immobilization from unacknowledged feelings. (Luterman 1987, 109)

This kind of notion of a "parent-centered" relationship seems not to exist in China: rather, the relationship is strictly hierarchical, controlled by the professional who provides information and advice to the parents.

When Chinese parents attend "parents' schools," or short training courses that teach them how to educate their deaf child at home, they are expected to behave as students; the rehabilitation professional is their teacher. One article asks parents to consider themselves in a formal educational setting similar to primary school: "No matter what kind of education parents have, we will start from the beginning, we will require them to be like primary school students, to study carefully" (An 1993, 29). A session of a parents' school I observed at the CRR Center for Deaf Children in Beijing was conducted formally, with about thirty parents and grandparents sitting in rows of desks and listening to a lecture from the instructor. The rehabilitation professional is obviously in an active position of authority, while the parents are passive and subordinate.

However, parents of children enrolled in a rehabilitation center assume a more equal role. Parents share the responsibility of their child's education with their teacher: the model is one of cooperation in pursuit of a common goal (Zhang S. 1992). Initially the teacher is in the position of giving advice and guiding parents' work with their child at home—they have the authority—but this balance is seen to shift as parents gain experience. Chen Guiqin finds it characteristic in the rehabilitation of deaf children that the balance of teacher's and parents' roles changes with time:

> When a child is first admitted to the center, the teachers there are teachers of the deaf child and teachers of his or her parents as well. The teachers play an active and dominant role in teaching and giving guidance—"teachers > parents." In the middle of the rehabilitation process, when parents understand the content and techniques of deaf rehabilitation, parents work with teachers to find study and training methods suited to their child: teachers and parents are then equal in their roles, so "teachers = parents." In the later stages, with the child's enhanced sense of listening and speaking, his parents are also in command of a certain amount of rehabilitation knowledge and training methods. As far as their roles in the child's rehabilitation are concerned, parents may now take the active and dominant role previously taken by teachers, so at this stage "teachers < parents." . . . Whether in the early, intermediate, or later stages, teachers and parents should maintain a complementary, cooperative relationship. (1993, 31)

No such shift occurs in the relationships between the child and the professional or parent. There is much evidence to suggest that the requirements of the rehabilitation professionals and the desire of parents that their child should become normal through the rehabilitation process take precedence over the needs of the child. Arguably, the deaf child needs first and foremost to develop the ability to communicate, and to be able to communicate freely at home with parents and other family members. But the preschool rehabilitation campaign in China stresses drilling the child in a structured way and focusing on articulation skills; there is substantially less emphasis on comprehension of language, interactional communication, or cognitive development. At the CRR Center for Deaf Children in Beijing, when discussing Total Communication methods and why these had not been adopted in China, I was told that a "child-centered" approach was not considered suitable for China.

The interactive methods that give priority to the child's communication needs do not accord with Chinese educational values and techniques, which focus on providing systematic speech training to as many deaf children as possible in order to return them to "normal" society. The importance of achieving normalization is currently a much stronger pressure for professionals and parents than consideration of the best developmental path for the individual deaf child. (This is certainly the case in other countries too: China is not unique in pressing these values.) In sharp contrast, the deaf consultants interviewed by Alys Young (1995) in her study of family adjustment to a deaf child in the United Kingdom felt that deaf children's optimal intellectual, social, and language development depended on acquisition of sign language as their first language; speech and English should come later.

The role that parents are asked to play in relation to their children is modeled on the traditional, authoritarian teacher-pupil relationship. In turn, the professionals involved in rehabilitation are in a position of authority in relation to parents, and determine the demands to be made of both parents and children. The resulting rehabilitation model is neither parent-centered or child-centered, as these concepts have been developed in Western countries: the needs of both these groups are subsidiary to the requirements set by the professionals, which in turn are determined by rehabilitation policies emphasizing the desirability of "normality" and the assimilation of deaf children into the mainstream. Both the rehabilitation policies and the professional discussion associated with them reflect the authoritarian imposition of a centrally designed program that establishes a single consistent approach to preschool deaf education. The focus on normalization and emphasis on speech training appear to be associated with a dearth of informed discussion of the full effects of deafness on language acquisition and on the emotional and social development of preschool-age deaf children.

CHAPTER FIVE

URBAN FAMILIES WITH DEAF CHILDREN

The information summarized in the previous chapters shaped both the questions I asked parents and grandparents of deaf children and my understanding of their answers. The interviews I conducted in the fall and winter of 1994 focused on obtaining a comprehensive picture of each family's circumstances and parents' perceptions of these circumstances. Most of the questions were open-ended, giving respondents greater freedom to present their own accounts of their experience in their own way (the questionnaire is reproduced in the appendix).

Questions covering basic information on the family's structure and circumstances provided important context; I paid a considerable amount of attention to the circumstances of the diagnosis, parents' reactions to the identification of their child's deafness, and their decisions on what course of action was the best response. I also asked about their access to information concerning deafness and their experience of contact with deaf people, as I expected that these would significantly affect parents' perceptions of the implications of deafness for their child. It was important to explore the routines of daily life, including children's activities outside school hours, to fully understand the effects of the children's deafness on the family. In examining the children's home life, I looked particularly closely at parents' views on discipline and on communication, as the preschool period is crucial both for learning socially appropriate behavior (and thus for children's subsequent emotional and social development) and for acquiring language. Parents were also asked for information on children's degree of hearing loss and use of hearing aids, which was very relevant here. I tried to determine parents' attitudes toward their children's education, investigating parents' relationships with the teachers at the rehabilitation center as well as the extent to which they themselves were able to teach their child. I included questions on their views on the relative importance of literacy skills versus speech and on the role of sign language in the education of deaf children. Finally, I looked at the special adjustments that a family with a deaf child makes—from moving nearer a rehabilitation facility or giving up a job to changing their social activities, whether because of lack of time, feelings of depression or shame, or a desire to spend time with other parents with deaf children. In China, parents of a deaf child are granted exemption from the one-child policy, if they choose; this additional dimension of their situation was also investigated.

After writing the questionnaire in English, I very carefully translated it into Mandarin Chinese (*putonghua*) with the help of a mainland Chinese woman who works as a medical interpreter. My aim was to ensure that the questions were clear, straightforward, and unambiguous so there would be no confusion over their meaning or scope (McNeill 1990). I was also careful to make the content and language of the questions appropriate to the Chinese context. I was unable to conduct a pilot study with the questionnaire; under such circumstances, Croll (1994) recommends adjusting the questions while carrying out research in China, but I felt that maintaining a systematic and consistent approach throughout the series of interviews was necessary.

To be sure, some areas would have benefited from further investigation. It would have been useful, for example, to obtain further details about the loans provided by family members and friends that enabled parents to search for a medical cure for their child's deafness; additional information on grandparents' role in looking after their deaf grandchildren in infancy would also have added to the overall picture. Conversely, some questions could have been omitted: for example, questions concerning the degree of the child's hearing loss were unnecessarily detailed in view of the fact that most parents had audiogram results; and specific information relating to the children's work and progress in school could perhaps have been more usefully obtained from the nursery teachers. In a few cases, questions reflected my inadequate background knowledge. For example, I asked, "Do you still take your child for regular hearing tests?" but soon realized that any such tests were arranged by parents; there was no follow-up system to bring them back to the hospital, as my question had assumed. Another problem was caused by my failure to fully understand the connotations in Chinese of the word *du,* "to read," as used in the question "Do you think reading and writing are important for your child?" *Du* can mean "reading aloud," the traditional way of learning to read in Chinese classrooms, and this was how several parents interpreted it. If their child was severely or profoundly deaf, a typical reply was "He can't hear, he can't speak, but we feel that writing is important." A better term for "reading" would have been *ren zi* or *shi zi,* "to recognize characters": parents themselves used the phrase frequently in this sense.

Certain types of questions that often appear on questionnaires are known to be problematic. These include hypotheticals, as well as questions that invite socially acceptable responses; neither type was entirely avoided in this study. For example, I asked, "Do you have any advice that might help other parents with deaf children?" One mother pointed out there were no families with deaf children living near them for her to help and give advice to; another respondent was dismayed at the thought she might be expected to help other parents financially, although she pointed out that generally she was the kind of person who was willing to help her neighbors. The question departed too much from the immediate context, and perhaps struck Chinese parents as strange: they, more than Western parents in the same position, seemed to feel it odd to give advice to people they did not know. The grip of convention in determining social norms and public behavior in China makes one expect that a number of topics would encourage socially acceptable answers. Croll (1994), who tries to compensate for this tendency in her own field methodology in China, describes how "normative" answers can distort the data: sensitivity to this source of error can help the researcher take steps to counteract it. One father in this study, who talked to me after I had finished interviewing his wife, spoke at length about the excellence of the rehabilitation center and its teachers, as if to make sure I recorded favorable impressions about the programs available. But because the majority of my questions sought straightforward information and parents' views on quite practical matters relating to their deaf child, normative bias was generally not a major problem.

Arrangements for the interviews with parents were made by the principal and the senior teacher of the rehabilitation center in Nanjing. During the day I observed the children in their classes at the center; during the evenings and weekends I visited their homes and conducted the interviews, taping them all. In each family, I spoke to either a parent or a grandparent: in all eight mothers, three fathers, two grandmothers, and one grandfather. The choice of interviewee was made by the senior teacher and the family: in seven of the fourteen families, the family member perceived to be closest to the child and most involved in their care was selected;[1] in six instances, the family member was one of two or three in the family who were all close to the child; and in only one case did I interview a family member who spent considerably less time with the child than another adult did. Although only one respondent was interviewed for each family, they provided information about all the family members. In addition, by visiting the homes of the parents and grandparents of the children attending the rehabilitation center I was able to see the general circumstances of the families and to gain some idea of their different lifestyles. The activities of family members and visiting friends, their personalities, and their interactions with the deaf child all helped contextualize information obtained from the interviews.

In visiting the parents' homes I was accompanied by one or more teachers from the center, including the child's class teacher:[2] usually we made our way there by bicycle. Visits were arranged for the evening or at weekends, when parents and teachers were free. Following some initial conversation after our arrival, I sat with the family member who was going to be interviewed at the kitchen table or in a bedroom, while the teachers talked to the rest of the family in another room. Each interview was between one hour and two and a half hours long; when it ended, everyone sat down to a meal together. The parents welcomed this chance to talk with the teachers about their children, and the conversation over the meal provided further opportunities for gaining an understanding of family preoccupations and concerns.

Pupils were drawn from all over the city of Nanjing, and cycling or taking a bus out to parents' homes made me realize how far some parents had to travel each day to reach the nursery school. Although a few families lived a short journey away from the center, several could be reached only after an hour and a half's cycling through the city. The housing of most families was quite compact, if not cramped, by Western standards; two families lived in just one room (see table 4). Eleven of the fourteen families lived in apartments

TABLE 4: FAMILY HOUSING

Type of Accommodation	Number of Families ($N = 14$)
Apartment with one bedroom	7
Apartment with two bedrooms	4
Single room off corridor	2
Rural-style house	1

allocated by their work units.[3] One of the families had decided to move from the apartment provided by the husband's work unit to one belonging to the wife's work unit so as to be nearer the preschool.

In a typical apartment, a small entrance room or hallway contained the table where the family had their meals; a small kitchen, bathroom, bedroom(s), and living room opened from this. Seven families lived in one-bedroom apartments; four families, each of which comprised four or more family members, had two bedrooms. The interiors of the apartments varied, according to family income: some were dingy, with poor illumination at night, while others were smart, with good furniture and bright lighting. The stairwells to the apartments were always pitch black at night, and flashlights were used to negotiate the stairs. It seemed strange that the children we met during evening visits did not seem to mind the dark—one deaf five-year-old spent the evening on the dark landing, seeming to find entertainment in gazing in on his family and guests. Parents or teachers never discussed the lighting, and whether it was sufficient for the deaf children: in this respect, they seemed to lack "deaf awareness."[4]

Two families lived in single rooms in a building owned by their work unit. Each couple and their one child had one room for living and sleeping, with shared cooking and toilet facilities along the corridor. The one room belonging to the family, which was by no means large, contained a double bed, a table and chairs, a cupboard, a cabinet displaying an array of flashy ornaments, a television set, a refrigerator, and a washing machine.

The one deaf couple in the study lived in a typical rural-style dwelling, along with their deaf daughter, the maternal grandparents, and the wife's younger brother, also deaf. Although still within the city, their house was in a group of rougher one- and two-story houses off a dusty, litter-strewn alleyway. It consisted of three large rooms: a central room for cooking and eating, a room on one side for storing vegetables and tools, and a room on the other side where all the family members slept.

My visits gave me a better understanding of living patterns, particularly the sleeping arrangements. Most of the children slept with their parents, or else their grandmother, as is usual for small children in China: when children reach kindergarten or primary school age, they generally move into their own bed. Three children in this study who had their own beds were still in the same room as their parents or a grandparent. Family members made no comments or complaints about children sleeping badly (respondents were not questioned directly on this subject). One mother said her daughter had been sleeping on her own but was frightened, so she was moved into the parents' bed. It is possible that sleeping so close to other family members provides Chinese deaf children with an added sense of security; in Western countries, where children usually sleep apart from their parents, deaf children may suffer more sleep disturbances.

Because they were interviewed in their own homes, parents probably felt more at ease, more inclined to discuss their own circumstances freely, and less obliged to produce socially acceptable statements. If the interviews had taken place in a room at the nursery school, for example, parents might have felt constrained to repeat what they had heard from teachers rather than their own views. Nevertheless, they treated the interview as a somewhat formal occasion; they seemed concerned that I obtain accurate information and understand what they were trying to say, sometimes amplifying or explaining further when they felt I needed to know more about something. But in general, apart from one mother who was quite talkative and provided a lot of detailed information in her answers, most respondents tended to give brief, straightforward replies that were to the point. Two respondents, with a son and grandson respectively who were profoundly deaf, seemed very depressed at the time of their interview: the children had been diagnosed as deaf only recently and their families were clearly still suffering from shock and grief. It seemed helpful in these instances to be asking questions that mostly required simple factual answers, which people could elaborate on if they wanted to; respondents were not pressed if they seemed reluctant to discuss a particular topic in detail or at all. One mother seemed rather curt and hostile, as if she were ashamed to talk about her deaf daughter; hers was the only family in which the couple had decided to have a second child.

The nature of my relationship with the parents and grandparents who permitted me to interview them is quite difficult to describe, and it is perhaps tempting for a researcher to give his or her role in such interactions more significance than it really has. The parents were persuaded to agree to the interview by the principal, to whom they felt to some degree indebted; thus they felt they were under an obligation to help me obtain information for my research, and they wished to fulfill that obligation as best they could. One or two parents were interested in finding out more about facilities for deaf children in Britain, but they only asked about this after the interview was finished, as if that had to be dealt with properly first. One mother invited me to go out dancing in a karaoke bar: this turned out to be a family outing, which included her deaf son, and was very enjoyable; I think part of her reason for extending friendship was that I might have information that would be helpful to her son. I also saw the parents and grandparents whom I interviewed when they brought their children to the nursery school in the morning and collected them in the evening; discretion seemed the best course, and I was careful to respect information that had been given privately in the interviews as confidential and, in general, to stay in the background. Thus although I saw these parents fairly frequently over a period of several months, our interactions were constrained to some extent by the situation. One other consideration seems relevant—I think that the relationship between myself and the parents would have been different if I too had been the parent of a deaf child; parents probably would have been more voluble and more inclined both to confide in me and to find out about my experiences as a parent. Nevertheless, the parents took a good deal of time and trouble to provide me with a great deal of useful information.

After all the interviews had been carried out I returned to England, where all the taped material was fully transcribed and translated with the help and advice of a postgraduate student from mainland China. In fact, she was from Nanjing, and this proved particularly helpful in translating the interview of one respondent who had a pronounced rural dialect. The responses to each topic were collated and compared by using a simple "cut and paste" procedure; the findings follow.

TABLE 5: PARENTS' LEVEL OF EDUCATION

Schooling Completed	Couples	
	Number	Percentage
One spouse technical college graduate, one spouse senior middle school graduate	2	14.3
Both parents senior middle school graduates	7	50.0
One spouse senior middle school, one spouse technical middle school graduate	1	7.2
One spouse senior middle school, one spouse junior middle school graduate	2	14.3
Both parents junior middle school graduates	1	7.2
Both parents deaf school graduates	1	7.2

THE FAMILY OF THE DEAF CHILD

Parents and Grandparents

All the parents were married and living with their spouse. Thirteen of the fourteen couples were hearing; one couple was deaf. The average age of the fathers was 34.2 years (range 28 to 45 years); the average age of mothers was 32.9 years (range 27 to 40 years). The deaf couple were several years younger than the other couples; one couple was markedly older than the rest because the husband was in his second marriage. Excluding these two couples, most were in their early thirties (the age range for fathers lies between 31 and 36, and for the mothers between 30 and 35).

Education is a particularly useful indicator of socioeconomic status, and table 5 shows the level attained by the parents. Students in China begin with five or six years of primary school education, followed by three years of junior middle school. Some then go on to three years at a senior middle school or technical middle school. At the tertiary level, there are technical colleges offering three-year courses as well as universities. For 12 out of the 14 couples in this study (86 percent), at least one spouse was a senior middle school graduate—that is, had received twelve or more years of education. For China as a whole, around 75 percent of children who finish primary school enter junior middle school, and 44 percent of

TABLE 6: OCCUPATIONS OF PARENTS

Occupations	Couples	
	Number	Percentage
Both parents government officials	1	7.1
Both parents in other nonmanual jobs	3	21.4
Father in full-time nonmanual job, mother working part-time or out of work	2	14.3
Both parents workers	6	42.9
Both parents doing half-time/temporary work	1	7.1
Both parents peasants	1	7.1

these go on to senior middle school (Lewin et al. 1994, 41, 68). While many in the urban workforce may achieve this level of education, the parents in this study are still a relatively well-educated group.

Parental occupations were categorized as nonmanual, manual, half-time/temporary contract, and rural (farming). They are presented, by couple rather than by individual, in table 6. Nonmanual employment included working as a government official, a secretary, a store manager, sales personnel, and hotel staff. Manual work—employment in a factory—covers a range of jobs from skilled to relatively unskilled work; however, when asked for their occupation, individuals in this category usually said "worker" and did not expand further. Two mothers had ceased full-time employment in order to devote more time to their deaf children: one was working half-time as a sales assistant, the other had taken unpaid leave from her work unit. The couple whose employment was least satisfactory and least stable were the deaf husband and wife, primarily because they lacked an urban residence permit. He had a half-time job as a carpenter and she worked full-time on a temporary contract in the warehouse of a steel factory, meaning that she was paid only the minimum basic wage without the pension or other benefits linked with permanent, stable employment.

In order to assess parental income, I asked respondents to give an overall figure for the combined monthly income of husband and wife, including bonuses and other extra payments as well as their

TABLE 7: MONTHLY INCOME OF PARENTS

Income	Couples Number	Percentage
High (more than 1,000 yuan)	3	21.4
Middle (500 to 1,000 yuan)	9	64.3
Low (less than 500 yuan)	2	14.3

TABLE 8: EDUCATION OF GRANDPARENTS

Level of Education	Grandparents Number	Percentage
University	4	14.3
Senior middle school	5	17.9
Junior middle school	4	14.3
Primary school	6	21.4
No education, illiterate	9	32.1

basic wages. The couples were then divided into three groups according to whether they had a high, middle, or low income (see table 7). The majority of parents had a combined monthly income of 500 to 1,000 yuan (about $75 to $150). Two couples in the study had a combined income of less than 500 yuan per month; one was the deaf couple, who lived with the maternal grandparents and paid nothing for their food or accommodation, and the other couple had a low income because the wife was not working.

The educational background of 28 grandparents (half of the total number of the grandparents) was ascertained (see table 8). The grandparents had a considerably lower level of education than did the parents: while most of the parents had attended senior middle school, fewer than one-fifth of grandparents had gone this far. Nearly a third were illiterate, and only a quarter had gone to primary school. Members of this generation were children in pre-1949 days when education was available to only a small percentage of the population. Yet while none of the parents were university graduates, four of the grandparents were. All the grandparents were hearing.

Retirement age in China is sixty for men and fifty-five for women. Most of the grandparents were in their sixties and seventies and were no longer employed. One grandfather worked as a warehouse watchman, although he was over retirement age. One grandmother, who lived with her two deaf children and looked after her deaf grandchild, was still getting up at four in the morning to work on her plots of land.

The Children

The study included nine boys in the preschool and five girls. The youngest child was 3.8 years old at the time the parents were interviewed, and the oldest was 7.0. The average age at the time of the interviews was 5.8 years.

Three of the children had siblings, though all the families were in compliance with China's strict family planning regulations. One deaf girl had an older half-brother, her father's child from a previous marriage. Another deaf girl had a hearing older sister: she came from a rural family, and her parents had exercised their right to have a second child since their first child was a daughter and they both were only children. In only one family did the parents exercise their right to have a second child because their first was disabled; both children in this family were girls.

The children's degree of hearing loss was ascertained from audiograms kept by their parents. Two children were moderately deaf (hearing loss in the better ear between 56 and 70 dB); four were severely deaf (hearing loss in the better ear between 71 and 90 dB); and eight were profoundly deaf (hearing loss in the better ear over 90 dB). None of the children had any other handicaps in addition to deafness.

The Family of the Deaf Child

The types of family structure in each household are shown in table 9. Nine of the children lived with their parents: two of these children had siblings, but in one of these families the younger, hearing child was being looked after by her grandparents in their home. Three children lived in a three-generation family, with their parents and one or two grandparents in the same household. Two children lived with their grandparents instead of their parents: in one case,

TABLE 9: FAMILY STRUCTURE

Type	Number of Families
Parents and child	9
Grandparents, parents, and child	3
Grandparents and child	2

the child's retired grandparents had more time to look after and educate him; in the other, the child had left her parents in the countryside to attend the rehabilitation center while living with her grandparents in the city.

The Role of Grandparents

Most families were in close contact with grandparents. Some grandparents, as we have already seen, lived with their children; others lived in the same or an adjacent apartment block. State enterprises, which often employ the children of present and former employees, can arrange their accommodation so that young married couples are living near their parents: this makes it easier for grandparents to help with child care and for younger people to look after their elderly parents.

For the families in this study, frequency of contact depended on how far away grandparents lived: if they lived nearby, they were seen daily or several times a week, if they lived on the other side of Nanjing parents might visit them once every one or two weeks. If grandparents lived in the countryside, their children were able to see them only occasionally. Table 10 shows how frequently the deaf child was in contact with his or her grandparents (if they did not live in the same household) — usually the child was taken to visit the grandparents by their parents. For those families with grandparents still alive who provided information, three-fourths of the grandparents saw their deaf grandchild at least every two weeks, and in some cases much more often. There seemed to be somewhat more contact with maternal than paternal grandparents. In only one family did something other than proximity play a role. One deaf child who lived with her deaf parents and maternal grandparents was taken by her father to see his parents only very occasionally, as they had

TABLE 10: CHILD'S CONTACT WITH GRANDPARENTS

Proximity, or Frequency of Contact	Paternal Grandparents ($N = 28$)	Maternal Grandparents ($N = 28$)
Child lives in same household with GPs*	3	6
GPs live in same/adjacent building	4	4
GPs seen at least weekly/fortnightly	5	14
GPs seen once a month	0	2
GPs seen infrequently	8	2
GPs dead	6	0
No information	2	0

*GPs = grandparents

disapproved of his marriage to a woman whose deafness was obviously genetic (she had a deaf brother): they made it clear that they had no interest in seeing their granddaughter because she was deaf.

In addition to their interactions with and influence on their children and grandchildren through frequent family contacts and visits, grandparents played important roles in the care and the education of their deaf grandchild. In several families, grandparents had looked after their grandchildren when they were too young to go to preschool; one profoundly deaf boy had lived with his grandparents until he was three, when he started at the nursery school. As already mentioned, the parents who had a second child because the first was deaf looked after their older daughter, while the maternal grandparents looked after the second child, who was three years old at the time of the interview. In this family, the grandparents looked after the older child as well on Sundays when the mother was working. In at least one other family, grandparents looked after grandchildren on Sundays when one or both parents were working.

Grandparents in three families were responsible for the home component of their deaf grandchild's education. In two cases, the deaf child was living with the grandparents and had little contact with his or her parents; in the third case, the deaf child was living with her deaf parents but her (illiterate) grandmother took on this

TABLE 11: CHILDREN'S PERSONALITIES

Characteristic	Number of Children So Described
Bad tempered	7
In relationships with others:	
sociable	6
obedient	4
considerate to parents	1
Likes learning/achievement	3
Lively	3
Intelligent	2
Happy	2
Confident	1

Note: The right-hand column totals more than 14 because most respondents mentioned several characteristics.

role because she was hearing and could communicate with the teachers in the rehabilitation center. In each of these three families, one grandparent (two grandmothers and one grandfather) was much more actively involved than their spouse with their grandchild. Their educational level is relevant here: two of these grandparents were university-educated and confident in their ability to teach their grandchildren, while one had never attended school and was concerned about her ability to teach her granddaughter.

Because grandparents have extensive contact with their children and grandchildren, their influence on the deaf child, whether informal or in the context of a teaching relationship, must be given considerable weight in evaluating the child's development in the family.

Views of the Deaf Child

Respondents were asked to describe their child's personality; this question was intended to reveal which personality characteristics parents were most preoccupied with and also to ascertain how parents might relate the child's deafness to other aspects of their character. Table 11 shows the characteristics of the deaf child that were mentioned. The characteristic most frequently mentioned was having a bad temper—half the respondents commented on this. In two instances the irritability was specifically associated with the child's deafness:

> Because she can't hear well, she tends to lose her temper easily—we can't understand her very well because her speech isn't clear, and then she loses her temper.
>
> *(grandfather, family 12; girl, age 7, severely deaf)*

> He gets angry very easily. Generally speaking it's not easy for him to hear what we say to him because his hearing isn't all there—he loses his temper and you need to coax him, humor him.
>
> *(mother, family 13; boy, age 6, profoundly deaf)*

But three respondents ascribed the temper tantrums to the child's wishes being thwarted, without reference to their deafness, as in the case of this child:

> He's quite stubborn. You have to do whatever he wants, otherwise he's quick to lose his temper.
>
> *(mother, family 6; boy, age 5, moderately deaf)*

Social convention dictates that parents might tend to speak deprecatingly of their children rather than draw attention to their good qualities: parents with hearing children might also say their child had a bad temper or was spoiled. But these parents did seem to be speaking honestly, providing concrete instances of bad behavior or temper tantrums. Whatever the level of children's actual misbehavior, it was clear that parents saw their inability to control their tempers as a problem that caused some concern.

The next most frequently mentioned group of characteristics concerned the child's relationships with others. Most parents who brought up their child's sociability made positive comments; only one father said his son was shy with strangers. Obedience was mentioned by four parents, and one respondent thought her son was considerate to his parents. After social relationships, the mental liveliness and intellectual capability of the deaf child were mentioned most often—parents may have placed particular emphasis on their child's intelligence because they wanted to point out that although their child was deaf, he or she was not stupid. Very few parents commented on their child's happiness or self-confidence.

In these descriptions, it is striking how rarely deafness came up. Apart from being mentioned by two parents as an explanation for their child's bad temper, deafness was referred to only by one mother who said that her severely deaf six-year-old son "plays with normal children, even though he has the hearing barrier, and other children play with him." Parents saw the children as children first and foremost; their deafness was extraneous. One father told me firmly that he treated his profoundly deaf son "as a normal child": this declaration has a number of implications, including his intention to give the deaf child the same value as a hearing child, but it clearly focuses on and emphasizes the child's nondeaf identity. At first, their representations seem to be incompatible with the evidence of discrimination against deaf people in Chinese society; depiction by Chinese professionals of common parental attitudes toward their child's deafness of denial, apathy, and rejection; and the shock and grief with which these same parents responded to the diagnosis of deafness. But parents come to make a distinction between the "childness" of their child and his or her impairment, deafness. In analyzing English parents' adjustment to their deaf child, Alys Young (1995) noted a number of ways that parents expressed this distinction. First, they focused on the child while deliberately choosing to disregard his or her deafness; second, they emphasized how their child was no different from other children the same age; and third, parents stressed how they chose to treat their child the same as they would a hearing child. Young found that parents in her study did perceive that in the realm of behavior (and their own response to it), as well as in language development and ability to communicate, there were differences between their child and hearing children due to their deafness; however, they maintained a *strategy* of focusing on the child without the deafness. The Chinese parents in this study appear to be taking a similar approach.

Although generalizations are dangerous, given the comparatively small number of parents interviewed, the parents' relative emphasis on these different parameters of personality corresponds to the value attached in Chinese child rearing generally to impulse control, appropriate social behavior, and educational potential and to

TABLE 12:   ARGUMENTS AGAINST HAVING A SECOND CHILD

Reason Given	Number of Respondents
First child would be neglected	8
Not enough money	5
Too much time and/or trouble	3
Fear second child would be deaf	1
Action would be socially irresponsible	2

Note: The right-hand column totals more than 11 because some respondents gave more than one reason.

the lack of overt emphasis on a child's happiness or self-confidence. It appears that in this particular context, parents are perceiving their child as they would a hearing child and judging them against the same expectations that they would have of any other children.

Having a Second Child

China's family planning policy limits couples living in urban areas to one child. However, if the child is disabled, parents may obtain permission to have another one. The 1995 eugenics law (the Maternal and Child Health Care Law; see chapter 2) states that a couple who have already had a child with a serious defect should have genetic counseling; hearing couples who already have one deaf child may not be able to obtain permission for a second if the cause of their child's deafness is unclear, as is often the case. The prohibition against having a second child extends even to deaf couples with a risk of transmitting hereditary deafness.

I asked parents if they wanted a second child, phrasing the question as follows: "I've heard that, according to China's family planning policy, if you have a handicapped child with a hearing problem, you can get permission to have a second child. Do you yourselves want a second child?" As mentioned above, three families already had two children (and in two of these families the deaf child was the second child) so only eleven respondents were asked this question. All replied that they did not want a second child, for the reasons summarized in table 12.

The majority of parents felt that having a second child would lead to neglect of the first. The following response was typical:

> If we were to have a second child, our attention would be focused on him. And our elder son would be bound to be neglected. Because our time and energy would be taken up with the new baby, and there'd be no one to care for and no one to teach our other child. We would feel bad about it, we'd feel we'd let him down. At the moment, with things the way they are with him, he's got all our love and attention, and as time goes on we can create good opportunities for him.
>
> *(father, family 1; boy, age 6, profoundly deaf)*

One mother mentioned how resentful the older child would feel if she had a second child:

> The elder one wouldn't get enough attention. Or the second one wouldn't get enough attention. My son would feel bad psychologically; when he grew up he would say, Oh, you don't like me because I have a hearing problem, you like the normal one. I don't want another child. I give all my attention to this one.
>
> *(mother, family 6; boy, age 5, moderately deaf)*

Another respondent emphasized the extra teaching time the deaf child needed, and how difficult it would be to keep up the teaching if there were another child:

> Because this child has a problem, we need to spend much more time on him, many times more than on an ordinary child. I couldn't do this if there were another child.
>
> *(grandmother, family 7; boy, age 3, profoundly deaf)*

Two mothers suggested that their feelings toward their deaf children would be adversely affected by having a second child, whom they would love more because it was "normal":

> If we had a second child, there would be some discrimination against the first, we wouldn't be so good to her, we'd have some prejudice against her.
>
> *(mother, family 2; girl, age 6, severely deaf)*

> If we had a second child, we wouldn't pay so much attention to him [the older child]. If the second child is very clever, and can speak, it will make the parents very happy and charm them. So we would not pay as much attention to our first child.
>
> *(mother, family 9; boy, age 6, severely deaf)*

Much as parents may have longed to have a "normal" child, they generally felt the only decision that was fair to their deaf child was not to have a second child.

Five parents mentioned the financial difficulties that a second child would entail. One mother said they could barely manage to bring up one child on their wages. Another parent made the same observation, and added that he and his wife wanted to save their money so that their deaf son would be well-provided for later. A second child would also be a burden in terms of time and trouble, according to several parents. As we have seen already, with both parents working full-time, often with time-consuming and inconvenient commutes, the daily routine was already hard enough without an additional child to care for. One father stressed that he and his wife could not afford to lose their jobs. The idea that a second child could be an onerous responsibility was clearly expressed by one respondent:

> The burden would be too heavy. The emotional burden, the financial burden, the burden of looking after the child, all of this would be very heavy.
>
> *(grandmother, family 7; boy, age 3, profoundly deaf)*

For the deaf couple in this study, the fear that the second child might also be deaf was paramount. The maternal grandmother was emphatic that a second child was not an option under the circumstances, explaining that her daughter had already had an abortion:

> She already had a chance for a second child. She had an abortion. She's worried that it would be like this one. She's afraid the second would be deaf as well. She definitely doesn't want another one.
>
> *(grandmother, family 4; girl, age 4, severely deaf)*

Though the cause of deafness in several of the other children may have been genetic, no other respondents mentioned fear of having a second deaf child—if this worried them, they were reluctant to discuss it. Two of the mothers said their work units had given them permission to have a second child (in one case, the cause of deafness in her profoundly deaf child was unclear and may have been genetic); both claimed they had no wish to do so.

Two mothers gave reasons beyond their immediate situation. One asserted that she did not want any more children because China's population was so big already; although this answer was normative, she sounded sincere. Another said that if she and her husband had another child, the welfare of their deaf son would fall on other people:

> We would not pay as much attention to our first child, and some of the responsibility would pass to society.
>
> *(mother, family 9; boy, age 6, severely deaf)*

Such a response again emphasizes the idea that parents—at least those in cities—have sufficient personal resources to cope with only one child.

Parents in this study were prepared to devote their efforts and energies to their deaf children's education and future. They reasoned that they could not bring up two children with the same degree of care: a second child would inevitably dilute the money, time, and attention that they could give to their first. Perhaps in places where adequate education is not provided for deaf children, when parents feel there is no way they can invest usefully in their deaf child's future, they may reason differently and make different decisions. I found that unlike the children in this study, most children attending the Beijing Third, Nanjing, and Chongqing schools for deaf children have a younger hearing sibling—or one or two younger deaf siblings, when parents tried for a hearing child but the deafness was genetic. Parents with deaf children who attend the rehabilitation centers may become a group who do not have second children even when they are permitted to do so, thereby demonstrating that early intervention programs are supporting the government's aim of population control. Perhaps this choice also will depend on whether their children can gain access to mainstream primary schools and succeed in an integrated situation. Parents who initially resolve not to have a second child may of course change their minds later, especially if they are disappointed by the results of their efforts to rehabilitate their deaf child.

Chinese parents who already have a deaf child appear to view this issue differently from many Western parents. While Western parents, like Chinese parents, apparently tend to limit their intended family size on the grounds that the deaf child requires more time and attention (see, e.g., Gregory 1976), they seem to place less emphasis on the fear that the deaf child will be neglected if another, hearing, sibling is born. On the contrary, evidence from personal accounts suggests that these parents perceive they risk neglecting *hearing* siblings because they are absorbed in meeting the needs of the deaf child, especially in regard to development of language (Spradley and Spradley 1978; Shaw 1985; Fletcher 1987; Robinson 1991). The Chinese parents seem to recognize their society's discrimination against deaf children, which they have to some extent internalized. They also are much more conscious of material constraints that would prevent them being able to bring up two children well: families cannot rely on support from the state if they run into financial difficulties.

The Diagnosis of Deafness and Parents' Reactions

The period when parents suspect their child is deaf, and subsequently have their suspicions confirmed by medical diagnosis, is as traumatic and distressing for Chinese parents as it is for Western parents. However, some features of the route to diagnosis and parents' behavior following the diagnosis are unique to China.

TABLE 13: DISCOVERY OF DEAFNESS

Pattern of Discovery	Number of Children
Early suspicion (age 6 to 10 months)	2
Notice of change before/after illness	4
Suspicion because of speech delay	8

How Parents Realized Their Child Was Deaf

In the absence of systematic screening for deafness in children, the parents' role in suspecting deafness and having their child's hearing tested becomes very important. In the sample of families interviewed, three main patterns of discovery were found (see table 13). Two parents whose children were born deaf, or deafened shortly after birth, took them for a hearing check because they realized they were not responding to sounds. In four families, a change noticed in their child after an illness led parents to take their child to a doctor. The respondents recalled:

> Before the fever she could sing songs, like the song on that TV series *Jigong,* but afterward she suddenly stopped.
>
> *(mother, family 10; girl, age 7, profoundly deaf)*

> Before she was deaf, if you raised your voice near her, she would start crying. But afterward she didn't hear anything—no matter how loudly you spoke, it didn't have any effect on her.
>
> *(grandfather, family 12; girl, age 7, severely deaf)*

In eight families, speech delay prompted parents to seek professional help; in four families, the children were over two years old. The child with deaf parents was not taken by her grandmother for a hearing test until she was well over two years old; although her grandmother had had two deaf children (as well as two hearing children) herself, she was slow to suspect that her granddaughter was deaf—or perhaps she did not think it so urgent to ascertain whether the child was deaf or not. In one family, parents thought the defect lay exclusively in speech production, so the child was taken first to a speech therapist. In another family, with a moderately hearing-impaired child, it was the child's nursery teacher who picked up the child's deafness and suggested to the parents that she should have a hearing test.

The accounts parents gave of how they first suspected or discovered their child's deafness showed considerable variation, probably due in part to differences in age of onset of deafness as well as in severity of hearing loss. Nevertheless, it seems significant that more than half the parents became concerned only when their child failed to acquire speech in the usual way—or at least took action only at this point even if they had suspicions earlier on.

Parents' Reactions to the Diagnosis

When asked about their reactions to the diagnosis of their child's deafness, the parents' answers tended to be frank but brief. Their terseness in recollecting feelings that must have been strong and conflicted at the time probably reflects their desire to control their emotions. The specific context also must be considered—in interviews, they were speaking to a relative stranger, an outsider to whom they were unlikely to reveal their innermost feelings. The following statement is characteristic, though longer than some:

> After the doctor told me, I came out of the testing room and burst into tears. And then I felt as though I couldn't stand up. I thought I would pass out. Because after all it was my own son who had suffered this blow, and what had happened to him was quite terrible. I just felt destroyed. When I got home I cried for three days. I couldn't go to work.
>
> *(father, family 1; boy, age 6, profoundly deaf)*

It is striking that respondents describe the physical manifestations of their grief—for example, crying or being unable to eat or sleep properly through worry—but show little introspection: they do not discuss feelings or thoughts in detail or use language related to the emotions.[5]

Most parents in this study emphasized how shocked and sorrowful they felt when they were told their child was deaf. One mother implied that the defect of deafness marred her idea of her son:

> I felt very upset. I cried a lot. I felt it was such a pity about my son. Such a nice boy and he's deaf.
> *(mother, family 6; boy, age 5, severely deaf)*

Five parents linked their feelings of grief with a pessimistic view of their child's future, expressed in terms such as the following:

> We thought she was finished. If she couldn't hear anything, then she wouldn't speak later. She was done for.
> *(mother, family 2; girl, age 6, severely deaf)*

> We were very worried, because if her hearing wasn't good it would affect her personal development. It would even cause her to become disabled, useless.[6]
> *(father, family 14; girl, age 5, moderately deaf)*

Searching for an explanation for their child's deafness could become a distracting preoccupation. One mother, who had considered very carefully whether there could possibly be any family history of deafness, consulted many doctors to try to find out the cause as well as to find some treatment.

One father specifically related his grief to the government's one-child family policy:

> We were very upset. We were very pessimistic . . . because nowadays the government one-child family proposals mean that a couple can have only one child—because our child was deaf we were extremely worried.
> *(father, family 3; boy, age 5, profoundly deaf)*

When parents are permitted only one child, it is not surprising that they hope that that child will be healthy and whole. As we have seen, if there is doubt about the exact cause of the child's deafness—if there is any possibility that the cause is genetic—then parents may not be able to take advantage of the special exemption allowing parents with disabled children to have a second child.

Disbelief was the response of one parent to the diagnosis of deafness in her son:

At that time I didn't really believe it. I thought there was probably something wrong with his hearing, but I didn't think it was that bad. Well, after that I went to see lots of people. I went to many hospitals to get his hearing checked. But the results confirmed it was definitely that severe. I was in despair.

(mother, family 5; boy, age 5, profoundly deaf)

In another family, lack of knowledge concerning the consequences of deafness clearly mitigated the initial response to their second daughter's deafness:

At first when we found out she was deaf, we thought she would just learn to speak later than normal, but as time went on we realized that wasn't going to happen, and it wasn't any good.

(grandfather, family 12; girl, age 7, severely deaf)

Several respondents expressed resigned acceptance of the situation. One of these was the grandmother who had already had two deaf children. From her point of view, the negative consequences of deafness in terms of education and employment may not have been so clear-cut: while she had a poverty-stricken childhood without the opportunity for even basic education and was still having to do hard manual work, her deaf daughter had been to deaf school, could read and write, and was in paid employment in a factory. Her pragmatic acceptance of her granddaughter's deafness was probably related to her familiarity with deafness and its implications.

Two mothers described how their emotions had changed: after the initial shock of the diagnosis, when they felt extremely upset, they had gradually accepted the situation. Generally speaking, however, the interviews did not yield enough information to make it possible to trace changes and development in parents' feelings over time.

Reactions of Grandparents and Other Family Members to the Diagnosis

As well as coping with their own emotional responses, parents had to impart the news to other members of the family and deal with their responses. Disbelief was sometimes the initial reaction:

Her grandparents didn't believe it at first. They couldn't really believe it. They said there wasn't anything wrong with her. Because when she was very little, she was quite lively. You would never have thought she was defective. . . . No one suspected she had a hearing problem; . . . the older generation think some children learn to speak early, some late, and it doesn't matter if a child is late with their speech. So they didn't suspect anything. Even after the hospital tests, they didn't believe it at first. Then we showed them the results of the hearing test and said, You have to believe this, this is reality. Then they accepted she had a problem with her hearing.

(father, family 14; girl, age 5, moderately deaf)

Grandparents and other family members did more than share parents' grief. They discussed the situation, suggested solutions, provided the impetus for parents to take action, and gave practical help in the form of money so that parents could seek treatment for their child. Grandparents could also help construct explanations of the deaf child's behavior, linking it to the newly discovered fact of deafness:

They were all very concerned. They said, that explains why he's so demanding and loses his temper. Because whenever you speak to him, from his point of view it's as if you haven't said anything. He didn't understand what you were saying and he'd sit on the floor and have a tantrum.

(mother, family 6; boy, age 5, severely deaf)

In addition, they suggested various solutions to the problem of their grandchild's deafness. One suggestion was that the parents should have another child. But many grandparents focused on the deaf child and urged parents to take steps to get treatment for the deafness, or to start rehabilitation:

When my parents got to know . . . they were very upset as well. They cried as much as I did. After a while they told me my son ought to have treatment quickly, urgently, to get through this. But at that time we'd only been married a bit

TABLE 14: CAUSES OF DEAFNESS

Cause	Number of Children
Aminoglycoside antibiotics	9
Hereditary	1
Middle ear disease	1
Cause unknown	3

more than a year, so we didn't have much money to spare. So my parents, my brothers, my elder brother, and my sister all gave me money to take my son for treatment outside Nanjing or here in Nanjing.

(father, family 1; boy, age 6, profoundly deaf)

The people in our family said to teach her, teach her really well. . . . They encouraged us.

(mother, family 2; girl, age 6, severely deaf)

Causes of Deafness

The parents and grandparents of the children at the rehabilitation center were asked the causes of their child's deafness (see table 14 for their responses). Injection of aminoglycoside antibiotics to treat illnesses in early childhood was by far the commonest cause of deafness given. Parents specifically mentioned the drug gentamycin in five cases, kanamycin in one. The injections were given for neonatal jaundice, fevers, and a cold. Some parents do not distinguish between deafness caused by the injection and that caused by the illness or fever: they say the deafness was caused by "injection-and-fever." Ototoxic antibiotics seem to be blamed too readily for a child's deafness when in fact its cause is not clear. For example, two children had injections of aminoglycoside antibiotics shortly after birth;[7] although they could already have been deaf for genetic or other reasons, doctors and parents both blamed the drugs.

In the case of the deaf child whose mother and maternal uncle were deaf, it was clear that the cause of deafness was hereditary. But no other parents raised the possibility that their child's deafness might be genetic. When the cause was unknown, a number of possibilities were suggested. One mother gave three possible causes—a threatened miscarriage, a mysterious "allergic" rash when she was six months pregnant, and an antibiotic injection given her not long before she gave birth. Another mother attributed her son's deafness to birth injury. While the cause of a given individual's deafness is often obscure, the parents' total silence about genetic causation was striking. In part, this may be explained by parents' (and doctors') lack of awareness that genetic deafness is relatively common and is often unaccompanied by any family history of deafness; but there also seems to be a strong element of wishful thinking in parents' denial. Not only do eugenic family planning policies prevent parents from having a second child if the deafness of the first is genetic (and indeed, parents do not want to have a second deaf child), but parents perceive genetic deafness as stigmatizing the family and possibly harming the prospects of all family members.

Serial Consultation of Doctors and the Search for a Cure

After their children were found to be deaf, all the families went on to consult more doctors. As one parent said, "You can't just go to one hospital" (father, family 1; boy, age 6, profoundly deaf). Parents went from one consultation to the next, not only to confirm the diagnosis and the extent of the hearing loss but also to ascertain the cause of deafness: for the reasons given above, parents had specific reasons for wanting that information. In addition, they needed to find out if there was a cure. Most of the parents went to several hospitals in Nanjing, and also consulted doctors in cities such as Shanghai and Beijing, where, they assumed, they could find the best and most advanced medical advice. In describing their course of action, parents emphasized the high reputation of the hospitals they went to and of the doctors they consulted. One father's account is typical:

> I went to quite a few places because of my child. Where we're living—Nanjing—all the big hospitals in Nanjing. I saw all the ENT hospital doctors, specialists, and consultants. I went to Shanghai. In Shanghai there's an ENT hospital that has a very good reputation in China. I went there as well. In Beijing there's a hospital called Tongren Hospital.

TABLE 15: TREATMENTS FOR DEAFNESS

Type of Treatment	Number of Children
Acupuncture	9
Intravenous treatment	7
Qigong	4
Herbal medicine	3
Variants of acupuncture	2

Note: The right-hand column totals more than 14 because some children underwent more than one form of treatment.

> There's a professor there called Z—— X——, who even has some reputation abroad. We went to see him as well.
>
> *(father, family 1; boy, age 6, profoundly deaf)*

Doctors practicing Western medicine tell parents there is no cure for sensorineural deafness; parents respond by turning to various Chinese traditional medical treatments in the hope they will effect a cure. Table 15 shows the treatments for deafness tried by the respondents in this study; the most common was acupuncture. A course of acupuncture might last several months or as long as a year. Despite the readiness of most parents to try this method, and to persist with it, none of the respondents reported any permanent improvement in their child's hearing. One parent had this experience:

> My son was diagnosed deaf at seven months. When he was just over eight months old, we took him to the Provincial Chinese Traditional Medicine Hospital for acupuncture. At the hospital there is a well-known professor specializing in acupuncture, Professor S—— C——. My son had acupuncture for somewhat less than a year. After this he had the brain trace again and this showed his hearing deficit had been reduced by 5 dB. But when we stopped the acupuncture treatment it went back to what it was before. So we stopped the acupuncture.
>
> *(father, family 3; boy, age 4, profoundly deaf)*

Seven children at the center had had an "intravenous" treatment. At least three of these children had received a special experimental therapy devised by doctors at the Railway Medical College in Nanjing. Children could receive one course of treatment a month. According to one mother, it involved her child staying in hospital and having an intravenous infusion for four or five hours every day. Three of the seven children who received the intravenous treatment appeared to show significant, even dramatic, improvement: for example, one girl's hearing loss apparently diminished by 10 dB with each of five courses of treatment, improving overall from a deficit of about 80 dB to 30 dB. I believe that the treatment may have been effective because it ameliorated a component of conductive deafness in these particular children—or else the deafness cleared up for reasons that had nothing to do with the infusions. The other four children showed no improvement.

Qigong, the traditional Chinese therapy that employs physical movements and exercises to maintain health and cure disease, was tried by four families to cure their deaf children, but none found it effective. *Tuina,* a special form of massage therapy that aims to improve the patient's condition by redistributing the balance of *qi* via the massage of acupuncture points, was mentioned by one parent. This parent also tried a traditional therapy that involves placing studs of traditional medicine around the rim of the outer ear and pressing them three or four times a day to stimulate the *qi*. But apparently neither of these treatments was effective.

Three respondents mentioned their use of herbal medicine. Since traditional herbal medicines are very commonly used in China for ailments of all kinds, it is likely that most if not all of the parents resorted to them from time to time, either as an adjunct to other treatments such as acupuncture or administered on their own. Indeed, they are so taken for granted that those interviewed probably saw their use as routine rather than as special treatment worthy of mention. Herbal medicines have notable advantages: they are relatively cheap and, unlike other treatments, do not disrupt parents' work routine or children's schooling. It is generally held that herbal medicines work gradually and actually cure the illness or condition rather than simply relieving symptoms. However, none of the three respondents who mentioned using herbal medicines reported any benefit as far as the child's hearing was concerned, although one girl apparently showed improvement in her general health.

Hearing tests were used to measure changes in children's hearing losses before and after treatment. Parents also relied on their own impressions of changes in their children's hearing ability:

> After every treatment we took him for a test, and the results showed some improvement, but looking at him, there didn't seem to be any change.
>
> *(mother, family 5; son, age 5, profoundly deaf)*

The costs of treatment were high. On average, parents spent between 10,000 and 20,000 yuan (about $1,500 to $3,000 — more than a year's earnings for some families) on treatment. This covered the expenses of doctors' consultation fees, tests, courses of treatment, and also travel and accommodation if parents traveled out of Nanjing. Children might also require special nutritional supplements—for example, if they were having the intravenous treatment—and these were not cheap. A single course of the intravenous treatment cost 1,000 yuan: one couple, whose combined monthly income was 660 yuan, put their savings toward treatment for their daughter; she had another course whenever her parents managed to scrape together the money. Clearly there was a connection between parental income and spending on treatment: in the poorest family, in which the deaf parents had a combined monthly income of 300 yuan, the deaf daughter had only a few acupuncture treatments.

Those parents employed by wealthy work units had their medical expenses reimbursed—up to 70 percent in one case, and almost totally in the case of another couple who were both government officials and already had relatively high incomes. Four parents complained that their work units did not make any special allowances for them—either failing to reimburse them to any significant extent or forcing them to take unpaid rather than paid leave when they had to take their child for treatment. Their inability to receive significant reimbursement for medical treatment compounded the financial problems of parents receiving lower salaries in poorer work units. In some cases treatment in a particular hospital was covered (e.g., the army hospital for one family in which the father worked in the army system), but since all the parents were determined to seek help from a range of hospitals, they were obliged to pay the full fees for medical care in other facilities. Several parents responded to the question "What do you think the Chinese government could do to help families with deaf children?" by saying they felt strongly that their medical and other expenses for their deaf children should be adequately reimbursed by their employers: their financial problems were a pressing concern.

In addition, some of the interviewees saw the speech training that their children were receiving at the rehabilitation center as a form of treatment. They viewed their child's beginning to speak a few words and phrases as evidence of an improvement in hearing. Thus one mother answered the question "Is your child's hearing getting better or worse?":

> I think it's getting better. Because of what the teacher at the rehabilitation center teaches them. When we first sent him there, he couldn't say anything. He hardly said anything the first month. Then the teacher gave him some instructions, and he started speaking.
>
> *(mother, family 9; boy, age 6, severely deaf)*

Parents persisted in their hope that a cure could be found. Several of the children were still undergoing treatment five or six years after diagnosis, although some parents sought it less actively once their child started at the nursery school. They described reading books and scanning newspapers in the hope of hearing about a new approach:

> What I'm really interested in is finding out how to restore a deaf child's hearing and speaking, those kinds of books.
>
> *(grandfather, family 12; girl, age 7, severely deaf)*

For a few parents their hopes were fulfilled — their children did respond to treatment, and they therefore felt that their continual quest and refusal to give up had been justified. This improvement also strengthened their belief that it was possible to cure deafness:

> We didn't give up hope. We tried hard to get her treatment. We think that deafness caused by medicine is not in fact incurable, something can be done about it. We think, generally speaking, it's possible to regain hearing with treatment.
>
> *(father, family 14; daughter, age 5, moderately deaf)*

Seeing one child cured would certainly have raised the hopes of other parents and encouraged them to persist in having their own children treated. But the continual search for a cure could be a dispiriting and painful experience: one respondent, who was very depressed when interviewed, seemed to be particularly despondent about the range of treatments on offer, some of which she had tried (unsuccessfully) for her deaf grandson. She worried:

> If there is any possibility, I still want to get him treatment. There's nothing I can do. I don't know these treatments. If there is some new treatment, we'll have it. . . . But I've heard of so many cases where people have been cheated.
> *(grandmother, family 7; grandson, age 3, profoundly deaf)*

These accounts reveal the responsibility placed on parents to make decisions about the range of treatments available for their children, some of which were traditional therapies, some more recently devised experimental "cures." Because the treatments were not regulated and properly tested, families were obviously vulnerable to exploitation by unscrupulous practitioners. Yet their desire to somehow eradicate their child's hearing defect was very powerful, and to that end they were prepared to keep trying a succession of treatments and spend relatively large sums of money. At the same time, in clinging to the hope that their child might one day be cured they were strongly denying the idea of their child as a deaf child, thereby preventing themselves from accepting the reality of his or her deafness.

Knowledge of Deafness

Parents' Previous Experience of Deafness

Only four of the fourteen respondents said they had previously known deaf people. One mother reported contact with two deaf people, an aunt deafened in childhood and a "deaf-mute" in her husband's work unit: this experience had strengthened her determination that her daughter should master speech, since she did not want her child similarly to have poor speech or be mute and suffer in consequence:

> These people can't hear . . . they don't know how to speak; psychologically it's very hard for them, I think. So I must teach my child very well, I must teach her the best I can.
>
> *(mother, family 2; girl, age 6, severely deaf)*

Another respondent, a grandfather who said he had been in contact with deaf people of all ages—children and middle-aged adults as well as elderly people—denied that this experience had affected his attitude toward his granddaughter. But the rest of his interview revealed a negative attitude toward deafness, deaf people, and sign language, suggesting that this denial in fact represented his refusal to consider the possibility that she would grow up to be like those deaf people.

A third respondent reported that she had not known any deaf people in the past. However, only a few days previously a deaf man, Mr. Liu, had moved into their apartment to help her and her husband by taking their son to the rehabilitation center and back; it was also understood that he would teach their son in return for his room and board.[8] During the interview visit to the family home, which took place on a Sunday evening when the whole family was there, I was able to observe the interaction between Mr. Liu and the profoundly deaf child. Their communication was lively and the child was thoroughly enjoying himself, naming all the pictures in a pack of flash cards using signs that Mr. Liu had taught him. Mr. Liu also took it upon himself to persuade the highly active child to behave better (e.g., at table). Their rapport seemed excellent and the relationship appeared to provide very valuable communicative opportunities for the child. But when his mother was questioned about the deaf man she tersely replied only that she hoped he would help them look after their son. In fact the arrangement broke down within a few weeks because Mr. Liu "couldn't teach" the little boy— in other words, he could not teach the child to speak or to read and write. When I asked the teaching staff at the nursery school, they explained that the parents "didn't like" Mr. Liu. The parents probably did not place much value on the friendly relationship between the deaf man and their son, or even on the development of language since this was in sign; and they may well have felt threatened by Mr. Liu's presence and what he represented in terms of their son's future.

One respondent had already had the experience of bringing up two deaf children; now she was looking after her deaf granddaughter. When asked "Because your daughter and her younger brother are deaf, does this change your view of N's deafness?" she replied:

> I look after her as best I can, because she can't speak, and I can't let her be neglected. She needs to be able to read characters, otherwise it'll be no good for her. As for being able to read: her mother can read, so she's got a light job.
>
> *(grandmother, family 4; girl, age 4, severely deaf)*

In sharp contrast to the other interviewees, the respondent felt that a deaf person was to be emulated—in this case, because she had a particular skill, reading, that enabled her to get a nonmanual job. This grandmother, given her experience raising two deaf children, had a realistic grasp of the possibilities open to her deaf granddaughter, and some of these possibilities were positive opportunities.

Parents' Access to Information

It became clear from parents' responses that information was not provided in any systematic way at the time of diagnosis: they were not necessarily given the advice they needed or suitable written materials concerning the medical and educational aspects of deafness; they were not routinely provided with information about rehabilitation facilities, either. Parents were left on their own to obtain further information and advice. One father described his efforts to find help for his son:

> When our son turned out to be in such a serious situation, I went to a special center—the Nanjing Speech Hearing Rehabilitation Center—to get more information. They explained things to me. Then they introduced me to some teaching material I could buy. The main thing was that as far as deaf people are concerned, there simply isn't any cure, so you need to do oral training or lipreading to learn to

speak. So they taught me various methods. After that I went home and taught my son.

(father, family 1; boy, age 6, profoundly deaf)

The different ways parents found out about the Amity Rehabilitation Center illustrates the ad hoc dissemination of information. Five respondents said they found out about the nursery from a newspaper article placed by the principal; three had been told by friends; and one had heard about the nursery from a hospital audiologist when he took his granddaughter to have a hearing aid fitted.

With official channels providing little help, informal sources — friends, family, and colleagues at work — played an important role in seeking out and passing on information to parents. The parents themselves demonstrated different levels of interest: several said they looked out for any books, magazines, newspapers, or television programs that might contain relevant information, while others were less active (and one respondent was illiterate). Some parents were most interested in finding out about treatments for deafness; others concentrated on educational methods. Some parents were most concerned with helping their children learn to speak, while others mentioned the importance of finding methods to teach their children to read characters. Thus to some extent parents made their own decisions about their own priorities and what methods they would use with their children at home, based on the information available to them and their own sense of what was important or feasible.

When their children were enrolled at the nursery school — by which time they were at least three years old — parents gained more access to information and materials. This rehabilitation center was reported by parents to provide a reading list, and it made available copies of the book written by the principal about how he had educated his deaf daughter as well as sundry magazines containing articles about disabled children. The center also held regular parents' meetings, which the respondents mentioned as a very useful source of information about treatment, hearing aids, and, in particular, methods of teaching their children at home.

In essence, parents described a situation in which the official information provided was piecemeal and inadequate — especially at the time of diagnosis, when parents most needed help and guidance. It improved later, when the center that the deaf children attended disseminated materials and held meetings for parents at which questions could be asked and information exchanged. Characteristically, parents' search for information had a do-it-yourself quality: they used their own initiative, depended on personal contacts, and set their own priorities for what they wanted.

Technology Available: Hearing Aid Use

Parents' first actions after diagnosis were directed toward finding a cure for their child's deafness—for most parents, buying hearing aids came second. At the time of purchase, parents were often given inadequate information about the benefits and limitations of hearing aids, leaving them with unrealistic expectations and increasing the possibility of disappointment—particularly for parents of profoundly deaf children. Some reported difficulty in getting their children to wear their hearing aid.

Children did not start wearing hearing aids regularly until they started at the nursery school, and even then more than half of the children using them wore them only for school and homework. Since the majority of parents thought that the hearing aids were ineffective, they seemed to view wearing them as necessary simply to satisfy the demands of teachers. Overall, attitudes toward the use of hearing aids were negative, in part because parents were unwilling to use equipment that marked their child as deaf and in part because they lacked adequate information about how hearing aids could help their child.

The three children who had responded successfully to the intravenous treatment, and now had moderate or severe hearing losses (40 dB, 60 dB, and 85 dB respectively), were the only ones who never wore hearing aids, either at home or at school. They were all in the first class at the nursery, with relatively good oral skills. Their parents said either that a hearing aid would damage the child's residual hearing or that while children were having treatment they should "exercise their hearing" rather than rely on a hearing aid. Two parents said they were advised in this decision against using hearing aids by a doctor; but a third family rejected the doctor's suggestion and made their own decision:

At the beginning, the doctor suggested we should have her wear a hearing aid. But we considered it, and we felt the hearing aid would affect her hearing. Her hearing isn't that good; if we damage her residual hearing, we could impair it permanently. We took positive action to give her treatment from the first: we didn't have her wear a hearing aid.

(father, family 14; girl, age 5, moderately deaf)

This example illustrates once again the considerable degree of responsibility exercised by parents in making decisions about their child's deafness: they did not necessarily take the advice of doctors, especially when it seemed to conflict with their desire to see their child recover his or her hearing. It also reveals that they are implicitly making an either/or assumption: to remedy deafness, the child can either undergo treatment or wear a hearing aid. This father, who was clearly thinking only in terms of his daughter's treatment and cure, did not consider how his decision might affect her language development. Overall, although staff at the rehabilitation center were able to get most of the children to wear hearing aids, parents showed a considerable lack of enthusiasm for them.

Contact with People outside the Family

With parents typically working full-time, children attending the nursery school for most of the day, and weekends often spent with grandparents and other relatives, the family members in this study devoted most of their time to family life, work, or preschool. But many also had time for a social life, whether going out to visit friends or entertaining them at home. Parents also encountered people outside the family in casual interactions such as shopping, when they were faced with other people's reactions to their deaf child.

Social Contacts

Most respondents denied feeling different from other families with a hearing child. Only one mother said she and her husband felt diminished because they had a deaf daughter. Their rejection of difference or social devaluation appeared to be closely connected with assertions of the deaf child's normality:

> I feel just the same. I feel it doesn't matter . . . someone else's child has their good points, my child has his good points.
>
> *(mother, family 9; boy, age 6, severely deaf)*

> We don't feel we have a handicapped child, and we don't feel awkward. I don't feel that at all.
>
> *(mother, family 6; boy, age 5, moderately deaf)*

> I thought along those lines earlier on. But now I feel the only difference between these two groups of children is that their hearing is not so good. In other respects they're the same. So I make a big effort to minimize this distance.
>
> *(mother, family 11; boy, age 6; severely deaf)*

One father rejected any acknowledgment of difference between their family and other families as defeatist:

> Because our child has this handicap, we try positively to find a solution, to get her some treatment. It's not necessary to think negatively, that there's a distance between you and other families, no, I don't think so.
>
> *(father, family 14; girl, age 5, moderately deaf)*

Some parents, with profoundly deaf children, did see a difference, but they did not perceive themselves as socially stigmatized — rather, they focused on their intense concern and worry about their deaf child:

> There are differences between families with disabled children and normal families. Because families with disabled children are under stress. Because when they see other people's children, happily going to school, and their own child can't go to an ordinary school, it makes them feel very worried.
>
> *(father, family 3; boy, age 4; profoundly deaf)*

Most parents took their child out with them to visit friends and relatives, or often had visitors at home. However, two respondents, both very distressed about their profoundly deaf children, limited their social contacts to close relatives or very close friends and were unwilling to discuss their child outside this circle. Another explained that their social life as a family had been curtailed because they had to spend so much time with their daughter (she too was profoundly deaf):

> Compared with other parents, we spend much more time with our child. Life is hard. We have almost no free time, for example to go dancing. After work, I just stay at home with her, get her to do writing and drawing, look after her. We can't go out and do other things.
>
> *(mother, family 10; girl, age 7, profoundly deaf)*

In casual social contacts outside the circle of friends and family, respondents said they did not experience discrimination. Nor were other people embarrassed: parents simply intervened if they tried to talk to the deaf child and were not understood.[9] When parents were out shopping it was common for shop assistants or passersby to comment on their child, usually in a sympathetic and caring manner:

> They say my son looks intelligent and lively, that it's a real pity. They want to find out about the situation — can he speak, is his hearing getting better. Generally speaking, people are very caring.
>
> *(mother, family 9; boy, age 6, severely deaf)*

Interest, sympathy, and curiosity were all mentioned by parents as characterizing other people's behavior toward them in public. One mother did mention that people could show prurient interest; if she felt this was their motivation in discussing her child, she refused to continue the conversation. Another mother regularly used the opportunity of casual conversations to warn others about the dangers of certain medicines to children's hearing:

> If anybody asks me, I will tell them about my son. I tell them to be careful when having any medical treatment. I

remind them to pay attention to any medicine their child might be given.

(mother, family 6; boy, age 5, moderately deaf)

Parents were asked about their reaction when their child made strange noises in a public place. For some children, especially the older ones, this did not seem to be a problem: one mother pointed out that once deaf children had had formal training, they did not make such noises. Some parents did feel self-conscious, and tried to make their child be quiet so that people would not stare. But one father felt he should not feel embarrassed about his son:

> Now that my son is older it doesn't bother me any more — whatever other people do, if they stare or whatever . . . just because my son has a hearing problem, he shouldn't be discriminated against. So at the beginning I was embarrassed, but now I don't take any notice.
>
> *(father, family 1; boy, age 6, profoundly deaf)*

Respondents reported that some people were rude about their child. The most common observation was that children called out "Mute kid! Mute kid!" Even when this behavior upset them, parents saw it simply as heedless and thoughtless and the children just in need of reproof:

> There are some children who are very naughty, they don't understand. They might say something like, "Oh, he can't speak." Sometimes my husband and I feel angry when we hear this; but we know those children are only young, they don't understand. If they did understand, they wouldn't say that.
>
> *(mother, family 9; boy, age 6, severely deaf)*

One or two parents mentioned similar behavior from adults, which they ignored.

Generally parents did not depict themselves as being devalued by having a deaf child, or as experiencing discrimination from others. They felt that people within their circle of friends and relatives "understood" their child's situation. According to parents, most casual social contact was marked by sympathetic interest. When children or occasionally adults were rude and upset them by calling their child names, respondents generally interpreted this behavior as ignorant and uninformed rather than malicious. For these particular families, living in a large city, other people's behavior toward them and their deaf child caused little anxiety compared to their immediate practical concerns over their children's education and future.

In discussing their interactions with people outside the family, most parents preferred to emphasize their similarity to other families and their children's similarity to other children. Perhaps this topic particularly accentuated their determination to maintain optimism and a sense of self-respect, so that they may have given a positive and upbeat account of their feelings when in fact at times they felt very low. Here their perception of me as an outsider may well have been relevant: if I had been a parent of a deaf child, they might have been more willing to admit to experiencing feelings of despair or difficulties with strangers' questions and reactions.

Children's Friends

The question of children's relationships with other children was particularly significant as only three of the fourteen children in this study had siblings — and even these siblings had little contact with the deaf child. One girl had a much older brother who got home very late from work; one girl had an older sister in the countryside whom she only saw in the holidays; and one girl had a younger sister who lived with their grandparents.

Many respondents spoke of the deaf child's playing with first cousins. Typically, children met their cousins when they went to see their grandparents on the weekend. However, two families lived so close to their in-laws that their children played with their cousins every evening. A cousin might be the only playmate the child had outside the nursery school:

> When other children come to play with her, she doesn't want to play with them. She plays with my other granddaughter, but not with other children around here. If her cousin doesn't come, she will play by herself at home.
>
> *(grandmother, family 4; girl, age 4, severely deaf)*

It is possible that this grandmother discouraged other children from playing with her granddaughter out of protectiveness, preferring to restrict her contacts only to other family members. Whatever the reason, her cousin was the only hearing child her granddaughter was in close contact with. Most urban Chinese children nowadays do not have siblings, although they may have one or more first cousins. If China continues with its one-child policy, then in the next generation even these first cousins will disappear. Presumably links to more distant relatives, as well as nonfamily relationships, will have to assume greater importance and fill the gap.

Only three children in this study played with nonrelated neighborhood children during the week. A number of practical reasons were given for this. One was lack of time in the evenings—children came home from school, did their homework, watched television, and had little time for anything else. One mother pointed out that by the time they got home it was dark, so children could not play outside with their friends. Some parents said they did not know their neighbors, or did not have much to do with them, especially if they had recently moved into a new apartment block. Going outside to play was more difficult for children living in sixth-floor apartments than those in ground-floor apartments. Because the families of the children at the nursery school were widely distributed over Nanjing, it usually was not possible for children to meet and play with their schoolmates outside of school.

Only two respondents suggested their child's deafness was a factor limiting their relationships with other children, though other parents may have felt the same but were reluctant to discuss it. One mother explained that other children's inability to understand her son's speech when he spoke quickly was one of the reasons he had just two or three friends he played with several times a week. One grandmother, who was particularly upset about her grandson's deafness, said:

> There's a child living opposite who comes occasionally. But she has to go to school, there isn't the time. My grandson can't understand what people say, so we don't go to their home . . . and he's a bit of a handful, climbing all over the furniture. People would find him a nuisance. . . . He never plays with other children.
>
> *(grandmother, family 7; boy, age 3, profoundly deaf)*

This respondent avoided contact with people outside her family and close friends—besides feeling unable to control her grandson's behavior, she did not want to discuss his deafness with other people.

All the children mentioned as playmates, whether cousins or neighbors, were hearing. When asked how the children communicated when they were together, most interviewees replied that gesture was used; other means of communication mentioned were speech alone and gesture used to supplement speech. Two parents maintained the children did not "communicate" or "speak" much, perhaps not taking into account that speech is not the only way children can communicate with each other.

Some parents emphasized the importance of familiarity and described the strategies adopted by the hearing child to communicate better with the deaf one—the playmates mentioned below were both first cousins of the deaf children:

> N sometimes uses gestures with him, and little by little he [N's male cousin, who is a year older] has come to understand them. He knows and understands my son's gestures very well.
>
> *(mother, family 5; boy, age 5, profoundly deaf)*

> The two of them play together very well. I like it when she comes. She understands his hearing isn't good. She speaks loudly, near to his ear. They play together very well and they talk a lot together.
>
> *(mother, family 6; boy, age 5, moderately deaf)*

The children in this study apparently had a limited number of friends outside school, in part because of practical constraints on children getting together that apply to hearing children as well. Children were more likely to have the time and opportunity to play with friends on the weekend, often at their grandparents' homes and mainly with relatives.

ISSUES OF CONTROL

Because hearing parents find it difficult to communicate with a deaf child, they have problems controlling the child's behavior: they are unable to warn, explain, or threaten using speech. Of particular interest in this area is how the different values and techniques that characterize child socialization in China affect parents' attitudes toward and actual practice in managing the behavior of their deaf children.

General Management and Discipline

There was a range of opinion on whether a strict or an easygoing approach was better for the deaf child. On the one hand, some parents said they did not want to be strict because they felt sorry for their child; similarly, others believed that because of the hearing loss parents should be more tolerant and understanding of the child's difficulties. One father said:

> Generally I'm quite easygoing with him. Why, because we feel he's already got a problem as regards his hearing, so we shouldn't be too hard on him. Basically if he wants something we give it to him as far as possible. We do have limits where we get firm. But if he wants something, or needs something, we do our best to get it for him.
>
> *(father, family 1; boy, age 6, profoundly deaf)*

On the other hand, some parents felt that since their children did not understand what was said to them, it was important to be more strict to prevent their children's behavior from becoming too willful. Several emphasized the importance of being strict over relationships with other people—showing consideration to their grandparents, or playing well with other children:

> In everyday matters we are quite easygoing, but in his behavior toward other people we are more strict . . . if he's playing with other children, and there's some conflict, if it's because of him we'll tell him off. If it's because of another child, we tell him he should forgive him.
>
> *(mother, family 11; boy, age 6, severely deaf)*

One father, whose daughter was only moderately deaf and was going on into mainstream schooling, felt he had to supervise her schoolwork more rigorously now that she was approaching school age, especially since she would find things more difficult than other children because of her hearing loss. Both of these parents are following a pattern familiar in Chinese child rearing generally: they stress that children must show concern for harmonious relationships with others and respect for their elders; and they become stricter and more demanding in their educational expectations when children enter primary school. Several respondents, including two with profoundly deaf children, did not explicitly acknowledge that their child's deafness affected their views on discipline at all; instead, they spoke of disciplining their child as they would a "normal" child. Here again we see the parental strategy of focusing on the child's "normality" while disregarding his or her deafness.

Parents described a variety of strategies for dealing with children when they were badly behaved. One approach was to avoid confrontation by giving in and letting the child have or do what he or she wanted. For example, if the child demanded a toy in the shops, the mother or father would buy it. Another strategy was to move the child away or offer another distraction. Coaxing was mentioned by several parents — one father explained how he dealt with his son's temper tantrums:

> If I want to get him to quiet down, I coax him and give him a hug; I say, Now you should listen to Daddy, shouldn't you. Although he can't hear I coax him and hug him, and he quiets down.
>
> *(father, family 1; boy, age 6, profoundly deaf)*

This father calmed his son by relying on physical contact and, by implication, the sympathetic expression on his face.

Praising her child worked well for one mother, whose son had sufficient hearing to hear and understand what she said:

> If you're angry with him, it's not a good way to stop him. It's better to be gentle, speak nicely to him, praise him and say how good and clever he is — and then he will do what you say.
>
> *(mother, family 6; boy, age 6, moderately deaf)*

But parents also used negative strategies to secure control. When children had sufficient residual hearing, a shout from a parent might be enough to tell them they were being naughty; several children had enough hearing so that parents could give them a good scolding and get across some explanation of what they were doing wrong. But some parents, if their children were severely or profoundly deaf, relied on their facial expression to convey disapproval. Threats, expressed either verbally or with raised hands (or, in the case of one respondent, a big stick) were sometimes used to persuade children to behave.

Smacking was resorted to by all but two respondents, although some parents maintained that they took this action only occasionally. Typically, it happened when children had done something particularly naughty, or when they paid no attention to gentler means of discipline and parents just got beside themselves: several parents said they smacked their child when they had lost their tempers. Sometimes it was specifically difficulties in communication that led to this parental frustration:

> Actually I don't want to hit him, but I get so angry sometimes. Sometimes he wants something and I don't know what it is he wants, and he keeps on asking, and in the end I just get so fed up I smack him.
>
> *(mother, family 8; boy, age 4, profoundly deaf)*

Despite their own behavior, half of the respondents said they believed it was wrong to smack a deaf child. Typically, they felt strongly that it was both wrong to punish a disabled child physically and unfair to use force just because communication is so difficult:

> I think you shouldn't smack these kinds of children if at all possible. Why, because their hearing is defective, they're already disabled, because the parents feel sympathetic and pity them. If they want to say something and you don't understand, or you say something and they don't understand, and you smack them, both the child and the parents will feel very bad about it, so generally I feel you shouldn't smack these children more than can be helped.
>
> *(father, family 1; boy, age 6, profoundly deaf)*

The two respondents who never smacked their children—two grandmothers—gave different reasons for their dislike of corporal punishment. One said she would not smack any child: it was important to talk to children nicely and be gentle with them. The other grandmother, who had had many brothers and sisters and whose own childhood had been very poor, believed that if there was only one child in the family then it was shameful to hit him or her—in her eyes, an only child was more valuable and deserved to be looked after more carefully. Furthermore, she said that because her granddaughter was deaf and could not speak, "you can't hit her."

All the respondents reported that their children lost their tempers; several said it happened frequently. The attributed cause in most cases was that the children could not get what they wanted: for example, they wanted to buy something but their parents would not get it for them, or their parents stopped them from watching television. Only two respondents spontaneously pointed out a link between children's temper tantrums and their difficulties in communicating—although when asked directly whether their children sometimes lost their temper for this reason, most agreed this was so. There are obvious dangers in asking such leading questions; nevertheless, it appears that although parents did not perceive their child's deafness as the key problem, the majority saw it as a contributing factor, at least on occasion.

Two parents, both with profoundly deaf children, discussed the way their close familiarity with their child enabled them to understand what he or she wanted so that such losses of temper were less frequent; one father said:

> He hardly ever loses his temper with me, because I'm with him quite a lot. He knows us; because when he loses his temper is when he wants to say something, express something, and he's afraid people won't understand him . . . But I look after him quite a lot. Usually when he speaks I know what he's trying to say . . . if you can understand what he says, he won't get angry.
>
> *(father, family 1; boy, age 6, profoundly deaf)*

Parents dealt with temper tantrums using strategies similar to those used with other kinds of misbehavior: by giving in to what children wanted, by persuading them, or by coaxing them, as well as by using threats or smacking them.

Safety

I had expected that when parents discussed the two issues in this section—whether the children understood that hot water and the hot stove were dangerous, and whether they understood road safety—they would also express their views concerning the amount of independence they were prepared to allow their deaf children in everyday life. Instead, parents gave quite specific and limited answers. Nevertheless, these answers provided some insight into how parents taught children about danger.

In urban Chinese households, hot water is boiled up and put in large thermoses to be drunk in tea or on its own during the day. Children learned quite early on that a hot-water drink had to be allowed to cool before they could drink it. Respondents let the children know by gesture (flinching after touching the side of a hot cup) and by facial expression when water was too hot for them to touch yet. Another obvious source of danger was the gas rings used for cooking. Children learned by parents' gestures, parents' facial expressions, or their own bitter experience that the cooking rings gave off heat: some parents taught their children by bringing their hands near enough to the heat to feel it. One child would turn off the gas under the kettle when he saw the steam rising up, having watched what his parents did.

Especially in light of the long journeys that some children had to make on their way to school and back home each day, traffic posed a significant risk to them. During rush hours, roads are thick with bicycles as well as cars—two respondents recounted occasions when their children were nearly mown down. Not surprisingly, most parents said they held on to children's hands as they walked by the roadside. Most of the children, except the youngest, understood they had to look carefully before crossing; one respondent said his granddaughter had learned to do this by observing him.

Communication at Home

Parents were asked a series of questions to investigate the modes of communication they use with their deaf children at home. The hearing losses of these children varied—there were two moderately, four severely, and eight profoundly deaf children—so it was to be expected that the families would use speech, gesture, or both to differing degrees to communicate with their children. Their answers were usefully supplemented by my observations of the children's communication both at home and at the nursery: the two accounts were generally consistent. In some cases, observation clarified what might have been misunderstood from the parents' explanations alone. For example, one father described how his son would get his attention:

> He wants me to see what he's done—"Look at my writing!" "Look at my book!"
>
> *(father, family 3; boy, age 5, profoundly deaf)*

My observation of the family at home made it clear that the father had translated into speech the meaning of what his son had communicated through gesture.

Parents stressed the role of familiarity in enabling understanding. Family members often understood their child's speech when people outside the family could not, and they interpreted the child's needs and wants even when use of speech or of signs and gestures was minimal. It was also clear that familiar routines and contexts facilitated mutual understanding. For example, in the interview a mother might say her child understood when she said to him "It's time to eat," when in fact the child's understanding probably derived largely from smelling her cooking and seeing bowls of steaming food on the table.

Much basic communication took place through parents' ascribing particular meanings to their children's nonverbal behavior. One mother said:

> When he sees me come in from work, he's excited and he'll touch me, as if to say, "You're back!"
>
> *(mother, family 8; boy, age 4, profoundly deaf)*

Mothers or grandparents were described as communicating most with children—only in one family was the father depicted as closest to and communicating most with his child.

Getting Attention

Generally speaking, parents called their child by name if he or she had sufficient residual hearing, and otherwise used touch. One father with a profoundly deaf child called his son's name into his ear—although he seemed to think his son responded after feeling his breath rather than hearing anything. One mother said she sometimes clapped her hands to attract her daughter's attention when she was close by; if the child were further away, she would bang on a pot or metal pan.

When children were at some distance—for example, in another room—a few parents were able to get their child's attention by calling them: otherwise, parents had to go to their children and call them or touch them. Only one mother said she would hold up something such as a sweet to get her child to come over to her; otherwise parents did not mention waving as a way of attracting their child's attention. Unlike in the West, stamping on the floor was not used—but the floors were all hard, usually concrete, so they were not effective conductors of vibration. None of the respondents mentioned tapping furniture or flashing lights on and off.

If children wanted to attract their parents' attention, they called them or touched them. One child would bang on something if his mother did not respond to his calls. Some children with greater degrees of deafness were unable to say "mommy" (*mama*) or "daddy" (*baba*) and just made noises; one respondent insisted that his profoundly deaf child say "*baba*" before he would respond, using the situation as an opportunity to encourage his child to use speech. Similarly, one respondent who had a severely deaf granddaughter tried to get her to say "*yeye*" to him and "*nainai*" to her grandmother, rather than just pulling at them. One mother had to moderate her child's efforts to get her attention:

> Before he used to start hitting me—then I told him, you can't hit me like that; so now he pulls on my sleeve.
>
> *(mother, family 5; boy, age 5, profoundly deaf)*

TABLE 16: COMMUNICATION WITHIN THE FAMILY

Mode(s) Used	Number of Children ($N = 12$)
Speech only	4
Speech, with gesture if necessary	4
Speech and gesture at the same time	3
Gesture only	1

Modes of Communication Used

Parents were asked: "How do you communicate with your child—using speech, or signs, or both?" The word used in this question to refer to the use of sign was *shoushi,* which strictly translates as "gesture" but is used in everyday language to mean either gesture(s) or sign(s). Since only one of the families in this study, the family with two deaf parents, used conventional sign language, this question was intended to explore the extent to which families relied on, or deliberately chose or rejected, gestural communication. Their responses, which are shown in table 16, indicated that the respondents themselves understood the question in this way.

The children of the four parents who said they used speech to communicate with them were moderately or severely rather than profoundly deaf. These respondents expressed varying degrees of disapproval toward using sign with their child: "Generally speaking I don't want to see signs" (mother, family 2; girl, age 6, severely deaf); "I make a point of not using gestures with her" (father, family 14; girl, age 5, moderately deaf). One parent said that if they had difficulty explaining something to their child, they would write down characters for their child to read, or draw a picture, rather than resort to using gestures.

The parents of three severely deaf children and one profoundly deaf child said they usually used speech, but would use gestures if they had difficulty explaining something. But they preferred not to—one mother said, "I don't want him to learn this bad habit from us" (mother, family 13; boy, age 6, profoundly deaf). One respondent in this group emphasized that he would rather use written language to supplement speech than use gestures with his granddaughter.

Three respondents used speech and gestures at the same time to communicate with their children, who were all profoundly deaf. One subject pointed out that if she did not use gesture her grandson would not understand. Finally, one mother said she used gestures only, without any speech, with her profoundly deaf son. She stated that the family could not speak to him because he could not hear. This family had been told there was no chance of their child learning to speak.

In her study based on interviews with 122 mothers with preschool-age deaf children in England, Gregory (1976) found that 72 percent used gestures with their child, although teachers advised them not to do this; and most of these mothers supported their use. By contrast, although two-thirds of the Chinese parents in this study used gestures with their children, none expressed approval of this form of communication — in fact, half explicitly disapproved, and it was clear that those who used gestures did so only because they saw no alternative. This group of parents both strongly valued speech as a means of communication with their children and firmly disavowed the value of sign.

Several parents mentioned using written characters to communicate with their child when they could not make themselves understood through speech. Others mentioned drawing as a way they could get through to their children. In both cases this was depicted as a one-way process — from parent to child — and the lopsidedness of the interchange was particularly clear in the case of writing, as the children had not yet learned to write more than a few simple characters.

Children's Understanding of Spoken Chinese

Respondents were asked: "When you speak to your child, what things can he/she understand? Could you give me some examples?" Two parents had already told me that their children understood only if gesture were used, or gesture and speech together were used; thus the answers considered below are drawn from the other interviewees. Parents knew from their children's response whether or not they had been understood.

Respondents emphasized their children's understanding of "everyday language":

> For example, getting up in the morning—"Fold up your quilt and tidy things" (*ba zhi dongxi bai hao*) . . . "N, time to go to school" (*gai shang xue le*), "Time to get up" (*gai qi chuang le*). . . . Then sometimes we say: "N, we're going out together" (*women yiqi chuqu wanr*). He understands simple phrases and everyday language.
>
> (*mother, family 11; boy, age 6, severely deaf*)

What is striking is that parents perceived that children "knew" what they called "everyday language," yet in fact the repertoire of words and phrases children could understand and respond to were very limited, and could be largely "understood" from their familiar context in the family's daily routine rather than through auditory clues or recognition of lip patterns. Furthermore, it is quite possible that children could understand these phrases only if they were spoken by someone with whom they were familiar—a close family member or perhaps their teacher.

Children recognized their own names, as well as words such as "teacher," "granddad," "grandma" (*laoshi, yeye, nainai*), and names or words representing other members of the family. These could be useful clues when parents were trying to explain to their children where they were going: one father said his son would not understand if he said they were going to school, but if he said to his son they were going to see his teacher, then his son understood because he recognized the word *laoshi*. Parents with children who were less severely deaf gave examples of more sophisticated language that their children could understand. One respondent said his child, who had a moderate hearing loss, could usually understand everything.

Parents considered lipreading important in helping their children understand speech, and some described the efforts they made to make this easier for their children. This is discussed further in the next section.

Communication Strategies

Parents who used speech with their children were asked: "When you speak with your child, do you speak as you would with a child with normal hearing? Or, for example, do you make sure you're face-to-face, do you speak more slowly, or perhaps more clearly?"

One father responded to the first part of this question:

> Basically yes. Because although he can't hear, I don't treat him as if he's deaf. I treat him like a normal person.
>
> *(father, family 1; boy, age 6, profoundly deaf)*

The father seemed to feel that his son's worth was increased by being treated as a hearing child, a treatment that included acting as if he could communicate as if he were a hearing child.

Several parents said they made a point of being close to their child when they spoke. Two parents specifically said they spoke near their children's ears, in fact one was careful to speak into her daughter's "better" ear. Some parents spoke face-to-face with their children — two parents explained that they wanted their child to lipread. Other strategies used by respondents were speaking slowly, articulating the words more clearly, and speaking more loudly. One mother pointed out that she would speak at greater volume at home "where there were no restraints" — presumably in public places she felt more inhibited about speaking loudly to her son.

In addition to adjusting their speech, parents had thought of other ways to improve communication between themselves and their children. Repeating phrases or sentences was mentioned as one strategy. Another method used was to place in a sentence single words that the child could recognize: for example, "teacher" or "grandparents," when parents wanted to talk about going to school or going to visit the grandparents.

Children developed strategies to clarify meaning as well. One boy would ask his mother to repeat what he had not understood. Another child would repeat back what he had heard to check that he had understood.

Respondents described a number of situations where they had trouble communicating necessary information. For example, explaining where they were going was difficult, as one parent found:

> If I want to take him out to play somewhere, if I want to tell him we're going to the park, if I say "park," he doesn't understand. If I say we're going somewhere by bike, he also

doesn't understand. In these situations I don't know how to explain, because you can't tell him, you can't explain to him; so I go and get a piece of paper and a pen and draw a park, a picture of the outside of the park, to tell him where we're going. Sometimes he understands, sometimes it seems he doesn't. When this happens I try to think of a way to make him understand. So I say: We're going to take photos, and then he knows we're going out to play. But he doesn't know where we're going. We've no way of explaining . . . if we're going to see some friends, or some people from work, and I want to bring him with me . . . he doesn't know people's names, so there's no way to explain. The only way is to take him.

(father, family 1; boy, age 6, profoundly deaf)

Parents also found it difficult to explain that they wanted to go out somewhere and their child was to stay at home, that they did not have enough money to buy toys in the shops, and that their children needed to go to sleep because they had school in the morning. In some cases they simply gave in to the child rather than struggle to get across an opposing view:

Sometimes he wants us to get something for him — if he was an ordinary child, we could explain to him that he already had one at home, or he can't have this. But for him, it's difficult to explain, so to make him happy we just buy another for him.

(mother, family 11; boy, age 6, severely deaf)

Children's Speech

It was not easy to determine the extent and nature of children's oral skills from the respondents' accounts: here, my notes and observations made at the nursery school and at home provided a particularly useful supplement. As might be expected, there was a range of skill: one child with moderate deafness demonstrated a good knowledge of language and a relatively wide vocabulary, and several profoundly deaf children could say only a few words, and these very unclearly.

Just as they did in discussing their children's ability to understand speech, parents repeatedly emphasized the use of everyday phrases to demonstrate the children's ability to speak:

> He can say the basic things: "go to school," "come home," "have supper," "I want to have my supper," "I'm hungry," "I'm full," "I don't want any more" (*shang xue le; hui jia le; chi fan le; yao chi fan le; duzi e le; chi bao le; bu yao chi le*). Sometimes he shouts to me if I'm busy, "*kan dianshi*," "*kan dianshi*"; he wants me to come and turn on the TV so he can watch the cartoons. He says, "*shui jiao le!*" when it's time to go to bed.
>
> *(mother, family 9; boy, age 6, severely deaf)*

Another respondent reported that his daughter could say "all the everyday things," and that "her speech now is almost the same as normal children's."

It appeared that as far as parents were concerned, being able to say everyday phrases indicated mastery of language appropriate or adequate for their children's age. But these phrases, referred to by the parents as "everyday language," are in fact very rudimentary in their vocabulary and syntax; hearing children of the same age have a vocabulary of hundreds if not thousands of words, are able to generate complex sentences, and also are able to understand and use a range of intonation to mark shades of meaning. The parents, however, did not seem to perceive the paucity of their children's language skills, particularly the inadequacy of such skills if their children were to enter mainstream schools and have any hope of succeeding in that language-intensive environment.

Most respondents said people outside the family would not understand their child's speech because it was not clear enough. Several parents stressed that their own comprehension was due to familiarity:

> We are used to his speech; generally we understand him. Perhaps people outside the family might not understand him, but in the family we understand what he means.
>
> *(mother, family 6; boy, age 5, severely deaf)*

Sometimes parents said that despite their own inability to understand the child's speech, they understood their child better than outsiders—experience enabled them to know what their child wanted. Once again, the role of routine and negotiated understandings, often not based on speech, was crucial.

Use of Sign/Gestural Communication

As we have already seen, many of the parents took a dim view of the use of gestures at home: they wanted their children to learn to speak. Yet some respondents acknowledged that they relied on gestures at home because communication was not possible if only aural/oral means were employed.

Three respondents suggested that at times it was their children who initiated and preferred using gestures. In one case, the child was described as not wanting to speak: "He doesn't usually speak much. He doesn't want to speak . . . he likes using signs" (father, family 3; boy, age 5, profoundly deaf). Some children used gestures that were not understood by family members:

> Sometimes she uses gestures we don't understand, and we try to guess, we ask her what she means by them. Several times she's used gestures I can't make out, and I've asked her teacher, but she doesn't understand either. I don't know what she's asking for—it's unclear to me. Even now I don't know what those gestures mean.
>
> *(grandfather, family 12; girl, age 7, severely deaf)*

This respondent went on to say that the difficulties of making herself understood made his granddaughter angry and frustrated.

A number of points were raised about the informal signs used at home, which parents viewed as having dubious legitimacy. They associated the use of "proper" sign language with the instruction of deaf children in deaf schools. The preschool staff did not teach the children sign language, one parent told me, thereby not only explaining their lack of access to sign but also suggesting that sign language as a proper means of communication had to be "taught" rather than simply acquired casually. One parent worried whether the gestures they used at home were "right" or not: she did not feel confident about her family's creating their own system of home signs, because she felt it was not as good as standard sign language. Another parent similarly implied a sharp distinction between the casual gestures that they used at home and "those formal gestures" that deaf people used and that neither her son nor other family members knew. None of the parents had tried to learn sign language themselves or to find ways of giving their child more access to it.

Signs used at home represented activities such as eating, drinking, and sleeping. There were also signs for people, which tended to reflect some aspect of their appearance—in one family, the sign for "father" was the fingers held to the eyes in circles to indicate glasses; the sign for "grandfather" indicated his beard; and the sign for "mother" outlined her shoulder-length hair. Another parent mentioned signs for "bus," "bicycle," "soap," and "drawing things," among others. Generally speaking, these home-signs were very simple and were used to communicate the most basic events of family life and routines.

In one family, of course, there were good models available for the development of communication at home using sign language: this was the family with deaf parents and a severely deaf child. Yet even though the girl's deaf mother thought it would be easier for her daughter to use sign, she explained that her daughter was not taught sign in the nursery school and she wanted her to learn speech.[10] It would have been extremely interesting to know what the communication patterns in this family actually were: the deaf daughter surely developed some understanding of signs and their meaning when she lived in such close proximity to three signing deaf adults (her parents and her mother's younger brother). Nevertheless, the main care of the child, and the responsibility for developing her language, was formally in the hands of her illiterate grandmother, while her educated deaf parents were, officially at least, not supposed to be signing with her.

Parents' Views on Their Child's Use of Sign Language

Parents were asked later in the interview about their views on the usefulness of sign language for their children, and about its role in their children's education. This question specifically used the word *shouyu*, meaning "sign language"; in the context of their children's education, it seems to have been understood as primarily referring to the sign language taught in deaf schools, which is in fact a form of manually coded Chinese—signs used in the order of spoken Chinese.

Half the respondents saw no need for their child to sign; some were emphatic that their children should not use sign language at all. For example, one mother felt the use of sign would prevent her child from developing good speech—despite his degree of hearing loss, he did have relatively good oral skills:

> If he uses sign language or gestures, he won't speak. If he doesn't speak, he'll be mute. I want him to speak; using gesture isn't good for him, speaking is best for him.
>
> *(mother, family 13; boy, age 6, profoundly deaf)*

Six parents felt sign language did have a role to play in their child's development. They knew that their children would be going to deaf school at age seven, and they of course knew that sign would be the main medium of instruction there. But some of these respondents maintained they would not be using sign language at home, whatever went on at school:

> We want her to speak as much as possible, because she does have some hearing. In the school the teacher will teach them sign language, I can't ask them not to. I will teach her to speak as much as possible at home, such as how to pronounce, and how to read out loud. . . . I don't understand sign language.
>
> *(grandfather, family 12; girl, age 7, severely deaf)*

One mother thought that writing would be a useful way of communicating at home once her son was at deaf school—but not sign language. She said quite firmly that she did not intend to learn sign language later:

> Once our son goes to deaf school, he will pick up sign language quite naturally. Then at home, for communication, we can use characters and he can understand. For all the purposes of daily life—eating, sleeping, washing, having a bath—he can recognize all those characters. . . . If we write

down characters, he can understand. I don't intend to learn sign language. Because my son has a good memory for characters. We teach him characters. He can understand what they mean. It's enough to know these characters.

(mother, family 8; boy, age 4, profoundly deaf)

What emerges once again is a theme that is not ever stated explicitly though it runs through all these accounts: for parent and child to be able to communicate about basic wants—eating, sleeping, and so on—is enough, and this level of communication is natural, adequate, and appropriate as far as the parents are concerned. There appears to be little perceived need, at this stage at least, for language to support more than these simple, functional interactions.

There were three respondents, all with profoundly deaf children, who said they might learn sign language. One father was quite definite:

Thinking of my son's situation at the moment, if he's going to be going to deaf school I'll need to learn sign language, standard sign language. Because if I don't, then I'll have no way of communicating with him.... Now if my wife and I learn sign language, we'll be able to understand and speak [*sic*] with him, so this method is necessary.

(father, family 1; boy, age 6, profoundly deaf)

The other two respondents were less enthusiastic, however. One grandmother thought she might learn it later, "if conditions were right," meaning if there were classes she could conveniently attend. And a mother, acknowledging that sign language was useful for communication for children who could not hear, said she might learn sign language in the future, without expanding on her statement. It seemed in fact unusual and a departure from the norm for parents with children in deaf schools to make a deliberate attempt to learn sign language. One wonders what the situation would be in a few years' time, when children have acquired a large vocabulary of signs at school—would some parents pick up signs from their children, or even make a deliberate attempt to learn from them?

In addition to the parents and grandparents with children attending the nursery school, I was also able to interview several other parents: one of these was a mother whose profoundly deaf son had left the rehabilitation center the year before and was in his first year at the deaf school. Although she said her son was now able to communicate freely in sign with the other children at school, she told me quite emphatically that they did not use sign at home; in fact, they did not allow their son to use sign language at home, because she wanted him to keep up his speech, "to keep his tongue supple." She mentioned the case of a seventeen-year-old youth in Shanghai who had had an cochlear implant and who could now "hear and speak": she thought her son should continue to exercise his tongue and speak as much as possible, in case he ever had an implant in the future. Besides showing her resistance to learning or using sign language herself, she also revealed the persistent hope that her son might still miraculously be transformed into a hearing child.

According to senior teachers at Nanjing Deaf School, efforts have been made by the school to provide sign language classes for hearing parents so that they can communicate better with their children and help them with their schoolwork.[11] But the classes were difficult to keep going and were not well attended. Apparently, most parents did not want to learn sign language. Perhaps some families do develop their own systems of home sign, even incorporating some of the signs their children bring home from school. Many children in deaf schools have a younger sibling who is hearing; the principal of the Third Deaf School in Beijing told me that siblings are often excellent communicators in sign with their deaf older brother or sister.

The Relative Value of Reading, Writing, and Speech

Parents were asked their views on the relative importance for their children of learning to read, write, and speak. Half the parents thought that for their children, speech was more important than reading and writing. As one mother said:

> If she learns to speak, then later she'll be able to get along with normal people, she'll be able to have conversations. This aspect is what I want for her. If she can write characters, but can't speak, that's no good.
>
> *(mother, family 2; girl, age 6, severely deaf)*

Two parents pointed out that speech was more convenient for communication:

> Speaking is more important, of course. With speech you can express yourself. Writing is much slower. . . . If there's no other way you can have a conversation in writing. . . . But being able to speak is good—it's quicker.
>
> *(grandfather, family 12; girl, age 7, severely deaf)*

> Speech is more important. It's more convenient. Because it takes time to write things—also, we need a quiet place to sit down and write. It's not convenient if you're walking down the street. Speech is important—more important than writing.
>
> *(mother, family 11; boy, age 6, severely deaf)*

The remaining respondents took the opposite position, maintaining that writing was more important than speech. Five of the children concerned were profoundly deaf; one was the severely deaf child of deaf parents. Their parents explained that writing was more important because their children's hearing loss precluded their learning to speak. As one grandmother put it succinctly: "At the moment it's like this—he can't hear, so writing is more important" (grandmother, family 7; boy, age 3, profoundly deaf). Several explicitly linked the ability to read and write to the children's need to communicate. The grandmother who had two deaf children believed that literacy would give her granddaughter a better chance of getting a nonmanual job.

Whether the interviewees felt that speech or that character recognition and writing should be learned first depended on which they saw as more valuable. Only one respondent believed that speech, reading, and writing were of equal importance, although she said learning to recognize characters should come before writing. Her son was profoundly deaf, yet he was in the most advanced class and had relatively good oral skills. She thought that an emphasis on speech alone would affect his understanding, implying that written language was crucial for her son's overall language development.

The hearing of one child had improved gradually from a severe to a moderate loss, and her father felt that while she was still in the process of recovering her hearing, reading and writing were good for her:

> Yes, reading and writing have an effect. If a child can comprehend what they read, and can write, this will be very good for the development of their language.... The best thing is to learn to speak first. The best thing would be if she could speak like a normal child. Before she completely recovers her hearing, she can't speak clearly, she is at a disadvantage compared with normal children: at this stage, reading and writing are good for her — they help to develop her intelligence.
>
> *(father, family 14; girl, age 6, moderately deaf)*

Here again, reading and writing were seen as contributing to language development when a child's access to spoken language was inadequate. None of the respondents ever expressed the view that it was necessary for children first to acquire a language of ready communication (whether this was speech or sign), before learning to read and write.

PRESCHOOL EDUCATION

Choice of Nursery School

Most ordinary nursery schools are reluctant to admit deaf children. Three children in this study had attended ordinary nursery schools briefly; two had to be removed because teachers complained they would not do as they were told, while the third, previously undiagnosed, was discovered to be deaf by her teacher and subsequently removed. Two of these children underwent intensive treatments following their diagnosis that would have prevented their attending nursery school in any case. Other parents felt that attending an ordinary preschool would be difficult for their child because they would not be able to communicate with the other children: "I feel if he went to an ordinary nursery school, it would have a bad effect on him, on his personality, in all sorts of ways" (father, family 1; boy, age 6, profoundly deaf). Another parent pointed out that in ordinary preschools a few teachers looked after relatively large numbers of children—but in the rehabilitation center her child would get much more attention. Two children had attended another rehabilitation center in the city before changing to this one. Their parents felt the children were now happier and receiving more attention.

Several parents had enrolled their children at the rehabilitation center specifically because they hoped the teachers could train them to speak. Other parents approved of the structured education that the nursery school provided, in good habits and good behavior as well as speech training, reading, and other subjects. One respondent stressed his preference for having his son educated in the preschool rather than being left with grandparents while he and his wife were working:

> Both of us work during the day, so there's no way we could teach him. If he stayed at home and his grandparents looked after him, he wouldn't be taught very well either. I thought of putting him in the nursery school mainly because the teachers can teach him some things, increase his knowledge. The other thing is that he will receive a systematic education from early on. I want him to learn how to behave, a daily routine, good habits, he knows about keeping himself clean and tidy.
>
> *(father, family 1; boy, age 6, profoundly deaf)*

Some parents also felt it was beneficial that all the children in the preschool were deaf, perhaps feeling that in such an environment their children would not be singled out as "different" and come to think of themselves as inferior to other, hearing children.

Parents as Teachers

Like many Chinese parents whose children are attending preschool, the respondents in this study expected to teach their child at home every evening—a responsibility called "home teaching." This required close coordination with the child's teacher so that they might know what to cover in the child's homework and how to approach it (such cooperation is also emphasized in mainstream education). These parents, of course, were all trying to improve their children's speech, and the teachers at the rehabilitation center gave them specific advice on this as well as on other matters. Some parents were prepared to put a great deal of time and effort into teaching their child at home, contacting the child's teacher frequently to get as much help as they could. Often this was done informally, when parents collected their children at the end of the school day; there were also opportunities for discussions at parents' meetings.

Parents tended to work harder at home education if their child was in his or her final year at the nursery school and they hoped that mainstreaming was possible:

> Now he is almost school age, we have been increasing our contact with his teacher: we want to know what she's teaching them in class, and what the teaching scheme is. We want to know all these things. Then we can plan extra work to give him at home.
>
> *(mother, family 11; boy, age 6, severely deaf)*

The phrase she used here for the extra work was "supplementary education," an expression widely used in China to describe parents' additional input to their child's formal education.

Parents' Meetings

At the time the fieldwork interviews for this study were carried out, parents' meetings took place at least once a month at the preschool. Sometimes all the parents were invited, sometimes just the parents or grandparents of children in one class: in the latter case the principal, the class teacher, and the parents would be present. I was able to attend two of these meetings.

A wide range of topics was covered at the meetings. Useful medical treatments for deafness were discussed; the principal made specific recommendations for cures, although at most rehabilitation centers the staff follow the official line that such treatments are a waste of time. The principal also emphasized the need for the children to wear proper hearing aids, and their function and usefulness were discussed. Methods of educating deaf children were presented in theoretical and practical terms, and different learning techniques were recommended. The class teacher then outlined her teaching plan for her class and explained the methods she used in class to improve pronunciation or promote character recognition so that parents could follow the same methods in reinforcing the work at home. Parents asked questions, described problems they encountered with their children, shared experiences with other parents, and picked up useful pieces of advice.

In the interviews respondents talked most about information on educational approaches they had been able to learn about at parents' meetings, methods they could use to teach their child at home. One respondent, for example, felt advice she had been given about how to teach her three-year old grandson to recognize characters through play was very effective—she said he was making very good progress. One father explained the kinds of things parents learned at the meetings:

> The meetings are organized so we can have a good talk, about how to teach our children, how to get your child to lipread, what things to study, how to reinforce things by repetition . . . each person's teaching methods are different. So if someone else has a teaching method, and I think it seems good, then I can try it out. Being able to exchange ideas like this is very useful. . . . For example, using cards with characters written on. You put the card on a chair, for example, so the child can see that's a chair, and that's the character for chair. Or the washing machine—you put the card with "washing machine" on it on the washing machine, then the next time he sees those characters he knows they mean "washing machine." It's a very good method.
>
> *(father, family 1; boy, age 6, severely deaf)*

The parents seem as open to methods they learn from one another as to those suggested by the nursery staff—as they keep searching for what will work with their own children, they do not automatically accord greater legitimacy to a fixed set of techniques imparted by professionals.

Children's overall development, and not simply their education, was discussed at meetings. Attention was paid to their developing good moral behavior and good personalities—exactly the themes central to child socialization in mainstream preschool education in China, and qualities stressed as necessary if the children at the rehabilitation center were to join mainstream society. One particular area much talked about was how to be firm and prevent the deaf child from becoming spoiled:

> You shouldn't let him do just anything he wants to. There need to be rules. You need to teach the child to face up to setbacks — life isn't all plain sailing. He has to know how to deal with difficulties. You can't be accommodating him over everything.
> *(grandmother, family 7; boy, age 3, profoundly deaf)*

This is of course a major preoccupation of urban Chinese parents with hearing children as well.

When asked what they found helpful about the parents' meetings, respondents most frequently pointed to the usefulness of learning from other parents' experience:

> We can make use of other parents' good points to overcome our shortcomings. We can learn from other parents' experience, and they can learn from ours. We can talk and share our experiences.
> *(mother, family 9; boy, age 6, severely deaf)*

A couple of parents also mentioned the inspiration and encouragement they gained from the principal. Clearly he was able to persuade some parents who felt depressed or hopeless about their child's situation to adopt a more positive attitude. One respondent spoke of the emotional support that other parents provided:

> Once I know there's a meeting, I very much want to go. Because the parents — the parents of the children in the nursery — they all have the same feelings as me. At the meeting I don't feel under stress . . . the stress is less. I feel quite relaxed. We can talk together, make use of each other's strong points to offset our own weaknesses. I think it's quite good.
> *(grandmother, family 7; boy, age 3, profoundly deaf)*

Although she was alone in mentioning this benefit, it seems possible that other parents found the same sense of relief in sharing their feelings but preferred in their interviews to focus on more pragmatic aspects of the meetings and to avoid discussing their emotions.

Parents' meetings were clearly viewed as useful and worthwhile. Although organized by the preschool, with an agenda to some extent controlled by the staff, parents were still able to share and learn from one another's experiences. Although they found such mutual dialogue valuable, they did not have meetings independently of the preschool: there was no initiative toward self-help in this respect.[12] Parents would have practical difficulties finding another time and place to meet—and perhaps they have little incentive to do so, since their primary motivation for gathering is to communicate with teachers and obtain information that might help their children.

Children's Progress

Parents were asked what they thought of their children's progress at the nursery school. Their replies indicate that they used learning to speak as a major yardstick of achievement:

> He's made very good progress at the nursery school. The first month he was there, he didn't say anything. One day, after he'd been there a month, he was able to speak *pinyin:* a e i o u. I was so happy.
>
> *(mother, family 9; boy, age 6, severely deaf)*

Lack of progress in this area might be excused by respondents on the grounds the child had not been in the preschool long enough:

> At the moment he's still having problems with his speech, because he hasn't had much time. He's only had a month or so, two months, in the nursery school.
>
> *(grandmother, family 7; boy, age 3, profoundly deaf)*

However, this respondent was pleased that her grandson was learning to recognize characters at the preschool. Generally speaking, parents or grandparents of children with severe or profound hearing losses who were not progressing well with their speech tended to emphasize gains in character learning or arithmetic:

> He's doing better than we would have anticipated. He's learned a lot of characters. There are various things he can read aloud, although his pronunciation isn't very clear. . . . As far as arithmetic and math are concerned, he's reasonably quick at those. He can do one-digit and two-digit sums. He's quite quick at mental arithmetic. So I think going to the nursery school has been very good for him; whether he goes to an ordinary school later or deaf school, he's certainly getting a very good foundation.
> *(father, family 1; boy, age 6, profoundly deaf)*

THE CHILD'S FUTURE

Education

Parents were asked how far they thought their child would go in his or her education. Several found it difficult to say anything definite because their child was still so young; one respondent saw the issue as hinging on whether his granddaughter would be able to recover her hearing. However, most answers were strongly positive and specific, reflecting not only parents' high aspirations for their child but also their willingness to invest in and support their child's formal education as far as it could go:

> I finished college myself. I think my son should reach at least this level. The best thing would be if he could go further than that.
> *(mother, family 11; boy, age 6, severely deaf)*

> I want her to have the same education as a normal child. . . . I'd like her to do something good, some scientific research, and go to some good institute.
> *(mother, family 2; girl, age 6, severely deaf)*

It would be good if he could get as far as technical middle school or that level, as far as he can, university perhaps.

(mother, family 13; boy, age 6, profoundly deaf)

More than half the parents mentioned the possibility of their child going to college.

Employment

Some parents felt that it was too early to say what their child might do for a living; several pointed out that how their child developed would determine the answer to this question.

Parents perceived that in order for their child to enter society, he or she must have a specialist skill or training, such as dressmaking, painting, or word processing. Families who had a relative with a special trade or profession saw the possibility of a family connection making it easier for the deaf child to get a job. The father who mentioned word processing felt that it would be ideal for his profoundly deaf son because he would have little need for language to communicate—he could simply type documents. But depending on the language skills actually required for word processing, this might not be a realistic aspiration unless his son became competent in written Chinese. In general, parents were particularly anxious that their child should get a "light" job that was well-paid and nonmanual, a desire that deepened their concern that their child receive a good education and specialist training.

Parents were asked whether they thought their child would be able to look after them when they were old. Several parents interpreted this question as referring to general care and attention: they felt that because they had brought their child up to respect them, their child would care for them in their old age. Others understood it on a financial level: none were planning to depend on the support of their deaf child, and they told me that they would probably rely instead on work unit pensions and old age homes. At least at this stage of their lives, parents were concentrating more on saving money for their child's treatment, education, or other future needs than on the possibility that their child might support them financially in the even more distant future.

Parents' Worries and Hopes Concerning Their Child's Future

Parents were most concerned about their child's prospects of finding a good job and his or her ability to become independent and self-reliant. They were also troubled about their child's marriage prospects. Some parents specifically mentioned the difficulties that the children's hearing loss would cause in relations with other people—they would not be able to communicate properly, other people would not understand what they were saying, they would have difficulty making friends, and they might develop psychological problems.

Significantly, although the phrase "psychological problems" was never used in connection with communication difficulties or behavioral problems at home, parents envisaged their child suffering psychologically once he or she was out in mainstream society, in the world of work. This suggests that parents are worried not just about the practical problems posed by communication barriers but also about the social isolation and discrimination their children may have to face in the future outside the protective environment of the home.

KEY PROBLEMS

Parents were asked what they thought was the most difficult aspect of their child's deafness both from the child's point of view and from their own. Regarding the first, most pointed to the problem of communication:

> Communication is quite difficult. Because when he wants to express himself, we don't understand him that well. And when we want to tell him something, we find that even if we use gestures, there are some things we can't express.
>
> *(father, family 1; boy, age 6, profoundly deaf)*

However, parents differed in their emphases. As we have seen, some were concerned with more than the immediate difficulties of communicating at home: they worried about what their child's hearing loss and inability to speak intelligibly might imply more broadly for his or her life and future. One mother, who was overtly very hostile toward her daughter's deafness and any visible signs of it, said specifically that the main problem was her daughter's articulation, focusing not on the difficulty of communicating but on the obvious evidence of her daughter's defectiveness. Several parents emphasized the obstacles that deafness put in the way of their children's education by making them difficult to teach.

For themselves, parents cited a range of practical problems in addition to that of communication. These included the drain on the family's financial resources of paying for treatments, the stress of the long commute to the rehabilitation center every day, and the difficulties of teaching their child. One mother was particularly worried that when her son started primary school, she would be unable to give him the educational support he needed because both she and her husband had to work full-time. Most parents anticipated more difficulties in the future, when it would be much harder for them to ensure that their child got a good job, married well, and had a good standard of living than it would have been if their child were "normal." Clearly these are pressing concerns when families have to rely on their own resources and cannot expect any significant assistance from outside agencies.

The Influence of Cultural Context

The families in this study show many similarities in their structures and in the roles of their members. With three exceptions, the families were one-child families; all the parents were married, and most were in their early thirties. As a rule, both parents were working: only one mother had decided to stop working so that she would have more time to spend with her son, although one other mother had cut her work to half-time for the same reason. Parents were in close contact with grandparents, who were a valuable source of support; they often helped parents by taking care of their grandchildren.

The homogeneity of these patterns of family life seems remarkable when contrasted with the diversity that would generally be encountered in an urban area in the United States or Europe. One-parent families and stepfamilies are common in the United States and Great Britain; large cities may have large ethnic minority communities, with some families who speak a language other than English at home. Employment patterns are also different: in areas of high unemployment, some parents live on government benefits for long periods of time. Mothers of deaf children may choose to stay at home to devote more time and attention to their deaf child, but this attention must be shared if there are other children in the family. Grandparents may be at hand and may play a significant role in some families, but they do not provide support so reliably in Western countries as in China. The variety in family backgrounds, reflecting the more diverse social and cultural mixes in many Western countries, especially in urban areas, has significant implications. It may be easier in multicultural societies to frame deafness as a form of cultural difference based on language use and cultural affiliations, rather than as a medical defect; conversely, in countries such as China where there are much more clearly defined social norms and society is strongly monocultural, there may be less tolerance of difference. Some research into social attitudes toward deafness supports this hypothesis: a cross-cultural comparison of attitudes of South Korean and American teachers of the deaf toward Deaf culture showed that the attitudes were more negative in the monocultural society of Korea than in the multicultural society of the United States (Choi 1995).

A striking finding that emerged from the interviews with parents was their apparent lack of awareness of the importance of age-appropriate language development for a young deaf child. For example, their idea of what was adequate seemed far short of the language that children need to cope in a mainstream school. This tendency may be accentuated by cultural concepts that underplay the importance of informal verbal interaction at home. However, it has to be said that rehabilitation teachers in China do recognize the importance of early language development at home (though of course they emphasize speech over other forms of communication), and they advise parents to talk to their children as much as possible.

In June 1996, eighteen months after the original interviews, I was able to talk to most of the parents again and find out how their children were progressing. Six out of the fourteen children had gone on to mainstream primary schools: in some cases, their parents had to work hard to persuade a local school to admit their child. Their progress was closely correlated with the amount of their residual hearing, the ability of their family (usually the mother) to support their development of language, and their progress in oral skills when they were attending the preschool. Three of the six children seemed to have a good chance of holding their own in the mainstream school, according to the reports from their parents and the assessments of the preschool teachers. Of the remaining three, two had severe hearing deficits and inadequate speech and language skills: one mother said that her son was having difficulties with reading and writing because it was difficult to explain sentence structures to him. The third child had parents who were not very supportive and did not let her wear a hearing aid. She was quite bright and had significant residual hearing, but her teachers had little hope for her success in primary school.

Two children, both profoundly deaf, had gone on to Nanjing Deaf School. Three children, now six years old and still at the preschool, had begun some lessons in sign from a deaf teacher in the new bilingual class. Another six-year-old had been removed from the preschool because his grandmother could no longer cope with the daily journey across town to the center—and perhaps she did not think it was worth it, since he had made so little progress in speech: she was now teaching him at home, and he had learned dozens of characters and could read stories and retell them in home signs. Those four children were all due to start attending Nanjing Deaf School the following September. One girl had dropped out: after she had spent one year at the rehabilitation center without making any significant progress toward developing speech, her grandparents sent her back to her parents in the countryside, where it seemed unlikely she would have any further education.

The different fates of the children seem to rest on two main determinants: the child's degree of hearing loss and how much support his or her language development received at home. The rehabilitation center and its teachers also played a crucial role: without this facility, it is extremely unlikely that any of the children would have been able to gain access to mainstream primary schools. Those children who attended the center and went on to the deaf school arrived having had the experience of preschool, with language lessons and structured learning activities, in the company of other deaf children. My observations of their very organized daily routine suggested they had learned good and appropriate social behavior toward each other and toward their teachers. Whichever route the children took when they left the preschool, their experience there seemed useful and valuable.

CHAPTER SIX

LETTERS TO ZHOU HONG

In addition to the interviews I conducted, I was fortunate to obtain a collection of letters written by Chinese parents of deaf children. Their contents complement the information and views obtained from the interviews. The majority of these 168 letters are addressed to Zhou Hong, at that time principal of the preschool for deaf children whose parents were interviewed for my study. The remainder are addressed to Zhou Hong's daughter, Tingting (born in 1980), whose severe deafness was caused by ototoxic antibiotics when she was eighteen months old. The parents who wrote these letters were seeking advice concerning their own deaf children.

Zhou Hong has become widely known in China because of his success in educating his daughter. He taught her to speak and also taught her Chinese characters, so that she now reads and write proficiently. Rather than taking a traditional, formal approach to learning, Zhou Hong adopted an informal style of interaction with his daughter in order to make education seem interesting and attractive to her. At her father's instigation Tingting memorized the figure for pi to 1,000 decimal places, using a special mnemonic technique, when she was eight years old, and she recited it faultlessly in front of an audience of educators at a national conference. Her achievements were further publicized two years later when her father published an account of her education and upbringing titled *From Mute Girl to Child Prodigy*. Subsequently she was named one of the "Top Hundred Teenagers of China" and one of the "Top Ten Young Pioneers," and she and her father became nationally famous.

The first series of letters to Zhou Hong followed the widespread media coverage that began in 1991; and because Zhou Hong has encouraged journalists to continue producing articles about his daughter and his educational methods, people continue to write to him—particularly parents with deaf children. Their persistence in doing so, in large numbers, clearly reflects the scarcity of information and support available elsewhere, as well as the tendency of these parents to look for help from every possible source. Zhou Hong has responded to many of the letters, sending parents copies of his and his daughter's book as well as teaching materials and tapes that he has prepared himself. He has also organized meetings for parents who travel hundreds of miles to hear him speak and to discuss their problems with him. With money raised through the sale of books and other materials, Zhou Hong has recently opened a private school for deaf children in Nanjing, staffed by parents of deaf children.

Zhou Hong offered me the letters to help with my research on families with deaf children in China. It was not possible to write to all the parents to ask their permission, both because of the number of letters and because in some cases the return addresses were missing or unclear. Nevertheless, it seemed acceptable to use the letters as research data, in part because their contents offer few details that parents would wish to conceal from others. The letters do reveal the parents' extreme unhappiness and frustration, but these feelings are shared by a majority of the parents. Nevertheless, I have been careful to maintain their privacy by preserving their anonymity.

Eighty of the letters are dated between 1991 and 1993, eighty-one between 1994 and 1996. Zhou Hong handed over the first series without prior examination or selection, straight from his files; at my request, in the second series he looked for letters containing "details of the family circumstances and descriptions of parents' experiences." Careful reading of the letters reveals no obvious difference between the two series; in particular, no obvious bias was introduced as a result of selection except length and detail. All of the letters include praise for Zhou Hong and appreciation of his achievement in educating his deaf daughter, so these elements were unlikely to have influenced his choice. Therefore, I treated the two series of letters as a group and analyzed them together.

In three cases, the same person wrote more than once, and in such cases all the correspondence was counted together as one "letter." Four criteria determined which letters should be included in the final sample:

1. The letters should be written by relatives of the deaf child; this excluded people who, although sympathetic toward the family, were unlikely to have access to key information and might not have been aware of the family's main concerns.

2. There must be clear evidence that the child was definitely hearing-impaired and not delayed or limited in speech for other reasons, such as mental handicap; in fact, most children in the final sample had had some form of audiometric testing that confirmed their hearing loss.

3. The child should not have started either mainstream primary school or deaf school.

4. The child should not be over ten years of age.

Using these criteria, I excluded 33 letters from the original sample, and I was left with 135 in the final collection. I selected ten of these letters to show the range of parents' circumstances and experiences, and these are included at the end of this chapter.

Certain specific characteristics of the writers can be inferred from the letters and the context in which they were written. First, simply writing a letter implies a good standard of literacy, especially when an ideographic language such as Chinese is used. Second, the letters were written after parents had read newspaper reports or magazine articles, or in a few cases watched television programs, about Zhou Hong and his daughter Tingting: with this kind of access to news and events they were more likely to be relatively well-educated urban families than uneducated peasants living in remote rural areas. Third, parents or relatives who wrote to Zhou Hong for advice felt motivated to seek help and believed that something useful might come of their action: clearly parents who were apathetic or too ashamed of their children would not write. While these letter writers are not representative of *all* parents with preschool-age deaf children in China, one can reasonably assume that their attitudes and views are to a large extent representative of educated, urban Chinese parents with preschool-age deaf children who are active in seeking help for their children.

Whether the letters are brief or discursive, they follow a basic pattern. Each letter contains three elements, often in the following order: an initial section of one or more paragraphs describing how the writer came to hear about Zhou Hong and praising his achievements, a central section giving an account of the deaf child's situation and the parents' response to it, and a final section in which the writer requests help or asks certain questions (the letters at the end of this chapter provide typical examples of this form). The style of writing tends to be compact and economical. It is also very stylized in expression: that is, the parents use a limited number of phrases rather than a wide range of descriptors to relate their experiences. For example, they frequently use the metaphor "going into the soundless world" to describe the situation of deafness, and conversely "coming out of the soundless world"/"coming into the world of sound" to describe a deaf child's acquisition of speech.

The letters were all translated from Chinese into English before analysis. Each letter was read through and discussed with a native speaker of Chinese: letters 1 to 33 with a postgraduate student with a good knowledge of English, the remaining letters with an experienced medical translator. It became clear to me that I was in danger of overlooking some subtleties and connections that were more apparent to my Chinese assistants. For example, one letter about a deaf child living with his grandparents contains the sentence "His grandparents are unable to communicate with him." One of my Chinese colleagues commented, "The grandparents maybe don't like the child": on being pressed for further explanation, she responded, "It's hard to explain, but there is only one sentence; it seems like there might be a family problem here." Of course such conjectures are based on close familiarity with Chinese cultural behavior, including common attitudes toward deafness and its expression in language. In general, though, our perceptions concerning the explicit themes in the letters tended to coincide.

Key data about the parents, where available, were extracted from each letter: where they lived, and, in particular, whether they lived in an urban or rural area; educational level; and occupation. Key data concerning the deaf children were then identified: the child's age, age when hearing loss was suspected, age at diagnosis, and degree of hearing loss. I noted further details about each family, such as whether or not the family consisted of a married couple with one or more children, as well as the number of siblings, if any.

The letters were then read through carefully to identify the main themes. Once a theme was identified, it could be elaborated qualitatively with the help of descriptions in different letters. For example, a recurring theme in the letters (as in the interviews) is the constant search for a cure for deafness. When this behavior starts, what resources — time, money, effort — are employed by parents, how parents find out about treatments, what their experience of the effects of treatment are (beneficial or otherwise), what causes parents to cease searching for a cure: all these details can be explored by sifting through all the letters. No one letter refers to all these elements, but a nuanced picture can be supplied by the cumulative description. In a few areas, a quantitative analysis is appropriate, as in comparing the number of parents who request information about cures or treatments for deafness with the number who ask for advice on speech training for their child.

My purpose in analyzing the letters was to uncover key preoccupations and understandings of the writers, not to provide a detailed linguistic analysis. However, it seemed important to focus on the exact words parents used in writing of deafness and deaf people in Chinese in order to build a picture of how parents construct these concepts.

The Parents

The writers of these letters were all blood relatives of the deaf children concerned, except in the case of one family whose deaf child was adopted and a niece of the child's adopted mother wrote to Zhou Hong. It is possible that because relatives by marriage may feel less closely concerned with the child, or feel the child is not their responsibility, they do not take the step of writing for help.

A breakdown of the different family members who wrote the letters is given in table 17 (distinguishing between paternal and maternal relatives of the child was easy, as there are different words in Chinese for these relationships). In a few cases it was not possible to tell either from the name or from internal evidence whether the writer — clearly the child's parent — was the father or the mother. Considerably more mothers than fathers wrote letters, and among other relatives, too, those on the mother's side tended to write more frequently than those on the father's side. Perhaps the disparity reflects a feeling that the children concerned, all of preschool age, are at this stage mainly the responsibility of their mothers.

TABLE 17: IDENTITY OF LETTER WRITERS

Relationship to Deaf Child	Number ($N = 135$)
Father	47
Mother	67
Both father and mother	4
Parent (father or mother)	5
Paternal grandfather	0
Paternal grandmother	0
Maternal grandfather	1
Maternal grandmother	2
Paternal uncle	1
Maternal uncle	4
Paternal aunt	1
Paternal greatuncle	1
First cousin (mother's side)	2

Based on their names, the fact they were writing in Chinese, and the lack of any internal evidence to the contrary, I concluded that all the parents—even those writing from the autonomous regions, which have large populations of ethnic minority peoples—were Han Chinese.[1] This might seem unexpected, as China's national minorities constitute 8.3 percent of the population (Kormondy 1995), but the relatively low educational level of some ethnic minority groups might limit their access to information and possibly also affect their attitude toward seeking help; besides, they might not feel the same affinity toward a Han Chinese father of a deaf child as they would to someone of their own ethnic group. All the writers were hearing, and all but one of the deaf children concerned had hearing parents: she had deaf parents but had been adopted soon after birth by a hearing couple.

In only two cases do parents give clear evidence of their level of education: because one mother mentions her thwarted ambition to go to college, she must be a senior middle school graduate; another mother states she is an economics graduate (i.e., she completed a three-year program at a vocational college). However, parents' level of education can be deduced from their jobs, as well as from the language and handwriting used in the letter. It appears that the majority of parents are well-educated, having completed at least senior middle school — in other words, twelve years of schooling. Similarly, occupations are specifically mentioned in only twenty letters, but they can be deduced from the letterhead, which gives the parent's work unit. Such evidence indicates that parents are mostly professionals, such as teachers or doctors, or workers in factories. Very few are farmers.

The letters came from all over the country: twenty-six of China's thirty provinces are represented. Nearly half the letters (48 percent) come from the densely populated eastern provinces — Shandong, Jiangsu, Zhejiang, Henan, and Anhui. Another fifth (21 percent) are from the six southeastern provinces — Fujian, Guangdong, Guangxi A.R. (Autonomous Region), Jiangxi, Hubei, and Hunan. The rest are divided among the remaining provinces and municipalities, as indicated in table 18. Whether parents live in urban or rural areas is of crucial importance, as it determines their access to medical facilities and special educational programs such as the provincial rehabilitation centers for deaf children. Therefore I attempted to deduce this information about their residence, concluding that the majority of parents lived in urban areas (44 percent lived in municipalities, provincial capitals, or main provincial cities; 33 percent in small cities or county towns; 7 percent in rural areas; and 15 percent in locations that could not be identified).

The Children

All of the parents had a single deaf child; none had two or more deaf children. Sixty of the children were male, sixty-six female, and in nine cases the sex of the child was not mentioned and could not be deduced. It is possible that parents with female deaf children were particularly encouraged to write to Zhou Hong because he also had a deaf daughter and they identified with him.

The number of children falling into each age group is shown in table 19. The exact age of eleven children was not known, but evi-

TABLE 18: RESIDENCE OF LETTER WRITERS

Region	Number	Region	Number
Beijing municipality	2	Hunan province	6
Shanghai municipality	6	Guangdong province	5
Tianjin municipality	2	Guangxi A.R.	4
Hebei province	2	Gansu province	2
Shanxi province	3	Qinghai province	0
Inner Mongolia A.R.	2	Ningxia Hui A.R.	0
Liaoning province	4	Sha'anxi province	3
Jilin province	1	Xinjiang Uygur A.R.	2
Heilongjiang province	3	Sichuan province	5
Shandong province	10	Guizhou province	1
Henan province	12	Yunnan province	1
Jiangsu province	16	Tibet A.R.	0
Anhui province	11	Hainan	0
Zhejiang province	12		
Jiangxi province	1	Hong Kong	1
Fujian province	5		
Hubei province	5	Location unknown	8

dence in the letters indicates that they were all of preschool age. The average age of the remaining children was 2.6 years.

Parents of forty-seven children gave figures from hearing tests (in decibels) for their child's hearing loss. In a further twenty-five cases the degree of hearing loss was described as "severe" or "profound" on testing, and other phrases were used to indicate the degree of deafness, such as "completely deaf." When parents simply reported a "severe" hearing loss, it was not always clear whether this meant "severe" or "profound" hearing loss according to the audiological definitions, so these were put into a separate category of "severe/profound" (see table 20). Thus of those children whose hearing loss was stated, the majority were profoundly deaf. None of the children were reported to have disabilities in addition to deafness.

TABLE 19: CHILDREN'S AGES

Age (in years)	Number ($N = 135$)
0–1	1
1–2	25
2–3	41
3–4	31
4–5	14
5–6	7
6–7	2
7–8	3
Exact age not clear	11

TABLE 20: CHILDREN'S HEARING LOSS

Severity of Hearing Loss	Number of Children ($N = 135$)	Percentage of Children
Mild	1	0.8
Moderate	3	2.2
Severe	12	8.9
Profound	47	34.8
Severe/profound	8	5.9
Not given	64	47.4

Nearly two-thirds of the parents (eighty-four) did not refer in their letters to the cause of their child's deafness. Of the remainder, ten said doctors had told them the deafness was "congenital." One child clearly had hereditary deafness, since her natural parents were both deaf. None of the parents admitted to or even raised the possibility of a genetic causation—an omission that suggests a strong element of denial, aversion to the idea of genetic causation, ignorance concerning the mechanisms of inherited deafness, or some combination of those factors. Twenty-two parents said their child was deaf due to the effects of ototoxic drugs; a further eight parents gave this as a possible cause. Ten parents specifically stated that the cause of deafness was unknown.

Family Structure

Almost without exception, the 135 nuclear families represented followed the pattern of a married couple with only one child — the deaf child. The only parents who were not married were a father who referred to his "girlfriend" rather than his wife, but called his deaf son "their" child, and one mother who explained in her letter that she was a widow. In 3 of the 135 families the parents had a hearing child or children in addition to the deaf child. In one family, a boy who was deafened by ototoxic antibiotics had a hearing twin sister. In another family, living in the countryside, the father who wrote the letter explained he had two children: the younger one, a girl, was deaf. One family living in Inner Mongolia had four hearing girls and a deaf boy who was the youngest in the family.

Of the 132 families with only one child, only 4 mentioned the possibility of having a second child. This is probably because the letters were focused on obtaining help for the deaf child. In each case the parents wrote that they either did not want or were not able to have another child. In three instances, parents' rejection of the possibility is linked to their devotion to their deaf child:

> We never intend to have a second child, or give up searching for a cure for him [the deaf child]. (LZH, no. 98)

> Even if there is only a glimmer of hope I'll make every effort to find a cure for my son. . . . The leader of my work unit told me that since my first child is a deaf child, I can have a second child. But I don't want to. (LZH, no. 93)

> My mother-in-law, a warmhearted person who comes from a small village, said: "Don't worry, when the child is three I will take him to the village and he can be a shepherd. Then you can have a second child." When I heard this I was really upset — a shepherd? Is this the only choice for my son? Is this to be his fate? I wasn't happy with my mother-in-law's

attitude. We decided we wouldn't accept her help, we don't want our son to be an idiot and isolated from society. My grandmother told me my son was the cleverest boy she ever met. We must save money for our son, so he can go to primary school. (LZH, no. 16)

In the fourth instance, the mother wrote:

> Because of the current family planning policy, I can't have a second child. So I should concentrate my efforts on the treatment of my son's deafness. (LZH , no. 66)

She does not explain the "can't": she may lack the permission of her work unit to have another child, or perhaps the deafness is congenital and she feels or has been advised not to run the risk of having a second deaf child. In any case, she and the other three writers all seem to associate the idea of investing in the welfare of the deaf child, specifically his or her recovery from deafness and rehabilitation, with rejecting the option of having a second, "normal" child.

THE DIAGNOSIS

Some parents first suspected that their child did not react normally to sound when he or she was only a few months old. Other parents became concerned that something was wrong when it became evident their child was slow to speak. Many parents suppressed their suspicions for some time by finding explanations for the child's unusual behavior or assuming that he or she would grow out of it:

> When she was four months old, we discovered she was rather slow to react to sound compared with other children the same age. At first we thought it was just slow development. (LZH, no. 55)

> Last February I gave birth to a daughter. . . . Not long after, I found her hearing wasn't very acute. I thought maybe she was too young to concentrate her attention. I didn't consider she might have a hearing problem. Why should she? There was no possible reason. (LZH, no. 79)

One mother described her fear that her suspicions might be confirmed, which led to several months' delay before she took her son for testing:

> When I was pregnant I had premonitions that something bad would happen. When my son was born he looked so handsome and intelligent my anxieties were swept away. But when my son was six months old, he wasn't reacting to sounds. . . . I didn't dare test my suspicions. I couldn't bring myself to go to the hospital. I just prayed. I just waited for another miracle to happen. So day after day passed. Other children the same age as my son were saying "*baba*" and "*mama*." . . . Finally one day during Spring Festival, the year before last, we went to Hebei Medical University. (LZH, no. 1)

When parents did decide to consult doctors concerning their child's hearing, they might not have had access to good quality medical care or the necessary hearing tests. Several parents mentioned unsatisfactory encounters with doctors: examinations were perfunctory and inadequate, misdiagnoses were made, or parents were told to come back when the child was old enough to have a hearing test. Some parents responded by traveling to larger cities with better facilities where they could get a proper diagnosis. Even when parents did manage to get access to good medical services, several reported being given only the bare facts with little explanation or discussion of what deafness implied for their child.

The diagnosis of deafness came as a terrible shock to parents. When they recalled the time preceding the diagnosis, it was to remember the happiness they felt at their child's birth and contrast it with the misery they felt now—the following passage is quite typical:

> Last August I gave birth to a baby girl. With the arrival of our daughter, our whole family was full of happiness. My husband and I showed our love to her in every possible way. We devoted ourselves to her. But by and by we began to notice she wasn't reacting to sounds. So we took her for a checkup at our provincial hospital, and they diagnosed nerve deafness. When we got the result, my husband and I

> were stunned. We seemed to fall into a bottomless chasm. Now we are always anxious, we can't put our minds to anything. Her grandparents are also worried and depressed. The happy laughter of the early days has gone. (LZH, no. 108)

Parents were often bewildered because they could see no reason why their child should be deaf. They often seemed not to understand how genetic deafness can be transmitted:

> We felt greatly distressed. We had some doubts about the test result, because it seemed there were no possible causes for my daughter's deafness at all. During her pregnancy, my wife was very cautious and there is no hereditary factor. (LZH, no. 113)

Often "the whole family"—grandparents, parents' siblings, and other members of the extended family—is described as sharing the parents' grief and frustration:

> [My sister and brother-in-law] cry all day long and don't even want to eat or drink. Our whole family feels greatly distressed, but we don't know what to do. (LZH, no. 112)

Thus in addition to the shock of the diagnosis, bewilderment at the seemingly inexplicable misfortune, and the anxiety, worry, and depression experienced by the entire family in coming to terms with the knowledge of the child's deafness, parents record the added distress of uncertainty about what action can be taken. None of the families mentioned any previous experience of deafness; in the absence of a professional support system, parents had to devise their own strategies and courses of action for dealing with a completely unfamiliar situation.

Most parents appeared to have withdrawn into the family circle, absorbed in trying to deal with their own grief, and did not say much about contact with neighbors or outsiders. But one severely depressed mother expressed her unhappiness that she was now vulnerable to other people's contempt:

> Sometimes I think how much better it would be if it were only myself and my son in the world. Then we wouldn't be looked down upon by others, and wouldn't have to listen to those voices that sound like goodwill but are actually making fun of us behind our backs. (LZH, no. 60)

This mother felt so guilty about her son's deafness (caused by injections given to treat a high fever) that she had contemplated committing suicide; perhaps her depression colored her perceptions of other people. But she identifies another adversity faced by parents of disabled children in China, especially in the countryside—they become the objects of gossip, and they have to work harder to maintain their self-respect.[2]

In some families there were added twists to the shock of discovering deafness in their child. The national family planning regulations, in conjunction with a strong desire for male children, sometimes contributed to the difficulties. One man described the price his sister paid for wanting a son:

> My sister has five children. The first four are girls. They are all very healthy, lovely, and clever. They're all doing very well at school. However my sister wanted very much to have a son. For the arrival of a son she paid a high price. But now it turns out her son is a mute. They are heartbroken. I remember she had a scan [to find out the sex of her unborn child] when she was pregnant—I wonder if her son's deafness is related to that. (LZH, no. 112)

In another instance, a mother had had repeated abortions (presumably after ultrasound scans to determine the child's sex), and eventually gave birth to the longed-for son—only to discover when he was eight months old that there was something wrong with his hearing; testing at the age of one year showed that he was completely deaf.

The only couple among the parents to have adopted a child had to endure the irony that the girl they chose was deaf:

> My aunt—my father's sister—was married for many years, but never became pregnant. Because she was worried about having a baby at her age, she and her husband decided to follow the advice of some of their friends and adopt a baby.

> They adopted a little girl from another family when she was three days old. The girl is now four years old. Both her natural parents are deaf. They have three daughters altogether; the oldest and the middle one are very healthy, without any hearing problem at all, and are doing well in school. That's why my aunt and her husband agreed to take their third daughter, this little girl, thinking she would be as good as her sisters. Unfortunately the girl said not a word after she came to my aunt's house, from that day until today. They brought her to the hospital for a checkup, and after that they finally had to accept the truth of her illness. (LZH, no. 22)

In view of the numbers of baby girls in China that are apparently adopted informally (see chapter 2), there must be a certain number who appear healthy at the time of adoption but turn out later to have impairments such as a mental handicap or deafness. We might well wonder if these children are more likely to be abandoned after their disability is discovered if they are not related by blood to their parents. The account above also illustrates popular lack of knowledge about the mechanism of genetic inheritance of deafness: this couple believed that the deaf couple's third child was unlikely to be deaf if the first two children were hearing.

The diagnosis of deafness forces parents to revise their picture of their child's future. Some educated parents who had special aspirations for their only child found it particularly painful to face reality. One couple had dreamed of bringing up their child to be bilingual in Chinese and English, since they themselves knew English well. When the mother realized that her son might never master even one language, she became very depressed and could not continue her job as an English teacher. She began working instead in a bank, where she could make more money to spend on her son's medical treatments (see LZH, no. 16, reproduced below). Another mother had hoped that her son would achieve her own unfulfilled ambition of going to college: the knowledge that her deaf son was unlikely to realize this goal seemed to revive feelings of failure and disappointment about her own life (see LZH, no. 2, reproduced below). Given the national family planning regulations limiting families to one child except under special circumstances, parents must find the shattering of their aspirations for their only children particularly hard to bear.

Family Conflicts and Stresses

Some of the letters reflected particular stresses and conflicts in the family arising from or intensified by having a deaf child; these were mostly related to parents' work and the need to earn money. Despite their obvious concern and feelings for their deaf child, very few — 3 out of 269 — had given up work to educate their children: the needs of the young child conflict with the necessity for both parents to keep on working to maintain a basic income. In addition, there is a strong feeling that mothers may be sacrificing their own lives and hopes for the future if they give up their jobs or devote less time to them, as one mother stated quite clearly:

> Sometimes I feel so depressed. I know parents are responsible for their children's development, but that takes a lot of time, which means you can't put all your energy into your job, so you may miss opportunities and your chance for a good future. That's my situation and it makes me feel very uncomfortable. (LZH, no. 20)

Parents may feel added pressure to work hard and make money because of the cost of medical consultations and treatments for their child: as one mother wrote, "Our whole family wants to earn money, find money to help my son" (LZH, no. 16).

Current economic reforms have made new money-making opportunities available, but jobs in state-owned enterprises are increasingly poorly paid and no longer offer the same security and benefits that they once did. A common practice is for people to keep a foothold in their state job while moonlighting on some more profitable business venture. This leaves even less time for a deaf child. One mother who wrote works unofficially with her husband in a different province, periodically being called home by the leader of her work unit. Though she overtly expresses the wish that her work unit leader give her time off to spend with her son, her tone conveys her guilt at her neglect of him:

> Nowadays I have no time to go back to work [at her official job]. So my younger sister in Henan looks after him because we are seldom at home. His grandparents are unable to communicate with him. So these days I'm quite worried

about him, whether everything is all right for him. If my work unit leader could understand my situation, I would take some time off to go home. I feel I haven't looked after him as well as I should have. I wish I could look after him every day and make him happy, and then I would feel at ease. (LZH, no. 1)

Sometimes tensions arose because parents did not share the responsibility of looking after their child equally. Several mothers complained of having to work full-time as well as look after their deaf child while their husband did very little:

Xuejiao's father is very busy. He often travels to other provinces. He has no time to look after Xuejiao. Sometimes I feel very tense and angry about this. I feel Xuejiao is not just my daughter; she is her father's daughter as well. (LZH, no. 20)

Another mother, with twins to look after, had similar problems; and although her mother-in-law was helping her, she herself could not find time to teach her deaf son:

As you know I have two children, and I have to work. So I have quite a heavy burden. Besides which my daughter isn't very well. She gets laryngitis very often and I have to take her to the hospital for injections. My son goes to the rehabilitation center with his grandmother during the day, and stays with her in the evenings. I only have time to be with him a short time after work. My husband is very busy with his job. He has no time to look after the children or do housework. I know you work as well as teaching your daughter. I would be interested to know how you manage your time. (LZH, no. 86)

Some have argued that the large-scale entry of women into the workplace in Western society has had a substantial and very harmful impact on the language development of preschool-age deaf children whose mothers no longer stay at home with them. Certainly in China, where all mothers are expected to work full-time, it is very difficult for mothers—or fathers—to find time to give to their deaf children.

Under these circumstances the nature of parents' relationships with grandparents becomes even more important. Do the grandparents live nearby? Are they still employed, or are they retired and ready to assist during the day when parents are working? Are they well-educated and able to help parents train their child to speak, or are they illiterate and old-fashioned in their views? Do they support parents' ideas about how the deaf child should be brought up, or is there conflict over this or other matters? Some mothers-in-law, like the one who wanted her grandson to live with her in the countryside and become a shepherd, try to persuade parents to forget about the deaf child and try again for a "normal" one; others, like the primary school teacher discussed later in this chapter, both are supportive of parents' desire to devote themselves to their deaf child's upbringing and education and are able to contribute to this effort.

Parents' Fears and Hopes

The diagnosis of deafness in their child caused parents great anxiety for their child's future. Typical sentiments expressed were "We are worried about his future study and life" (LZH, no. 10) and "How can he go to school? How can he live when he grows up?" (LZH, no. 73). It was not clear to parents what the exact effect of their child's deafness would be on his or her future—and the uncertainty seemed to intensify their fears:

> We can't imagine how our daughter will live in a soundless world for the rest of her life. (LZH, no. 3)

> He is such an intelligent and handsome child, but when I think of his future I feel very depressed and anxious. (LZH, no. 16)

These feelings would be compounded by the lack of professional support and scarcity of information available to most parents.

As children approached school age, parental concern focused on whether they would be able to cope in an ordinary primary school. One mother, who was pleased with her daughter's progress in learning to speak, was nevertheless apprehensive about her starting school:

> When she speaks, her sentences are not clear, and there are a lot of mistakes. It's quite difficult for other people to understand her speech. She will be starting primary school this September. She will be studying with normal children. Her hearing and speech difficulties still exist and are still a problem. (LZH, no. 18)

The focus of her apprehensions also exemplifies how parents characteristically stress the quality of speech rather than considering more broadly the understanding of language that will be essential if the child is to be able to cope with the school curriculum.

When parents have already placed their child in an ordinary nursery school, and their child is unhappy, they may wonder how he or she can survive independently without the protection of the family:

> I am worried about my son. He feels inferior and has no self-confidence. When he was in the nursery school he was always by himself, he never spoke with the teachers or the other children. When the other children picked on him, he just cried; he didn't know how to fight back. I am worried about him: later on, when we get old, will he be able to be independent in society and to survive? When I think about this I get very upset; I don't know what to do about it. (LZH, no. 23)

The lack of any apparent solution for his son's problems must have exacerbated this father's distress.

Parents' hopes for their deaf child focused on two main areas. Some parents simply desired a "cure." But the majority of parents expressed the wish that their children could learn to speak, would be able to attend ordinary primary school with "normal" children, and would be able to live like ordinary people:

> We have only one thought—to work as hard as we can to teach him to speak, even if he only manages some words and everyday expressions. (LZH, no. 98)

> If our child could speak, that would be the happiest moment of our lives. (LZH, no. 16)

> How I wish [my daughter] could speak fluent standard Chinese so she could communicate with other people. (LZH, no. 65)

> My one aim and desire in life is to enable my son to speak and to live like an ordinary person. (LZH, no. 42)

Again, the parents focus almost exclusively on the child's learning to speak as the key to education and life as a "normal" person.

THE SEARCH FOR A CURE

Fifty-three parents (39 percent) of the 135 who wrote to Zhou Hong mentioned they had already tried various treatments, and sixty-five (48 percent)—including some in the previous group—sought information about cures. Clearly this was a course that many parents were very interested in pursuing. Nor is silence on the subject evidence of lack of interest; some of the parents who did not mention medical treatments may have tried them, or may have intended to when their child was older, but chose to focus on some other matter in writing to Zhou Hong—for example, advice about speech training.

Parents generally pursued any information or advertisement that seemed to offer hope; typically, they had tried many hospitals and many forms of treatment:

> My son is taking Chinese herbal medicine now, but there is still no effect after six months' treatment. In order to find a cure for him, whenever we hear of a therapy for treating deafness, we take him to try it. (LZH, no. 118)

> My son is now three years and three months old. . . . Whenever we heard about a treatment for deafness, we took him there for treatment. From when he was two and a quarter to now, we tried everything to treat him. He's taken medicine and had injections—he has his medicine now just like he has his meals. (LZH, no. 52)

They persisted despite having been told by ENT doctors that there was no cure for sensorineural deafness.

> My son is now seven years old. Since we found out our son was deaf when he was eight months old, we have been trying all sorts of medical treatments for him. At Shanghai ENT Hospital the diagnosis was nerve deafness, which is a severe deafness and difficult to cure. However, we still pay particular attention to information of this kind. (LZH, no. 36)

> We took her to the departments of neurology and otology at all the big hospitals in Shanghai for treatment, but we were told "there is no cure." When she was one and a half, she started *qigong* and acupuncture and moxibustion.[3] (LZH, no. 95)

One parent expressed the conclusion that many parents must have reached, before turning to Chinese traditional medical treatments:

> As we know, modern medicine doesn't have any effective treatments for congenital or acquired deafness. (LZH, no. 85)

He and others seemed to view this more as a regrettable failing of Western medicine, in contrast to Chinese traditional medicine, which offers potential cures. This father, a surgeon, wrote to Zhou Hong asking for information on how Tingting had regained her hearing,[4] saying that if his son's hearing could be restored through treatment, "they were willing to do anything at any cost."

Unfortunately, some parents who had previously been impressed by advice not to pursue treatment for their child's deafness were persuaded by reading Zhou Hong's account to investigate its potential:

> Originally we intended to take her to have acupuncture and moxibustion therapy at an army hospital in Shanghai. But the principal of No. 4 Deaf School in Shanghai told us acupuncture and moxibustion therapy didn't work. Almost all the students in his school had had acupuncture and moxibustion at some point, but the only effect was pain. So he advised me not to let my son suffer the treatment. However, after reading the report about Tingting I feel somewhat undecided. So I venture to write to you and would be very grateful if you could give me advice. (LZH, no. 126)

Twenty-eight of the parents who wrote of treatments did not specify what they had tried. Of the twenty-five parents who did provide details, thirteen had tried or were trying herbal medicine; five, *qigong*; and seven, various forms of acupuncture. Other treatments mentioned were high-pressure oxygen, "injections," desensitization treatment (used for deafness due to ototoxic drugs), another treatment for deafness due to ototoxicity (details not given), injections of an "energy mixture," and injections of ATP (adenosine triphosphate) and vitamins B and E. One father living in the countryside, having been told there was no cure for his son's deafness, followed advice to give his son a porridge made of walnuts every day, as this was said to improve hearing.

Parents sometimes traveled hundreds of miles to faraway provinces to seek treatment. One mother living in the eastern province of Anhui mentioned journeys to Beijing and Shanxi province in northern China, as well as to Changchun in the far northeastern province of Jilin (LZH, no. 91). For each trip parents would have to bear the expenses of travel and accommodation in addition to the cost of medical consultations and treatments. There was a high cost, too, in repeated disruption to their lives:

> During the last few months [my brother] has taken his son to all the major hospitals all over the country trying to find a cure for his son, but without any result. Seeing my brother and sister-in-law mentally and physically exhausted, I feel really sorry for them. (LZH, no. 90)

On the fifth of November my wife, my son, and I came back to Fujian by plane [from Nanjing]. The next day I went to work. A week later, I asked for leave again and took my son for treatment to a hospital in the south. As you know, even if there is just a glimmer of hope I will make every effort to find a cure for my son. . . . If the treatment in the hospital in the south has no effect, I intend to take my son to Shanghai next year for treatment. (LZH, no. 93)

The same parent mentioned the enormous sums he had spent so far:

Recently we took our son on a two-month trip to Tianjin, Beijing, Shanxi, and Nanjing for examination and treatments. The fees for examination and treatment, and the accommodation and traveling expenses, altogether cost us nearly 30,000 yuan. And then we also spent quite a lot on the treatment in the hospital in the south. Some of the money is borrowed from our relatives and friends . . . so you see my financial situation is not so good at the moment. (LZH, no. 93)

Most parents did not say exactly how much money they had spent searching for a cure, but one other parent detailed the huge amounts in relation to his income:

The monthly income of my wife and myself together is less than 500 yuan. Therefore our financial situation isn't very good at all. But for our son we took all our savings, less than 1,000 yuan, and borrowed 2,000 yuan from our relatives and colleagues. Then we took our son to Beijing for a checkup. . . . Because there wasn't enough money left, we had to go back to Shanxi. But the cause of my son's deafness still remained unknown, I couldn't just give up. So I raised more money every way I could, and got 8,000 yuan, and once again we went to Beijing. . . . After coming back from Beijing, we kept on looking for treatments for our son at the same time as paying back our debt. We tried traditional Chinese herbal medicine, Western medicine [e.g., injections of ATP and vitamins], even *qigong*. . . . Altogether we spent 20,000 yuan. (LZH, no. 44)

Some parents felt that the expense prevented them from embarking on courses of treatment they wanted to try:

> We often read about good therapeutic methods in newspapers and magazines, but we earn very modest wages and simply can't afford the expensive treatment. (LZH, no. 34)

Of the fifty-three parents who had tried treatments, six reported some improvement in their child's hearing (in two cases described as "slight"). The remainder (89 percent) said that treatment had made no obvious difference.

Some parents turned to the possibility of speech training their child only after they had exhausted their money and hopes in seeking a cure:

> We have tried traditional Chinese herbal medicine, Western medicine, even *qigong*. Every time we were filled with hope, and every time hope turned into disappointment.... But the chances of my son being cured were too small. So we had to accept the fact, and began to consider how to educate my son. (LZH, no. 44)

Others were pursuing both courses of action at the same time; as one wrote,

> We are determined to give him rehabilitation training while giving him medical treatments. (LZH, no. 89)

Although the decision to give their child speech training indicates a partial acceptance of their child's deafness, the impression given by these parents is that they have not yet surrendered the hope that the deafness can be eradicated and are still holding on to an image of their child as whole and "normal." In practical terms their resources and efforts are divided between two aims — eradicating deafness and eradicating its effects; in emotional terms they are still far from accepting the reality or the permanence of their child's deafness.

Hearing Aids and Cochlear Implants

Thirty parents out of 135 (22 percent) mentioned they had bought hearing aids. In all but two cases, only one hearing aid was purchased. Only two parents reported the cost of the aid: 750 yuan and 3,000 yuan respectively (the latter was imported). Six mentioned they had bought foreign brands; one mother said she had initially bought a box-type hearing aid for her son, and later a Chinese-made behind-the-ear model: otherwise there was no information on the types of hearing aids purchased. None of the letters contained information concerning ear molds.

Nine parents gave the age of their child when a hearing aid was obtained. The youngest was one year old and the oldest six at the time of fitting: the average age of this group was 2.4 years. Parents considered buying a hearing aid at different stages: after an extensive trial of medical treatments, after a brief period of treatment, or as the first option. Thirteen parents made no further comment about their experience with hearing aids beyond the fact of purchase, although two wrote that their children were making good progress with their speech, suggesting that they had achieved some success with hearing aid use and speech training.

Seven parents reported that the hearing aids they bought for their children were "ineffective": five of these children were profoundly deaf, with hearing losses of 100, 105, 120, 120, and 120 dB respectively; the exact hearing loss of the other two children was not clear, though one was described as "severe." Although most parents did not mention the price they paid or the type of hearing aid they bought, four of this group of parents did, as if to emphasize that although they had purchased an expensive or high quality foreign aid, the result was still unsatisfactory. Two parents were concerned that the hearing aid was not functioning properly, but they did not have access to any service that could check the aid for them.

Four parents reported that their children would not keep the hearing aid in their ear, thereby frustrating attempts at speech training. One, whose child was nearly three years old, wrote:

> She is very unwilling to wear her hearing aid. Even if she wears it, reluctantly, she can learn for only a very short time. (LZH, no. 91)

This parent appeared to have no strategies for dealing with this behavior. It is not clear from the letters whether parents expected their children to wear their hearing aid only when they were having formal speech training sessions or they tried to get the children to wear them throughout the day.

Five parents reported that the hearing aid their child wore was effective, but two had qualifications: "her hearing is a bit better, but her speech is still poor" (LZH, no. 39); "he is fairly sensitive to surrounding sounds with the hearing aid in, but his discrimination of sound is poor (LZH, no. 42)."

Some parents explained in their letters why they had not purchased a hearing aid for their child, at least yet. Their reasons included lack of access to centers selling hearing aids, or aids of adequate power; advice from doctors that their child's hearing loss was too great for a hearing aid to be useful; and their need for advice before buying an aid. In general, most parents did not exploit assistive technology appropriately or adequately, a failure that reflects not only their lack of understanding concerning the role and usefulness of hearing aids but also, and above all, of the dearth of professional services essential to support children's use of these devices. Expense may also have been a consideration for many parents. It is also possible, as the interviewees suggested in chapter 5, that some parents resisted because buying a hearing aid for their child would mean acknowledging to themselves the reality of their child's deafness or would provide others with a definite and visible sign of their child's deafness; but the letters are silent on this point.

Two parents brought up the subject of cochlear implants. One father, who had recently gotten a job in Malaysia and been told by a doctor there about the "artificial cochlea," was interested in passing on details to Zhou Hong, wondering whether such technology was available in China yet. And one mother had heard about a cochlear device available in China that she was interested in for her three-year-old son:

> I have some information for you. It is about an artificial cochlea. I've heard that the Beijing ENT Institute can do this kind of operation: Professor H—— D—— is the person to contact. I wrote to him, and he wrote back that they can do the operation for the single-channel device. But the opera-

tion is very expensive—it costs 50,000 to 60,000 yuan. I want very much to take my child to Beijing to have the operation, but I can't afford that amount of money. So I intend to sell one of my eyes or my kidney to raise the money for the operation. (LZH, no. 60)

Although cochlear implantation programs for children are beginning in China, the vast majority of parents cannot afford them. However, the implants were discussed and considered by these parents, who perceived them as a means of eliminating deafness; it seems that the actual benefits and drawbacks of cochlear implantation for children are not well understood in China (or indeed by many parents or nonprofessionals in Western countries, either).

Teaching Their Child

Three children of the 135 children in the sample had experience of "rehabilitation training" in a rehabilitation center; the speech training of the remaining 132 children was the sole responsibility of their parents. We should keep in mind that the average age of these children was 2.6 years, so many of these children might in the future attend rehabilitation centers, some of which do not accept children until they are three or four years old.

Parents' level of education appeared to affect the degree of confidence with which they undertook their child's education. This is clearly seen, for example, in the letters reproduced in their entirety at the end of this chapter. In number 80, the mother argues that because she and her husband are only workers and not very well-educated, they do not feel able to teach their daughter—she asks Zhou Hong if he will teach her. By contrast, the mothers in numbers 81 and 82 emphasize that they and their husbands are well-educated and therefore in a very good position to teach their child themselves. It may also be the case that better-educated parents are more likely to get an earlier start in giving their child speech training rather than persist in searching for a medical cure for their child's deafness; however, even well-educated parents seemed to show a marked interest in medical treatments.

The majority of parents were employed in full-time jobs. Only three parents, two mothers and one father, said they had taken leave from work or given up their jobs to stay at home and devote themselves to educating their child. One mother, who had spent three years at home with her daughter, said that although they were short of money, she was very pleased with her daughter's progress. She was now thinking about sending her daughter to an ordinary nursery school.

Most of the parents writing to Zhou Hong about speech training had experienced difficulties and discouragement. They felt it was difficult and were disappointed at the slow progress of their child:

> It takes a lot of effort for me to teach her to speak. (LZH, no. 83)

> After wearing a hearing aid for one month, Zixuan is able to say some words . . . but there hasn't been much improvement on that so far. I know we must have great patience and willpower with children of this kind. Sometimes I think—I am at the end of my resources, and my daughter still isn't speaking. (LZH, no. 46)

> We have given him some training, but there has been no effect. When my child was two and a half years old, he could say "*baba*" and "*mama*," but at three years old he hasn't improved on this. We intensified our efforts to train him. After three months' concentrated training, day and night, he could say a few words. But his pronunciation is poor, and he has difficulty saying some words. (LZH, no. 35)

> When my son was two years old we bought him a hearing aid and sent him to a speech training class to have speech training for an hour and a half every day. When he gets back home, we help him with his speech training. It is over one year now since he began training, but there is no obvious effect. (LZH, no. 56)

> I've been teaching my son to speak for over a month now, but he still can't produce a sound. What is the problem? How can I achieve the goal of enabling him to speak? (LZH, no. 93)

Parents often lacked confidence and they felt that they were not using the proper technique:

> Maybe our teaching method is wrong — the more we teach him to speak, the more unwilling he becomes. (LZH, no. 44)

> I wonder whether my method is wrong, or whether I am not strict enough with her. (LZH, no. 46)

> (*letter to Tingting*) We sent her to study in the language training center. Now she can say some simple words and everyday expressions. She can read *pinyin* and say several nursery rhymes by memory. How I wish she could speak fluent standard Chinese so she could communicate with other people, just like you! But she can't at the moment, because we don't know how to guide her correctly and give her training. (LZH, no. 65)

> He has been wearing a hearing aid for over a year, but the effect is not so good. He is already two and a half, but he can only say "*baba*." I think the training methods we're using aren't right. (LZH, no. 92)

Some parents described specific problems they had encountered, mentioning the children's inability to "remember" what they had already been taught to say; difficulties with specific sounds, such as distinguishing "*wawa*" and "*hua*" or pronouncing the retroflexive initials *zh, sh, ch,* and *r;* associating words they could say such as "*mama*" (mommy) and "*baba*" (daddy) with the right people; making sentences out of words; and understanding and formulating questions.

Parents were concerned their children would not be able to speak well enough by the age of seven, when they were due to start primary school:

> I simply have no idea how to teach him. I've no confidence that I can teach him so he can go to school some day. (LZH, no. 86)

> I think his progress is so slow. If he keeps going like this, I'm afraid he won't have the same ability to speak as normal children when he goes to primary school. In that case, how can he go to an ordinary school? (LZH, no. 115)

Parents saw the goal of speech training as their child's acquiring sufficient speech to attend primary school; when they realized that this goal might be difficult to achieve, they experienced pressure, frustration, and uncertainty. The apparent lack of results, despite their best efforts, clearly made parents lose confidence and feel hopeless; again, lack of professional support and advice greatly exacerbated their difficulties.

The Deaf Child and Ordinary Schooling

Some parents hoped that by placing their child in an ordinary nursery school they would stimulate his or her speech development and social interaction with other children. However, preschools in China, especially in urban areas, may have several hundred children and a high pupil:teacher ratio, making it difficult to give individual children special attention.

Four parents mentioned sending their deaf children to ordinary preschools. In one case, the child's grandmother was a primary school teacher and was able to stay with her granddaughter all day in the nursery class attached to her school. At the age of two and a half one boy was sent to nursery school where the teacher picked up his hearing problem, prompting the parents to get his hearing tested. The other two children experienced difficulties, which included being picked on by the other children. One father, as we have already seen, was deeply distressed about his son's treatment and inability to defend himself. Another parent wrote:

> I sent her to nursery school so she could play with the other children and learn from them. But she was left on her own there, she's even been bitten by the other children. When she came home, she showed us the marks, and it upset me. I went to see her teacher to ask her to take special care of her. (LZH, no. 26)

Parents' perceptions of how well the home environment satisfied their child's requirements seemed to affect their decision on sending him or her to an ordinary preschool. Other considerations, such as how protective parents felt, or whether there was a grandparent at home able to look after the child while they were working, must also have played a part. One mother explained:

> She is growing up in an atmosphere of love and affection at home. We haven't sent her to nursery school, so she is never hurt by others. (LZH, no. 82)

Another mother had stayed at home for three years to educate her daughter, and now wanted to go back to work; she was thinking of sending her child to an ordinary nursery school:

> I'd like to send my daughter to an ordinary nursery school next year. I don't know how it will turn out, and I would like your opinion. I know that Tingting did well through rehabilitation at home, in the family. But we have not got such a good family environment as Tingting. Sending [my daughter] to nursery school may be better for her. I don't know whether I'm right about this or not. You know much more than I do about deaf children. Have there been any successful instances before, as far as you know? If there has, then I will send my daughter to a nursery school. (LZH, no. 53)

Such letters reveal parents' uncertainty and anxiety when faced with decisions about their children's education. Informed professional advice, along with professional support in the mainstream educational setting, would do much to help parents make appropriate decisions on their deaf children's education: for now, however, most lack this needed assistance.

Requests for Help

The letters to Zhou Hong were written to ask him for help. Some parents asked simply for "help and advice." However, most were seeking specific information or materials; the nature of their re-

TABLE 21: PARENTS' REQUESTS FOR HELP

Specific Request	Number of Parents (N = 135)	Percentage of Parents
Information about treatment	65	48.1
Information about speech training	46	34.0
Information about both treatment and speech training	25	18.5
Help with child's pronunciation	13	9.6
Help with reading and writing	4	2.9
Information about educational methods	19	14.0
Materials and books	25	18.5
Admission to Zhou Hong's nursery school	12	8.8
Information about meetings	4	2.9

Note: The number of requests totals more than 135 become some parents made more than one request.

quests (listed in table 21) reveals how parents perceive their child's deafness and what they consider appropriate action to be. Nearly half the parents (48 percent) wanted information about treatments for deafness, substantially more than asked for information concerning speech training (although more than a third of parents who asked about treatments also asked about speech training methods). Thus, as a whole, these parents were more interested in medical than educational measures.

The reports and articles in newspapers and magazines about Zhou Tingting mentioned that she had had a number of treatments, including acupuncture, that had apparently resulted in a slight improvement in her hearing. For this reason many parents asked for the exact details, so they could go to the same hospital and have the same treatment from the same doctor:

> We know that with acupuncture and moxibustion therapy, even if the same acupoints are used, different manipulation by different doctors can produce a very different effect.

> Therefore we would like to ask about the following points: Which hospital did your daughter have treatment in? Which doctor gave her acupuncture therapy that had a good effect? Did she have hearing tests before and after treatment? How long is the course of treatment? (LZH, no. 95)

> We learned that Tingting once had acupuncture and moxibustion therapy. Although it didn't improve her hearing permanently, it did help for a little while. I am wondering if the transient improvement in her hearing had a significant effect on the accuracy of her pronunciation. Do you think long-term treatment is worthwhile, or not? (LZH, no. 82)

> (*letter to Tingting*) I'm writing to ask you — in which hospital did you have your treatments? What's the name of the doctor who treated you? How long did the treatment last? How much money did you spend? How could you endure the pain of the acupuncture? (LZH, no. 72)

Some parents felt measures that had been effective for Tingting would only be effective for their child if the two had the same degree of hearing loss, etiology, and age of onset of deafness. If so, they reasoned, then following the course that had helped Tingting should bring similar results for their child. While some parents were satisfied with the facts presented in the articles they had read, others wanted more precise information:

> From the description in the report of your daughter's condition when she was young, it seems to me it's nearly the same as my son's condition now. So I'm writing to ask for help and advice. (LZH, no. 101)

> I heard that your daughter was unable to speak before the age of three. So I'd like to know if she had some hearing or no hearing at all at that time. Could she say simple things like "*baba*" and "*mama*"? . . . Is her deafness congenital or acquired? Please let me know in detail. (LZH, no. 117)

> I'd like to ask about the following: How old was Tingting when you found she had a hearing problem? After that,

which hospitals did you take her to, and what kinds of checkups did she have? What were the results? Does Tingting have some residual hearing? What is her level of hearing? What caused Tingting's deafness, drug poisoning or some other cause? (LZH, no. 69)

In the article I read, it didn't mention the degree of your daughter's hearing loss. Did she have a BSER [brain stem evoked response] hearing test? What was the result? I'd like to know this because I read in the article that the treatment your daughter had had some curative effect. But my child's hearing loss is 100 dB—I don't know if treatment will have any effect. (LZH, no. 92)

Some parents sought information on speech training as well as or instead of advice on medical treatments. Usually they simply asked for general guidance. Any specific questions tended to focus on pronunciation and how to correct it. Thus the parents emphasized the correct articulation of speech rather than the acquisition of meaningful language.

Images of Deafness

Parents reveal their attitudes toward deafness in the imagery they use to describe it and the opposing states with which they contrast it.

Health and Illness

The deafness of the deaf child was often contrasted with his or her "health" before the diagnosis was made:

> Before he was one year old his health was very good (*ta de shenti hen hao*). Then we discovered his hearing was very poor. (LZH, no. 129)

Alternatively, the contrast might be made implicitly between a "normal" outward appearance—just like other healthy children—and the hidden defect of deafness:

> Fangfang looks pretty, intelligent, and healthy (*jiankang*); people are glad to see her. (LZH, no. 4)

Deafness was consistently perceived and spoken of as an illness or disease:

> I have a girl who is three years old. She suffers from deaf-illness (*long bing*) and has never spoken. (LZH, no. 132)

> Why did heaven give me such a lovely son but make him suffer from an incurable disease (*bing*) so he is unable to live like a normal person? (LZH, no. 44)

Because it is a disease, parents discuss their efforts to find a cure:

> Whenever we heard about a treatment for deafness, we would follow it up, in order to cure his disease. (LZH, no. 52)

> We want to do everything we can to cure her illness before she is seven, because after that age the organs for hearing and speech stop developing, so it will be more difficult for her hearing to recover. (LZH, no. 4)

> The doctor said there was no effective treatment for this disease at the moment. (LZH, no. 75)

In the second case, the father is aware of the critical period for language development during the early years: the search for a cure acquires a particular urgency as the child grows older.

The "disease" of deafness is portrayed as a malign force that disrupts family life, and some parents depict it as an entity that must be opposed and fought against:

> The rhythm of our life and work is disturbed by her sickness. (LZH, no. 3)

> At present we are greatly affected by my daughter's illness, which interferes with our work and life. (LZH, no. 55)

> We would like to learn from you, to fight the disease with all possible means, and create a miracle. (LZH, no. 100)

The word used to describe the speech training provided in preschool—translated into English as "rehabilitation"—is *kangfu,* which literally means "health restore/recover." This officially sanctioned term, which appears in such contexts as the name of the speech training centers (*kangfu zhongxin*), is also taken up by parents:

> We should learn from you and try our best to get Ruirui rehabilitated as soon as possible. (LZH, no. 105)

Here, the parents envisage that speech training will definitely end the deafness just as treatment cures disease.

Deafness and Muteness

The well-known saying about deaf people in China—that "out of ten deaf people, nine are mute" (*shi long, jiu ya*)—simply reflects the reality before special education programs began providing aural/oral training for deaf children. Deaf adults and children are frequently labeled *yaba* (mutes). The words for deafness (*long*) and muteness are frequently combined: for example in the phrase "deaf-mute school," *longya xuexiao,* or the colloquial phrase for a deaf-mute person, *longya ren*. The combination implies a link, and clearly for many parents deafness and muteness are synonymous:

> My brother's son is now three years old, but he still can't speak. So he had a checkup at a hospital, and they found he was a deaf-mute person (*longya ren*). (LZH, no. 90)

> I have a three-year old son who is also deaf-mute (*longya*). (LZH, no. 96)

> We've discovered he has a hearing problem. We are afraid he is deaf-mute (*longya*). (LZH, no. 109)

> My son is completely deaf and completely mute (*quan long quan ya*). (LZH, no. 134)

Some parents were surprised to learn that a deaf child can speak. The mother of a eighteen-month-old profoundly deaf child wrote:

> How shall I give my daughter training? Can I teach her to speak now? I've heard that children who can't hear can still learn to speak. (LZH, no. 79)

One mother asked, "Does deafness mean a mute child?" (LZH, no. 108). That a "deaf-mute girl" like Tingting learned to speak seemed miraculous and unusual:

> Tingting was completely deaf and completely mute at the age of three and a half, but now she has become a student of great character and scholarship. It is really a miracle. (LZH, no. 85)

> (*letter to Tingting*) I read about you—a completely deaf, completely mute girl who has learned to speak and studied in an ordinary school like normal children. I'm greatly inspired by your achievement. (LZH 131)

For some parents, acquiring speech somehow implies that the deafness vanishes, too.

The World of Sound and the Soundless World

The metaphor opposing the world of sound to the soundless world is very frequently found in writing about deafness, including professional publications. The worlds are envisaged as two separate places, into which a child goes or from which he or she emerges. Set apart, the child is painfully separated from his or her family and from other people. Teachers or parents who succeed in teaching the deaf child to speak are pictured as bringing the child out of the soundless world, into the world of sound. The letter writers used the same image, in various contexts:

> Seeing our child live in the soundless world, while other children live in happy laughter, we feel greatly distressed. (LZH, no. 110)

> We can't bear to see our child live in the soundless world all his life. We must do our utmost to help him enter the world of sound. (LZH, no. 117)

> You finally enabled Tingting to leave the soundless world. . . . I'd like to do my best to educate my child so that some day she also can live in the world of sound. (LZH, no. 105)

> [Zhou Hong] put in untold effort to teach his daughter, and finally brought her to the wonderful world of sound. . . . I'd like to follow his example and do my best to try to bring my child to the world of sound as well. (LZH, no. 135)

Some parents referred to their child's "returning" to the world of sound, even when he or she had been born deaf. One mother, with a daughter whose sensorineural deafness was detected soon after birth, wrote:

> I also have a deaf child. I really hope that someday she can be like Tingting, and come back to the world of sound and live like a normal person. (LZH, no. 94)

This metaphor is significant because it is so firmly rooted in the parents' perspective: when a child "enters" or "returns" to the world of sound by acquiring speech, the world is still "soundless" to *them* — although the parents may now have a child who produces speech and so is, in a superficial sense, participating in their world.

Being Deaf and Being Normal

Parents are first and foremost aware that their child is different; the contrast is most painful when they see other children speaking or laughing and playing. But they also distinguish a part of their child that is normal, or perceive that their child is entirely normal — except for his or her deafness. Typically, parents' pride in their child's perceived intelligence and quickness to understand is set against their grief over the aspect of the child that is defective.

As deaf children grow older, the gap between their achievements — in learning to speak and in their progress in school — and those of other, normally hearing, children becomes more obvious. When parents look to the future, they express the hope that their children will be able to "live like normal people," or "live a normal life." In this sense "normality" means following the main path; deaf children have fallen by the wayside, and unless they can get back on the road early in their life, they will never be able to keep up with everyone else. Normal education—in an ordinary nursery or primary school—is every parent's hope; the prospect of special education fills them with dismay. These parents, like those I interviewed, sometimes insisted that they treated their deaf child "as normal." They too meant that they do not treat him badly just because he is deaf; but here again, the phrase and the behavior seem to indicate a kind of wishful thinking—if the child is treated as normal, then he or she will somehow become normal.

Thus parents perceive deafness in a number of different ways, some of which are interlinked. Deafness is seen as a disease, non-deafness as a state of health. Deafness is a contrast to, and a deviation from, normality. Deafness implies muteness, inability to speak, which makes deaf children different from others and isolates them from their family and other people. In the imagery of the two worlds, with and without sound, deaf children are envisaged as being in a different place, as if they were physically removed from others; to return to their parents' world, they must acquire speech. In all these polarities of meaning, there is never any doubt that for parents deafness and its related meanings are negative, while not-being-deaf and its related meanings are positive. Furthermore, speech is the outward manifestation of normality; its opposite is the dreaded state of being "deaf-mute."

Parents' Search for Solutions

These letters from parents of deaf children underscore the difficulties they face in their efforts to educate their children. It should be emphasized that most live in cities or large towns, are well-educated, and are interested in seeking help for their children; parents living in the countryside far from medical and rehabilitation facilities, who have less education and fewer financial resources, or who feel less able or less willing to seek solutions would be able to do far less for their children. In the analysis of the letters, six main points emerged.

1. Diagnosis of deafness depended solely on parents' acting on their own suspicions. The quality of the audiological services they received depended on what was available locally or how far parents were prepared to travel to reach a hospital with the appropriate equipment for testing.

2. As it is for hearing parents in Western countries, the diagnosis was a severe shock to parents. However, while audiological centers in the United States and Britain routinely arrange follow-up appointments with parents to provide counseling and support, as well as to put them in contact with other parents of deaf children, no such support was available to these parents in China. In coming to terms with the diagnosis and deciding what to do, parents had to rely on their own resources, and those of their family and friends. Only one letter mentioned contact with other parents with deaf children—the kind of contact that might have led to more information and made possible mutual support.

3. Following the diagnosis parents typically engaged in "doctor shopping": they went from hospital to hospital to confirm the diagnosis and to ask doctors if there was a cure. When Western medicine failed them, parents turned to Chinese traditional medical treatments. Some parents long persisted in seeking cures— for years, in some cases—and expended substantial amounts of money. The decision to begin speech training occurred at different times for different parents; some parents continued to seek medical treatment even after their child had begun speech training.

4. Only a small proportion of parents (22 percent) had bought hearing aids, and those who had did not necessarily find them helpful. An often-cited problem was that children refused to wear their aids; parents also were not clear about the benefits of using them and how they might help in training deaf children to speak. Without information, materials, and qualified support, parents lacked confidence in what they were doing. In this area—establishing good practice in wearing hearing aids

and helping parents in their efforts to educate and give speech training to their children — there was obviously a very great need for professional advice and support.

5. The parents' concepts of deafness and the language they used to refer to it rely on consistently negative imagery, starkly contrasting with the positive connotations attached to "normality," its perceived opposite. None of the letters mentioned any experience of or acquaintance with deaf people. Thus parents' ideas about deafness were not informed by contact with deaf adults, and there was no suggestion that they felt such contact might be helpful in any way. Parents believed that their children could be restored to normality by learning to speak, joining "normal" children in ordinary mainstream schools, and leading ordinary lives.

6. Parents saw entry to primary school as the fateful moment in their deaf child's life. If children had not been cured by that time, or had not acquired sufficient speech through speech training, they could not be enrolled in mainstream schooling; the only alternative was to enter a school for the deaf. Some parents also realized that the preschool period was critical for the development of speech,[5] lending added urgency to the pressure on them and their children.

We can speculate about what will happen to these children as they get older. The evidence suggests that only a small minority will have acquired enough speech by the age of seven to enter mainstream schooling. Even if a deaf child has made good progress in the preschool years, parents may still find it difficult to persuade a local primary school to accept their child — many schools are reluctant to enroll children with special needs. The children most likely to gain entry are those who have some residual hearing, whose parents have access to and support from rehabilitation services, and whose parents (with other family members) have been able to establish an effective program of education and speech training at home. Their only other educational option is to go to deaf school; and since parents so strongly desire speech acquisition (by medical cure or not) and mainstream schooling for their child, they see deaf schooling as representing the utter failure of their efforts and the futility of their hopes for their child's future. Clearly, many of the parents who wrote these letters will be severely disappointed.

Government policies for the preschool rehabilitation of deaf children were initiated only in 1988, and the facilities and resources available even in the cities are still far short of what is needed. However, the system is being expanded and improved year by year, and in the future many more parents will have a much better chance of obtaining the advice and support they need. As the system develops, it will have to deal with a number of critical issues.

1. While parental initiative should continue to be respected as an important element in identifying deafness, effective screening programs should be devised to ensure that deafness is diagnosed at an early stage. If national or regional programs seem too expensive, then other, more cost-effective avenues can be introduced or reinforced, such as educating parents who attend mother-and-baby clinics about the importance of taking a baby to be tested early if he or she is not responding to sounds.

2. More systematic procedures need to be implemented at the time of and immediately after diagnosis. Parents should receive information, advice, and support from professional services; prompt fitting of hearing aids should be arranged by the center where the diagnosis is made; and medical and rehabilitation services in each area must be better coordinated. The experience of audiologists in the United States and other countries has shown that having a network through which parents can be introduced to other families with deaf children greatly helps parents come to terms with the diagnosis of deafness in their child.

3. The process of serial consultation of doctors and of trying different treatments to cure deafness wastes parents' financial and emotional resources terribly. It prevents parents from focusing on the constructive actions they might take to develop effective communication with their child, including establishing hearing aid use and speech training. As rehabilitation services become more widely available and more information is disseminated through books and the media, it is possible that the parents' tendency toward multiple consultations will diminish. The government could help reduce the abuse and exploitation of parents by

encouraging them to try treatments that are scientifically proven and accredited, perhaps through a licensing system.

4. There is a great need for trained, qualified personnel to provide support for parents with deaf preschool-age children, to help them establish proper use of hearing aids, and to assist them in developing their child's speech. Although the government recognizes that programs to train such specialized personnel are crucial, it lacks the resources to implement them fully.

5. At the moment government policy is focused exclusively on auditory and speech training in early intervention programs, but future preschool rehabilitation services might support some parents in developing sign communication with their children, particularly if the children are profoundly deaf or if the parents themselves are deaf. Increasing these options would make it more likely that individual families could effectively support their deaf child's acquisition of language.

6. As in Western countries, in China many hearing parents with deaf children have only negative ideas about deafness. The expansion of rehabilitation services should help nurture more constructive attitudes; but before long-standing prejudices can be erased, society as a whole must acknowledge deaf people as different rather than simply defective; the same, of course, is true in Western countries.

7. In the rehabilitation of preschool-age deaf children, the acquisition of speech by school age receives disproportionate emphasis, exacerbated by a system in which placements either in mainstream or deaf schools are made at age seven and are difficult if not impossible to reverse afterward. A major difficulty for children with special needs is that schools are exam-oriented, and children are moved up to the next class only if they pass regular tests. Successful integration of large numbers of children with disabilities, including deafness, will require major changes in the curriculum and in teaching techniques, as well as the training of teachers to support special needs children in the classroom.

8. As preschool services develop, more deaf children entering deaf schools will have first attended rehabilitation centers or had speech training at home; it will thus be feasible to expand aural/

oral programs at least in some deaf schools. This change will help erode the current sharp distinction between mainstream schools, where deaf children use speech to communicate, and the deaf schools, where sign is used to teach the curriculum. Such convergence might lead parents to feel more positive about deaf schooling as an option for their child and less inclined to see it as the end of their hopes that their child will gain a full education, social acceptance, and a good job. Of course, parental dismay at the prospect of deaf schooling would also be lessened if deaf people achieve better status and a higher profile in Chinese society, and if indigenous Chinese sign language is given greater recognition and currency as a language in its own right.

After reading the letters to Zhou Hong and his daughter written by parents of deaf children, one is left with the strong impression that the actions these families have taken to help their deaf child are of central importance. To a large extent, the family's financial resources are a key factor: urban, educated parents, in contrast to parents in the rural regions, are in a position to afford medical consultations, expensive tests, good-quality hearing aids, information and teaching materials, and the fees of a rehabilitation center. Parents' attitudes and priorities are also critical to the child's success: they must decide how much time and effort they are able and willing to devote to their deaf child's education. The letters that follow provide a glimpse into the burdens, conflicts, and decisions that parents face in preparing their deaf child for the future. They are presented in no particular order.

Selected Letters

(letter 43)
Principal Zhou:

Greetings. I am sorry to trouble you. I am a student at Anhui Education College. My name is C—— G——. The Mental Development Center at Wuhan University told me about you and your daughter. I feel very sympathetic about your daughter's misfortune, and very pleased and excited at her miraculous transformation. Thanks to your training and the treatments she received, from being a mute girl she has become a child prodigy.

I have the same suffering as you. My daughter Chen Yang is now two years old. She is a lovely child and very lively. She was just learning to speak when, about six months ago, misfortune befell her. She had a severe illness, and was given an injection of penicillin, gentamycin, and streptomycin. At the time we did not know how toxic these medicines could be. Then recently we realized something was wrong with her hearing, so we took her to a hospital in Hefei and had her hearing checked. The result of the test was that she is completely deaf in both ears. When I heard this I was very shocked. My dream of a child prodigy was shattered. What made me even more upset was that my daughter is only two years old and she was just beginning to understand the world, but soon she will lose this and become a disabled person for life.

I took her to see doctors everywhere, but they all said they had no means of curing her. Finally she was given a desensitization treatment at the hospital attached to Anhui Medical College, but there was no improvement. Then I wrote to the Mental Development Center in Wuhan to ask for help. They told me that your daughter had been in the same situation. So I am writing to you to ask for advice. Could you please tell me what treatments your daughter had for her deafness? Thank you very much.

With best wishes, C—— G——
29 November 1994
Hefei, Anhui province

(letter 4)
Principal Zhou:

Greetings. I am the father of a three-year old deaf girl, Fangfang. My name is X—— F——. When Fangfang was one year old, we discovered she wasn't able to say "daddy" and "mommy" and so we tried testing her hearing—we stood just behind her and clapped our hands and shook some toys. She didn't respond to these sounds, and we knew then she was deaf.

Several big hospitals said Fangfang's ears looked normal and they could find no reason for her deafness. Eventually, when we went to the Beijing Deaf Children's Rehabilitation and Research Center [China Rehabilitation Research Center for Deaf Children], we were told she had "severe sensorineural deafness in both ears." At that time we bought a high-quality Swiss hearing aid, but it didn't seem to make much difference.

When Fangfang was between fifty days and one year old, she had several high fevers and had between three to six injections. We have forgotten the name of the medicine—perhaps it was a toxic drug such as kanamycin or streptomycin.

Fangfang is pretty, intelligent, and healthy. People are always happy to see her. She reacts to the sound of fireworks 100 meters away, and if there's thunder she covers her ears and says "pong!," imitating the sound of the thunder. So we think she still has some hearing left. We have given her a great deal of speech training, and she can now say "daddy" (*baba*) and "no" (*bu*) quite well. But she can't pronounce "mommy" (*mama*), "grandma" (*nainai*), or "airplane" (*feiji*) clearly, although the shape of her mouth is right. She relies mainly on gestures to communicate with people. She is an intelligent girl.

I read your and Tingting's story in the magazines *Guide to Family Life* and *Life* recently. I was very moved, and feel there is some hope of solving Fangfang's problem. So I'm writing this letter to you, and look forward to hearing from you as to where and how we can get Fangfang good treatment, or any other useful information. We want to do everything we can to cure her illness before she is seven, because after that age the organs for hearing and speech stop developing, so it will be more difficult for her hearing to recover. I hope you can give us some suggestions and help. Thank you very much.

        Best regards,
        X—— F——, Center for Agriculture and
          Science,
        13 November 1995
        Ningchen county, Inner Mongolia

(letter 80)
Comrade Zhou Hong:

When I write to you I feel the pen in my hand is as heavy as lead. I know very well how busy you are. I feel compelled to write but importunate in bothering you. Perhaps you can understand my feelings.

Lately I have begun to feel more and more distressed and worried about my daughter, because she is getting older and will soon be school age. But she can't speak at all. I feel completely helpless. I'm out of my mind with worry. I think only you can help us save our daughter, and I am confident you can effect the miracle of teaching our daughter to speak. So I intend to rent a house in Nanjing or live in a hotel. I beg you to spare several hours each day to give my daughter individual coaching. I am sure you know the right method to teach her. The question is whether you will accept her. As you know, both my husband and I are workers and we are not very well-educated. We really don't know how to educate her. Therefore we have to turn to you for help. As well as that I'd like to ask you to help me get in touch with the doctors who gave your daughter medical treatment. I would like my daughter to have medical treatment while she's having speech training. As for payment, I don't mind how much it costs, so long as my daughter can be cured or can learn to say some words and expressions for everyday use. I'm prepared to go to any lengths and spend any amount of money. How I wish my poor girl could get her hearing back and become a lovely, intelligent, and healthy child.

Comrade Zhou, I beg you to give us help and save our child. I will feel very indebted to you even if you just agree to a trial period at first. I am very much looking forward to your reply.

> With best wishes,
> W—— H——
> Jiangsu province

(letter 81)
Teacher Zhou:

We received your letter after an anxious wait. We're so pleased to hear from you.

Our child is now over two years old. He is lovely, intelligent, and always eager to learn. He particularly likes playing chess. He can recognize all the pieces and arrange them on the board, and knows how to play a little. Of course we spend a lot of time and put in a lot of effort teaching him. He is very interested in drawing now, and he can write the numbers 1 and 2. We teach him to write and draw every day. We find it very difficult to give him speech training. When we try and teach him to say "mama" he can only produce the sound "ah." He won't wear his hearing aid, so we have no way of knowing how useful it is.

We learned that you have put together a set of materials based on Tingting's study from when she was a little girl up to now. We'd very much like to have a copy. We hope to obtain some advice and enlightenment from you and find a set of educational methods that is appropriate for our child so that he can be a second Tingting. Both my husband and I are teachers, one in arts, the other in sciences. So conditions are favorable for our child. As you said, if we make unremitting efforts, we are bound to succeed. We long for that day to come.

Teacher Zhou, we are both unfortunate people. For the sake of our children, I hope we can keep in contact. You live in a large city, so you are bound to be better informed than us. I hope you can give us help.

I am enclosing some money. Please mail us a set of materials and the book *From Mute Girl to Child Prodigy*. Thank you very much.

>With best wishes,
>Y—— G——
>10 April 1992
>Qinzhou district, Guangxi province

(letter 82)
Teacher Zhou:

Greetings. When I read your article, I felt my situation was similar to yours. So I am venturing to write to you to ask for further advice and help.

I also have a lovely daughter who is deaf. She is now two years and seven months old. After she was given a checkup and found to have a hearing problem when she was nearly two years old, I bought her a hearing aid and began to teach her to speak. Her deafness is very severe. She has had two brain stem potential tests, and the reports showed hearing losses of 100 to 105 dB in the right ear, and 110 to 117 dB in the left. But I have doubts about these results. From our own observations at home, I think her hearing loss is less, about 80 dB. She refuses to wear her hearing aid, so to teach her to speak we have to speak loudly near her ears. She can say more than twenty words now. I also try to teach her to recognize the characters for these words. I think maybe this is helpful, but I have some questions to ask you about this. First, when I teach her to read, should I teach her *pinyin* first and characters later, or vice versa? Second, how did you teach your daughter *pinyin* and how did you teach her to read? Could you please advise me from your experience? I am just starting to educate a deaf child, and I don't know how to go about it. I'm very interested in learning from someone who has succeeded in this. I know you must be very busy, but I hope you can spare the time to send me a short reply. Maybe you have written down your experiences and published them. In that case, I sincerely hope you can send me all your articles and your book *From Mute Girl to Child Prodigy*, as well as related materials. I'll mail the money to you soon after receiving them.

Just like you, I also love my daughter very much, and I am determined to teach her to speak. Not only that—I also want her to catch up with normal children. Both my husband and I have received higher education and my mother-in-law is a primary school teacher. All of us feel the same way about my daughter's education, and we work together very well. My daughter is very intelligent and eager to learn. And our financial situation is good. Our situation is favorable. So we are full of confidence. At the same time we know we will have to put in a lot of effort, and I am prepared for that.

I am sure that since you and your daughter became well-known you must have received many letters like this. I feel sorry to trouble you, but I think you can understand the feelings of parents with deaf children.

We are looking forward eagerly to your reply. Thank you very much.

>With best wishes,
>C—— X——
>31 December 1992
>Guangzhou, Guangdong province

(letter 44)
Teacher Zhou:

Greetings. To begin with, please give my best wishes to your family.

I am writing to you with tears in my eyes. It was a warmhearted aunt who showed me your article "From Mute Girl to Child Prodigy — A Miracle Created by a Father" published in the Shenzhen evening paper on 18 March. I burst into tears after reading it. I feel deeply moved by your courageous actions and sincere love for your daughter. I know very well how much love and hard work you must have put in to your daughter's upbringing. The same misfortune happened to me as well. I had lost all hope that my son could be cured. Your account led me to see some light amid all the darkness. It gave us hope again. My wife and I read the article again and again in tears. I think you are the only one who can help our Peng. Maybe you will be our son's savior.

A year after we got married we had a lovely son. We named him Peng, hoping he would have a bright future when he grew up.[6] I am a guard in a labor reform camp and my wife is a temporary worker.[7] After work I used to enjoy looking after our son. But unfortunately fate played a cruel joke on us. One day when my son was eight months old, I realized he didn't react to sound. Even when I shouted in his ears he still had no reaction. So we took him to have a checkup in Taiyuan, the capital of Shanxi province. The doctor said my son had lost his hearing, but they couldn't identify the cause. So they recommended we take our son to Beijing to have a thorough checkup. At that time it was not long after we got married, and we had just paid back the money we had borrowed from our friends to get married. The monthly income of my wife and me together is less than 500 yuan. Therefore our financial situation is not good at all. But for our son we took all our savings, less than 1,000 yuan, and borrowed another 2,000 yuan from our relatives and colleagues. Then we took our son to Beijing for the checkup. In 301 Hospital they found that he suffers from nerve deafness. They said they couldn't cure him. Later we went to another big hospital and the result was the same. Because there wasn't enough money left, we had to go back to Shanxi. But we still didn't know the cause of my son's deafness, so I couldn't just give up. So I did everything I could to get money, raised 8,000 yuan, and we went back to Beijing. Tongren Hospital and Xiehe Hospitals are said to be the two best hospitals, so we took our son there. In Xiehe Hospital my son was given a hearing test. His hearing is only 85 to 95 dB. They refused to take him into the hospital. They said they couldn't cure him, nor could any of the big hospitals in China. When I heard this I despaired completely and felt my heart was breaking. I just held my son in my arms and cried. Why has heaven given me such a lovely son but let him suffer an incurable disease and made him unable to live like a normal person?

After coming back from Beijing, we paid back our debts while still seeking treatment for our son. We have tried traditional Chinese medicine and Western medicine, even *qigong*. Every time we were filled with hope, and every time hope turned into disappointment. Altogether we spent 20,000 yuan. But the chances of my son being cured were too small. So we had to accept the fact and began to consider how to educate my son.

My son is now four years old. Following doctor's advice I bought him a hearing aid. It seems to make a difference when he's wearing it. He reacted when I tried shouting from next door. My wife and I began to teach him to speak. After countless repetitions, he gradually learned to say "daddy" (*baba*), "mommy" (*mama*), "no" (*bu*), and "go" (*zou*), and so on, but not very clearly, and he doesn't seem to understand what the words mean. He can't distinguish between "daddy" and "mommy." We found his hearing was better in the evening, so we arranged most of our teaching in the evening. Maybe the way we're teaching him isn't right — the more we teach him to speak, the more unwilling he becomes. He shows obvious feelings of resistance. He enjoys playing and eating, so it seems to me he is completely normal apart from the deafness. Later I bought some books to teach him to read, but he didn't want to look at them either. And he has a bad temper. Sometimes he cannot be coaxed to learn to read, even with the promise of play or treats to eat. Sometimes in order to avoid learning to write, he opens the drawer, takes all the things out, puts his workbook at the bottom of the drawer, and puts everything back on top of it. When he does that I feel upset and yet pleased as well — he is so unwilling to study, but sometimes he does things that seem more intelligent than other children his age.

Teacher Zhou, I have told you all this about my child in the hope you could give me help and advice. I want very much to try the methods you have summarized in *Methods of Learning the Mother Tongue through Play* and *Method of Learning the Mother Tongue through Family Education*. How I wish my son could gradually learn to speak, read, write, and go to school just like Tingting. I really want to send my son to the school where you work, and entrust you with his education. But I am heavily in debt, and I can't really afford it. Besides, I don't want to trouble you too much. I just have one small request — could you please send me the materials you used to teach your daughter? I will mail the cost to you later. I am sure you can understand my feelings. My child is now over four years old. If I don't devote time to him now, I will miss the best period for educating him. I earnestly ask for your help.

Just to be on the safe side, I mailed two copies of this letter, one copy to each of your work units. I hope you will give us advice as soon as possible.

With best wishes,
Z—— G——
19 April 1995
Shanxi province

(letter 87)
Tingting:

How are you? I read the account of you being elected one of the Ten Best Young Pioneers in *Chinese Children's Newspaper* on 16 October. The account inspired us and gave us hope. From the report we know that when you were three and a half you were completely deaf and mute. After various treatments you finally learned to speak and made great progress. We are deeply moved by your achievement. So I am writing to you to ask — (1) What kind of treatment restored your hearing? (2) How did you learn to speak?

I have a daughter who has just turned three. She has been diagnosed as having nerve deafness. We have taken her to see various doctors, but they all say they have no means of curing her. They said she would have to have special education. That means she will have to go to a deaf school and learn sign language. We feel very upset about this. Now, after reading your story, I'd like to find out from your parents, through you, about your treatments. We also want to give our daughter treatment early on so that she can be like you some day and go to an ordinary school and receive a normal education. Our whole family are eagerly looking forward to your reply. I hope you can spare the time to write to me after receiving this letter and tell us in detail about your treatments.

>With best wishes,
>W—— P——
>11 November 1991
>Industrial Chemicals Institute
>Wuhan, Hubei province

(letter 2)
Principal Zhou:

Greetings. I heard about Tingting some time ago—two years ago when I brought my son to Lianyungang for treatment for his deafness, at the Second Railway Convalescence Center. And now the magazine *Family* has published a detailed article about her—when I read it I felt very much encouraged. You bring us, the parents of deaf children, hope.

I am the mother of a deaf child named Zhu Tianyi. My son is three years old. He can't speak. The hearing loss in his left ear is 100 dB, and in his right ear 105. We feel very dismayed by this. There is a little bit of reaction to sound in his left ear. For two years we have kept on taking our son for treatments and have borrowed a lot of money—we have lots of debts. But the treatments have all been disappointing.

I failed the national exams for university. I used to be very good academically, but in the end I gave up because my health wasn't very good. I have to tolerate the pain of failing. Now heaven has sent me a deaf child, and that has shattered the dream I once had of my son going to college. When I talk to other people about my child, my eyes fill with tears, and my nerves are very weak.

Principal Zhou, I think you have experienced the same kind of pain. I admire you very much. So I decided to write to you. I would like to learn from your experience of educating deaf children, but because of our bad economic circumstances it is not possible for us to send our son to your school. So I have to teach him myself, but I don't know where to start. My son is very naughty. I used to try to teach him to speak and read words. But it didn't work. He can only say "daddy," "mommy," "grandpa," and "grandma," but not clearly or correctly. I don't know if it would be better if I bought a hearing aid for him. Which kind of hearing aid is best for children? When teaching, is it better to read the words, write them, or learn how to speak them—should they all be started at the same time? Or some other way? I used to try to teach him, but it didn't work. Even though we live in the countryside, I don't want to destroy my child's life just because I don't have enough money. I am eager to teach my son with your help, and hope you are able to write back to me.

Principal Zhou, I am really eager to hear from you, because I have had so many disappointments. I hope you can give some fresh hope to this mother in pain. My husband and I will pray for you, and look forward to hearing your news.

I hope you will take pity on our unfortunate son,

> With best regards,
> M—— Y——
> 16 November 1995
> I look forward very much to hearing from you.

(letter 16)
Principal Zhou:

Greetings. How is Tingting? She seems to be making even better progress than she was before. On 20 July, I saw you on the China Central TV program *Follow You*. Later I read about your experiences bringing up Tingting published in *Family Friend* in August. I was deeply moved, it is a real miracle! I so admired your story, and it gives me hope.

Yuanyuan,[8] my son, is three and a half today. We had so many dreams for him, and now they are all shattered. When he was six months old, he got diarrhea and it took him a long time to get better. While he was in hospital, a disaster occurred that destroyed his whole life [he was given injections of ototoxic antibiotics that damaged his hearing]. When he was eight months, we noticed something odd about his behavior. At ten months, we took him for a brain stem check in Lanzhou in Gansu province. The professor at the Air Force Hospital gave us the final and terrible diagnosis: deafness caused by drug poisoning. His hearing is 110 dB. He can't hear voices so he can't learn to speak. He is a deaf child. Everyone in my family took a long time to get over the painful news. He is such an intelligent and lovely child, but what sort of future does he have now?

I used to be an English teacher. My son's father is an English-speaking tourist guide. We had a wonderful dream of the future, which was that we would teach our child both Chinese and English. But the reality is so cruel. He has a mouth but he can't speak, let alone learn a foreign language. All he can say is, "A mama, a ba. . . . " Every day I would be teaching basic English to innocent students, but my mind would wander. I couldn't concentrate; when I thought of my son, unable to speak Chinese, I couldn't bear it. So a year ago I gave up teaching and got a job in a bank. Now I keep myself to myself and just work hard.

Our whole family wants to earn money, find money to help my son. We tried treatment with Chinese medicine made in Yuncheng in Shanxi province for over six months, but we are disappointed with the results. He is growing bigger every day, and our anxiety is increasing. We did go to several hospitals, but in the end we gave up. I think advertisements are just advertisements and the treatments are just experimental. I don't think these treatments can help him, and what is worse, they may cause even more damage. Language training should begin as soon as possible. It is you who inspired me to believe that we shouldn't depend only on medical treatment. But in our small city, renowned as it is for its Buddhist landmarks and hometown of the flying apsaras,[9] there is little in the way of education for deaf-mute children. I want to teach my son to speak, but feel confused about where to start. I bought a speech trainer from Beijing, a DJ-1000 Sirui speech trainer, which cost me 1,500 yuan. But he refuses to use it. I need your help. If only our child could speak again, it would be the happiest day in our life.

I look forward to hearing from you.

> Best regards,
> Yuanyuan's mother, S—— H——
> 18 August 1995
> D—— branch of the People's Construction Bank of China

(letter 37)
Teacher Zhou,

After reading "A Father's Love Makes the Iron Tree Blossom"[10] I am deeply moved by your sincere love for your daughter. I am so happy at Tingting's miraculous transformation, and greatly inspired by your success.

I am eagerly writing to you as soon as I read the article, because I also have a deaf-mute daughter just like Tingting. At a time when I despaired of my daughter getting better, you gave me fresh hope. So with renewed expectations of enabling my daughter to leave the silent world, I am writing to you for help. I sincerely hope you will be able to give me some advice.

My daughter, now seven years old, suffers from congenital deafness, resulting in both deafness and muteness. She has a little bit of hearing but reacts only to very loud sounds. As a mother, I have had similar experiences to yours. I took her everywhere to see various doctors, but without much result. I once tried teaching her to articulate sounds, but she could not understand what I said. Sometimes when she was in a good mood she would learn, but when she was unhappy she would not listen at all. So it is very difficult for me to teach her. From your article, I saw you had a method for educating Tingting, but it was not described in detail. I hope you can tell me more about your educational methods. I would greatly appreciate your help.

I hear that about 80 percent of deaf-mute children in the A—— Rehabilitation Center for Deaf Children have recovered owing to your educational methods. So I would like to ask about the center's conditions for accepting deaf-mute children and the environment of the center as well as how much the tuition fees are.

I hope you will write to me although I know how busy you must be.

I live in a remote mountain area in Sichuan province. I am not well-off, and my husband is dead. So I bear a double burden of financial and emotional stress. Nevertheless, for the sake of my daughter's rehabilitation, her future and her happiness, I will do my best to make her better whatever the cost. I am eagerly looking forward to your reply.

> I wish you success always.
> L—— X——
> 10 August 1995
> Chongqing, Sichuan province

CHAPTER SEVEN

Conclusions

In both the interviews and the letters that I have analyzed throughout this book, there is strong evidence that Chinese parents perceive deafness as disease, abnormality, and medical defect. Their efforts are devoted to trying to normalize their child—in other words, to make them more like a hearing child—by finding a medical cure or by teaching their child to speak. Parents focus their hopes and expectations for their young deaf child on two main goals: acquiring speech and entering mainstream schooling.

The Chinese parents in these two studies express views toward deafness that are congruent with a medical model of deafness; this is not unusual, as a medical perspective governs approaches to the prevention and treatment of deafness, and the rehabilitation of deaf children and adults, in many countries. However, the status of different forms of medicine in China, the nature of the provider-client relationship, and Chinese parents' understandings of the effects of deafness do result in some unique features:

1. Parents engage in serial consultation of doctors to confirm the diagnosis and find a cure.

2. Parents resort to traditional remedies such as acupuncture and herbal medicines.

3. The paramount concern for most parents is the search for a medical cure; usually it is only after a persistent and unsuccessful search that parents turn to rehabilitation through auditory and speech training in an attempt to eradicate the effects of deafness on their child.

4. Normalization through acquiring speech is conflated with the concept of cure, just as muteness and deafness are regarded as a single pathological entity.

In Western countries parents may be able to take advantage of educational approaches to deafness developed from different assumptions—specifically, the bilingual/bicultural approach—but in China diagnosis, treatments, and early intervention programs all reflect the medical model. Professional approaches to deafness are highly consistent with parents' views of deafness as deviation from normality.

The development of early intervention programs for deaf children in China through the national network of preschool rehabilitation centers has been rapid, purposeful, and systematic. Despite the constant and serious lack of resources, which severely limits the training of badly needed personnel as well as the setting up of new facilities, thousands of deaf children have already been given access to early auditory and speech training and their families provided with advice and support; by the year 2000 an estimated 7.5 percent of preschool-age deaf children will have access to rehabilitation services ("Eastern Red" 1998). In the following discussion of changes that would make services more effective and beneficial to families with deaf children, I reiterate some points made in earlier chapters; however, some of these deficiencies are already being addressed while others will be in the near future as the rehabilitation system expands and develops.

Deafness must be diagnosed earlier through screening programs, campaigns to increase parental awareness of the importance of early testing if hearing loss is suspected, or both. Once the diagnosis is made, an organized referral system must link parents promptly with rehabilitation facilities for information, support, and fitting of hearing aids. There needs to be more emphasis on auditory and speech training from the time of diagnosis, not just for those between three and six years old.

Beyond an official referral system, parents should organize for mutual support among themselves. Although they rely on informal support networks of family members, relatives, friends, and colleagues in responding to their child's deafness, they tend to have little contact with other parents of deaf children until their children are enrolled in a rehabilitation center. Then the rehabilitation staff organize meetings whose agenda is to a considerable extent controlled by the teachers. While these are valuable forums for exchanging information and experiences, the time when parents would benefit most from such exchanges would be shortly after diagnosis (see, e.g., F. Martin, Abadie, and Descouzi 1989), not several years later; perhaps contact with other parents of deaf children might help convince them not to waste their resources in searching for treatments for their child's deafness and encourage them to take appropriate and constructive action more quickly.

Official channels of action in China tend to be vertical: parents are supported and essential information is spread by educational institutions, from personnel to parents, and by government organs via the media to individuals. In this top-down approach, expertise is imparted from the professional to the consumer. Horizontal networks such as parents' organizations are less familiar in the Chinese context, but this should not rule out the possibility of their developing in the future. In the last few years a number of networks and organizations have emerged—for example, women's organizations—that have varying degrees of independence from official, government institutions and that function in various ways to support their members' interests (White, Howell, and Shang 1996). Advocacy—parents of deaf children pressing for improvements in provision—could become an important force for change. Just as we can expect that urban Chinese parents of girls will be unwilling to see their daughters discriminated against in access to education (Davin 1995), so it seems likely that the growing numbers of urban parents of deaf children in China whose children have attended the new rehabilitation centers will be expecting faster implementation of policies giving their children better access to mainstream schools and, once admitted, a greater chance of educational achievement.

For deaf children to achieve their full potential, early language development in the home—whether this is in speech or sign—needs even more emphasis. Rehabilitation personnel and parents must recognize the level of communicative competence a child requires and should be helped to achieve in order to be well educated, whether in the mainstream or in the deaf school system. Preschool rehabilitation is now often presented as being completed in two or three years; after this period, during which the child acquires speech, he or she can enter primary school as a "normal" or "near-normal" child. Subsequent support, termed "follow-up education," generally receives less emphasis. Yet deaf children need substantial support for language development throughout their education. At the moment China lacks the specialists needed to help deaf children in mainstream schools, forcing regular classroom teachers to learn how to assist any deaf children in their class. Furthermore, deaf children are held to the same academic standards as other children in the class.

When I spent a morning at a small primary school in Nanjing that in September 1993 had accepted five deaf children from Zhou Hong's nursery school, I saw some of the problems faced by deaf children in an integrated setting. The teachers, who were very positive about the children, made a point of seating them near the front of the class and kept a close eye on their progress. During their first year, all these children had either their mother or their father sitting with them in the classroom, effectively acting as full-time, unpaid classroom assistants. This experiment, by providing a very constructive and innovative solution to the problem of lack of classroom support, appeared to have contributed to the children's learning. However, the teachers would not permit it to continue into the second year because they found the parents' presence in the classroom distracting: they felt that the children paid less attention to the teacher and behaved worse when their parents were there. The children themselves were cheerful and positive about their school life, but they said they found their Chinese language lessons difficult; Chinese was their least favorite subject. The rehabilitation center staff considered it better for them psychologically to have several deaf schoolmates, so that no individual could be singled out as the only "different" child in the class; and indeed the children said they were all close friends.

Of the five children, four seemed to be coping reasonably well in the mainstream setting; however, one profoundly deaf girl who was struggling to keep up with her schoolwork continued to fall behind the others, and some months later she had to drop out of school. Her mother was very upset because the deaf school would not accept her daughter, who at nine was said to be too old. When parents run into difficulties like this, they often return to the staff in the preschool rehabilitation centers for help and advice, but there is little the teachers can do. Although all concerned are attempting to keep the children in school, any child who cannot overcome the communication barrier faces grave challenges. The problem of successfully integrating deaf children into mainstream primary classrooms is critical, and Chinese professionals and officials are currently devoting much thought and energy to addressing it: unquestionably, parents will continue to be an essential component of any solutions or programs that are devised.

Both the interviewees and the letter writers, as we have seen, perceived deaf people outside the family as of little relevance to their own situation; and when contact with deaf people did occur, it made them view deafness more negatively. Because their reactions reflect widespread social attitudes, changing those attitudes themselves would help parents accept the implications of deafness with more equanimity. Initiatives to raise the status of deaf people and affirm their value to society might include government publicity emphasizing employment opportunities for deaf young people, including those who have been educated in deaf school; government policies promoting the involvement of deaf personnel in the education of deaf children, whether in integrated or segregated settings; educational policies for preschool-age deaf children that include the use of sign language; and investment in research into indigenous sign language, in collaboration with deaf people.

Unfortunately China's moves over the last decade toward a market economy—particularly the recent decision to stop subsidizing thousands of money-losing state enterprises—have resulted in large numbers of workers being laid off. The welfare enterprise system, which in 1997 employed 940,000 disabled persons in 60,000 businesses nationwide (*Development* 1997, 10), is also suffering cutbacks and job losses: an estimated 8,000 welfare factories are in financial difficulties ("Amity Supports Workers" 1998), threatening the livelihoods of thousands of disabled workers. Although the government is also complementing the welfare enterprise system by promoting a quota system, whereby each work unit is expected to employ a specific percentage of disabled people (Luo 1997), employers feeling economic pressure resist taking on any extra employees, let alone people perceived as less productive. A member of the Beijing branch of the China Disabled People's Federation told me that most companies and work units currently prefer to pay fines rather than fulfill their statutory quota. When both sheltered and quota employment policies for disabled people are inadequate or actually disintegrating, and when disabled people have little hope of competing successfully in an increasingly tight job market, unemployment among disabled people is bound to rise sharply, creating hardships for them and their families. The social position of deaf people, along with that of other disabled people, will be undermined if they no longer have jobs that confer on them the status of productive citizens, contributing to society. Their status will be secure only if the economy improves and the government continues to pressure businesses to institute practicable employment policies for disabled people.

The refinement of preschool deaf education in China may help change how parents define "normality." Although government policy is likely to remain focused on auditory and speech training of children with residual hearing, the development of additional approaches that emphasize the importance for preschool-age children of effective communication per se — including those that incorporate sign language — could reduce the current emphasis on attaining speech, which is now absolute. Profoundly deaf children and their families could find this change particularly positive and beneficial. The possibilities offered by one such approach, a bilingual experimental project with profoundly deaf preschoolers, are discussed below.

The Bilingual Experimental Class

In November 1995, the Amity Foundation (a Chinese nongovernmental organization based in Nanjing), Nanjing Deaf School, and the Centre for Deaf Studies at Bristol University in the United Kingdom cooperated in an initiative to set up a "bilingual experimental class" within the rehabilitation center for preschool-age deaf children attached to Nanjing Deaf School. The idea was to give children already at the rehabilitation center a daily session of storytelling in sign language from a deaf teacher. The rest of the school day, they would receive auditory and speech training from their two hearing teachers, as before. The nine children selected to form the first bilingual class, which began in March 1996, all had severe or profound hearing losses (more than 90–95 dB) and all were expected to enter the main deaf school when they finished their preschool education. There were six boys and three girls; their average age was six years old. The deaf woman appointed to teach the new class was an experienced teacher who had taught art at Nanjing Deaf School for many years.

I observed the class for several days in June 1996. The teacher of the experimental class taught language through stories and simple language exercises. As a rule, signs were introduced with the written characters, usually presented to the children on the blackboard in the form of simple sentences. The teacher did not use books, games, or toys in her lessons but she did make maximum use of the blackboard, illustrating stories with expressive drawings as well as writing characters. At this stage, the children were expected to learn to recognize characters but not to write them.

Although the teacher used a number of simple signs to direct the children and keep them in order, the main content of several lessons was delivered in sign-supported Chinese closely connected to written characters presented on the board. The sentences and story lines on the board contained a substantial number of syntactically redundant items that were nevertheless faithfully signed by the teacher and reproduced by the children, following her model. But in other lessons, the teacher told the children a story in sign and then involved them in role play. Stories were illustrated by drawings on the blackboard labeled in written Chinese characters—"old man," "old woman," "dog," "cat," and so on. In these sessions the teacher emphasized storytelling in sign much more and the written characters less, although she did drill the children in the written vocabulary items. She relied heavily on mime because this group of children did not yet have enough vocabulary to grasp the story otherwise. While individual lessons varied considerably in content and style, the children were consistently exposed to sign language closely linked to written Chinese, as their deaf teacher intended. The children were absorbed in the class, enjoyed the stories and exercises, and rapidly learned the signs. Their teacher had established a warm and constructive atmosphere in the classroom and had excellent rapport with the children. Presumably, she represented a very positive role model for them as a deaf person.[1]

The class took place every day for forty to sixty minutes just before lunch. Thus the deaf teacher was not at the nursery school when parents brought their children in the morning or collected them in the afternoon: she apparently had no informal contact with them. Because she stayed for lunch at the nursery school with the children and the hearing teachers, she did interact with the other teachers (though outside the classroom).

A sign language class for parents was arranged, taking place on Saturday afternoons so that most would be able to attend; it was taught by a very experienced hearing teacher from the deaf school. Fourteen people were present at the class the afternoon I visited—only one, a mother, was a parent of one of the children in the experimental class. The sign language class was taught very formally; "students" were given a list of signs to learn by imitating them after the teacher had explained their meaning and demonstrated them. The parents had no opportunities to practice conversations with one another. At one point the teacher asked them to translate a text into sign-supported Chinese. In these circumstances—a formal academic atmosphere in which a hearing teacher used signs that followed the order of spoken Chinese—parents seemed to be learning little that would help them communicate informally with their children.

While based on a program for deaf children in the United Kingdom, a number of its elements have been changed. Bilingual education can be defined as "an approach to the education of deaf children which uses both the sign language of the deaf community and the written/spoken language of the hearing community" (Gregory 1996, 18). In the experimental class I observed, the form of manual communication chosen was primarily not the sign language of the deaf community but manually coded Chinese (though more natural sign language was used in some storytelling sessions). As chapter 3 outlined, in China indigenous sign language does not enjoy equal status with spoken language; furthermore, "sign language"—in its standardized form—is valued primarily as a tool in education to support the learning of the written language and to give students access to the deaf school curriculum. This view of sign language appears to be perpetuated in the experimental class: because parents show little enthusiasm in learning sign language or in using it to communicate at home, it is essentially being used to give preschool-age deaf children a valuable head start for their education in deaf school. Although contact with an adult deaf person as teacher may greatly benefit the children concerned, the Chinese hearing teachers frame this not, as would teachers in the United Kingdom, as her strengthening a positive deaf identity in deaf children but rather as her being more effective because, as a deaf person, she can "understand deaf children better"; they also note that of course she is highly proficient in sign language. The relatively low status of deaf people in Chinese society extends to deaf adults involved in the education of deaf children, who therefore may not be welcomed by parents; nor do hearing professionals adequately appreciate the significance for deaf children of their involvement.

Deaf professionals in China, however, seem to take a different view, as we saw in chapter 3. They see that by acting as an exemplary model, a deaf teacher can play a positive role in the education of deaf children. The deaf teacher involved in the bilingual experimental class described above very much agreed; much of her deep personal commitment to her teaching seemed to derive from her own sense of common identity and affiliation with her pupils.

The class has continued, with a second intake of profoundly deaf children in September 1997: six children, five boys and one girl. A major difference between this group and the first is that members of the current class are considerably younger, between three and four years old; in addition, my brief observation of the class led me to conclude that they were further ahead in developing language and communicating in sign. One three-year-old with deaf parents stood out as being particularly confident and expressive. A second deaf teacher has been appointed, who gave up a better job as supervisor in a welfare factory because she particularly wanted to teach the bilingual class (Carino 1998). The class has been assessed by local education officials and researchers as effective and beneficial, which should ensure its continuation, but a number of problems and uncertainties remain. Most obviously, no objective assessment of the children's language development has yet been carried out. Appropriate measures for evaluating children's receptive and expressive abilities in sign would need to be designed first; these could then be used not only to develop teaching content and techniques more systematically in the bilingual class but also to ascertain in what ways and to what extent spending one or two years in the bilingual preschool class benefits this group of children. The children could then be compared both with children going straight into the deaf school at age seven or eight without any preschool education and with children who have experienced only an aural/oral rehabilitation program. Such formal assessment is essential to increase understanding of language development in preschool-age deaf children and to underpin development of further bilingual initiatives.

In addition, a gap persists between hearing and deaf adults involved in the bilingual class, marked by tensions and difficulties in the working relationships between the hearing and the deaf teachers. Similar problems have been noted in bilingual programs in the United States and the United Kingdom. One set of issues involves the dominance of hearing teachers in influencing school policy and setting staff roles and responsibilities (Rinne 1997). Working relationships deteriorate if the needs of the deaf minority are ignored, yet the habitual use of speech by hearing teachers excludes deaf teachers from exchanging information and making decisions (A. Young, Ackerman, and Kyle 1998). Hearing and deaf teachers tend to perceive their respective roles in fundamentally different ways; not surprisingly, deaf teachers see themselves as role models and, therefore, vital components of the educational program. Chinese bilingual programs are prone to the same problems if they do not have a clear communication policy, or if the policy is not adhered to. Another gap evident in the experimental class in Nanjing is that between hearing parents of the deaf children and deaf adults, including the deaf teachers. The sign class for parents that started in 1996 has lapsed. Again, the difficulty that hearing parents have in learning sign is also an important issue in Western programs: considerable effort is required to find ways to encourage and support them.

Despite these difficulties, it is very important for parents and educators to persist in exploring options for profoundly deaf children in China, whose needs may not be met by government efforts to expand the network of rehabilitation centers. While it seems entirely appropriate that the government should focus scarce resources on supporting the many children with residual hearing who can benefit from the aural/oral approach, its emphasis ignores a need that could usefully be supplied by innovative new projects—some perhaps developed with assistance from institutions or organizations abroad.

Deaf education in other countries has offered models that have already led educators and other professionals in China to raise larger questions about the underlying values in deaf education and which can help in developing a consistent educational approach. A recent article in the *Rehabilitation of Deaf Children in China* summarizes the issues quite succinctly:

> Every model for an educational approach to deaf children's language rehabilitation, without exception, is confronted

with the following questions in establishing their basic concepts:

Which aspects should be stressed when looking at the similarities and differences between deaf children and normal [sic] children?

In considering deaf children's hearing loss, do you stress compensatory mechanisms, or other solutions?

As regards language, do you emphasize stereotypical acquisition or language as an instrument of social communication?

With regard to deaf children's potential for mastering language, do you emphasize oral language or sign?

With regard to the process of deaf children mastering language, do you emphasize natural speech, or intervention?

As regards criteria for deaf children's mastery of language, do you emphasize knowledge or ability, form or content?

As regards the process of deaf children's language education, do you emphasize "teaching" or "learning"?

As regards the relationship between deaf children's language development and their overall development, which aspect do you emphasize?

If the above questions are not answered, or cannot be answered, then we will not be able to clarify our educational aims, identify the essential precepts for guiding education, or formulate appropriate educational principles, with the result that we will not be able to produce a consistent philosophy for an educational approach for deaf children's language rehabilitation. (Li M. 1997, 13, 18)

Here Li Ming not only encapsulates the recurrent issues underlying different approaches to the education of deaf children but also addresses a crucial question affecting all children: whether education should be focused on the teacher and their teaching, or on the learning processes of the child.

His presentation seems to promote finding one consistent approach to the education of deaf children. While some questions could be resolved by applying a single model—for example, decisions about the extent to which a program should be teacher-centered or child-centered ("teaching" versus "learning")—others are more dependent on context. Some children (those with an acquired hearing loss and significant residual hearing) may benefit from an oral program, while others, if they were born profoundly deaf, would benefit from a sign-language-based program. Keeping a number of options available depending on the needs of the deaf child, and those of their family, requires that those designing programs and facilities appreciate the value of flexibility and plurality, perhaps moving away from a monolithic model for preschool intervention. Moreover, some of the questions posed by Li Ming have no absolute answers; their solutions depend on one's perspective and system of values. Those who believe that speech is a primary goal will develop educational programs based on an aural/oral approach; those who believe that early, age-appropriate language development is essential for severely or profoundly deaf children, or that a positive deaf identity is important, will develop programs incorporating sign and involving deaf adults. At the moment, preschool education in China does not encourage plurality of perspectives and appreciation of different value systems per se—but this could be a particularly constructive approach to take in the future.

Exchanging information with colleagues in other countries through publications, conferences, visits, and joint projects has significantly shaped the development of services for deaf children in China, especially the efforts in the last decade to establish early intervention programs for preschool-age deaf children. Assessing the language of deaf children, researching sign language, and developing community-based rehabilitation programs for families with deaf children in the countryside are all projects in which further collaborative work may be useful. The opportunity to work with Chinese colleagues should raise some reflexive questions about how we in the West organize services for deaf children in our own societies, and about the role of families in the early development of deaf children in our own cultures. But it is particularly important for professionals in the United States or European countries who may work with Chinese colleagues to develop educational programs for deaf children to understand and appreciate the Chinese cultural context, Chinese sociopolitical objectives, and the pressures shaping the development of special education programs in China. The work presented here is offered as one step in furthering that understanding.

APPENDIX

Interview Questionnaire

Basic Details of Child, Parents, and Household
1. Could you tell me your name?
2. How old are you?
3. And your husband's/wife's name?
4. How old is he/she?
5. How many children do you have?
6. What is your child's name?
   Does he/she have another name that's used at home?
7. What is your child's date of birth?
8. Is there anyone else who lives here with you?
   Relationship   Age
9. Apart from N, is there anyone else in your household who has a hearing problem?
10. (If child not in school or nursery school)
    Who looks after your child when you're at work?
11. (If attends school or nursery school)
    Who takes your child to school/the nursery school?

Parents and Grandparents: Education and Work
12. (Parents) How far did you go in your education?
    How far did your husband/wife go in their education?
13. (Parents) What is your job/occupation?
    What is your husband's/wife's job/occupation?
14. (Parents) How many hours do you work each day?

15. (Parents) What time do you leave home in the morning? What time do you get back in the evening?
16. (Grandparents living in household/caregivers) How far did they go in their education?
17. Are they retired, or not?
18. (If still working) What is their job/occupation?

Child—Personality, Health
19. What is your child like? Could you describe him/her for me?
20. What does he/she enjoy doing?
21. How is his/her health?
22. Apart from the deafness/hearing difficulty, does your child have any other long-standing problem with their health?

Diagnosis
23. Has your child been deaf since birth?
24. Do you know the cause of the deafness?
25. (If hereditary) Are there any deaf people in the family?
26. When did you realize your child was deaf?
27. How many doctors did you take your child to see because of the hearing problem?

    What did they tell you?

    What treatment(s) did they advise?
28. Do you still take your child for regular hearing tests?

Reactions to Diagnosis
29. When the doctor told you your child was deaf, what was your reaction? Can you remember how you felt at the time?
30. What did your parents, and other people in the family, say?

Child's Deafness

I would like to find out more about your child's hearing.

31. If your child isn't wearing a hearing aid, can he/she hear any sounds?
32. If your child isn't wearing a hearing aid, and you're next to him/her, can he/she hear you if you shout?
33. If your child isn't wearing a hearing aid, and you're next to him/her, can he/she hear you if you speak normally?

(If the child has a hearing aid)

34. When he/she is wearing his/her hearing aid, and you're next to him/her, can he/she hear you if you shout?
35. When he/she is wearing his/her hearing aid, and you're next to him/her, can he/she hear you if you speak normally?
36. Are there particular noises that attract his/her attention?
37. Has your child had a hearing test?

    What kind of hearing test?

    What were the results?

38. Is your child's hearing getting better or worse?

Experience of Deafness

39. Have you ever met any deaf people?
40. (If yes) Is your view of your own child's deafness different because you have been in contact with deaf people?

Information

41. Have you ever tried to find out more about deafness?
42. Have you read any books or periodicals about deaf children?
43. Have you seen any television programs about deaf children?
44. Have you found out about deafness from any other sources?

Hearing Aids

45. Does your child wear a hearing aid, or not?
46. When did you get it?
47. Did you buy it yourself?
48. Is it made in China, or foreign?
49. Many parents say it's difficult to get their child to wear their hearing aids at first. How was it with your child?
50. Is he/she willing to wear it now, or not?
51. Does he/she wear his/her hearing aids all day?
52. Are there any situations where he/she doesn't wear his/her hearing aids—for example, in the bus or on the street?
53. Do you have any difficulty keeping the hearing aids working properly?
54. If there's a problem with the hearing aids, where can you go to get them repaired?

Daily Routine

55. (If child not at school or nursery school)

    Could you tell me what your child does each day?

    Who looks after him/her?

    (If child attends school or nursery school)

    Who gives him/her breakfast? Who gets him/her dressed?

56. What does he/she do on Sundays?

    Who is he/she with then?

57. Does he/she watch television at home?

    (If yes) How many hours does he/she watch each evening?

58. What programs does he/she like?

    Does he/she know what time his/her favorite programs start?

    Does he/she know which day they are?

Friends

59. When your child is at home, are there any children nearby he/she plays with?

    (If yes) Do they play together often?

    How many times a week?

60. Do your child's friends have any problems with their hearing?

61. How do they communicate when they're together?

Childrearing—General Management and Discipline

62. Are you less strict, or more strict, with your child because he/she has a hearing problem?

63. Most children this age are naughty sometimes—what about your child?

    When he/she is naughty, what sorts of things does he/she do?

64. If you want to stop him/her being naughty, what do you do?

65. Does your child lose his/her temper?

    (If yes) Often?

    In what sorts of situations?

66. How do you deal with him/her when he/she loses his/her temper?

67. Do you think your child loses his/her temper sometimes because he/she can't make other people understand him/her?

68. Do you sometimes smack your child?

    (If yes) In what sorts of situations?

69. Some people say you need to smack deaf children more, because it's difficult sometimes to get your meaning across; some people say you shouldn't smack deaf children. What do you think?

Learning about Safety

70. Does your child know that hot water and the hot stove are dangerous?
71. How did you teach him/her this?
72. Does your child know that traffic is dangerous?
73. How did you teach him/her?

Attention

74. At home, if you're next to your child and you want to attract his/her attention, what do you do?
75. If you aren't near your child, and you want to attract his/her attention, what do you do?
76. If your child wants to attract your attention, what does he/she do?

Communication

77. How do you communicate with your child — using speech, or signs, or both?

(Comprehension of spoken language)

78. When you speak to your child, what things can he/she understand? Could you give me some examples?
79. How do you know he/she understands what you are saying?
80. When you speak with your child, do you speak as you would with a child with normal hearing? Or, for example, do you make sure you're face-to-face, do you speak more slowly, or perhaps more clearly?
81. Do you sometimes use gestures to help express your meaning?
82. Do you find there are some things you would like to explain to your child, but it's very difficult to get him/her to understand?

(Child's speech, if he/she uses it)

83. Could you tell me what sorts of things your child can say?
84. When he/she speaks, does he/she speak clearly, or is it difficult sometimes to understand what he/she is saying?

85. Can people outside the family understand your child's speech as well as you can?

(Use of gestures/signs)

86. At home, how many different signs do you use? Could you give me some examples?
87. At home, who communicates most with your child?
88. At home, who understands your child best?

School Education

89. When did your child start at the nursery school?
90. How did you find out about the nursery school?
91. Did you have any difficulty getting your child enrolled, or not?
92. Did you ever think of sending your child to an ordinary nursery school, or not?
93. Why did you want to send your child to this special nursery school?
94. How much does the nursery school cost per month?
95. Does the teacher at the nursery school give you advice on how to help your child at home?

What advice do they give you?

96. Do you find it difficult sometimes to follow the teacher's advice?
97. If you have doubts about how to teach your child at home, is there someone you can ask about this, or not?
98. Do you go to the school sometimes to find out from the teacher how your child is doing?

(If yes) Do you do this often?

99. When your child first started at the nursery school, was he/she upset when you left him/her there?
100. Do you know what he/she likes at the nursery school?
101. Do you know what he/she dislikes at the nursery school?
102. How do you feel your child is doing at the nursery school?

What sort of progress is he/she making?

Parents/Grandparents as Teachers
   103. Do you teach your child at home?
   104. Who spends most time teaching him/her at home?
   105. What do you teach him/her?

   What methods do you use?

Parents' Views on Their Child's Education
   106. Will your child go to an ordinary school later, or to deaf school?
   107. Do you think this school is best for him/her?

   or: Why do you think this school is best for him/her?
   108. Do you think sign language is useful for your child, or not?

   (If yes) What role does sign language have in your child's education?

   Do you yourself plan to learn sign language so that you can communicate better with your child, and help him/her in their education, or not?
   109. Do you think that reading and writing are important for your child?

   Or is learning to speak more important?

   Which do you think your child should learn first, reading, speaking, or writing?

Contact with Other People
   110. Some people say that if you have a handicapped child, it makes you feel very different, and distant from other families. From your experience, do you feel this is so?
   111. Do you often take your child to see friends and relatives?

   Do relatives and friends come and visit you?
   112. Some people, when they meet a deaf child, don't know what to do or say. Do you find this is so, or not?
   113. Generally speaking, do you think other people understand the difficulties deafness causes for a deaf child?

114. What is your child like when he/she meets strangers? Does he/she take out their toys and play with them, or is he/she shy?

115. Do you find that when people realize your child is deaf, they tend to start a conversation with you about him/her?

    How do you feel about this?

116. Deaf children sometimes make strange noises, don't they?

    When your child makes these noises, do you sometimes feel embarrassed, or not?

117. Are some people rude to you, or to your child, because he/she is deaf?

    (If yes) What do they do/say?

Mutual Support among Parents

118. I know there are parents' meetings sometimes at the nursery school. What do you talk about?

119. Do you find these meetings helpful, or not?

    (If yes) In what way?

Economic Effects

120. What is your basic income per month?

    What do you and your husband/wife earn together, including bonuses?

121. Has your child's deafness had an effect on your household finances?

    (If yes) How much have you spent on seeing doctors and getting treatment?

122. How much do you spend on books and toys for your child?

123. Have you or your husband/wife changed your job, or changed your work hours to make it more convenient to look after your child?

Having a Second Child

124. I've heard that, according to China's family planning policy, if you have a handicapped child/child with a hearing

problem, you can get permission to have a second child. Do you yourselves want a second child?

(If no) Why not?

Parents' Views on Their Child's Future
125. How far do you think your child will go in his/her education?
126. What sort of work do you think he/she might do later?
127. Do you have any particular worries about his/her future?
128. What do you hope your child's future will be like?
129. When you get old, do you think your child will be able to look after you?

The Central Difficulty (Parents' Opinion)
130. What do you think is the most difficult aspect from your child's point of view?
131. For parents, what is the most difficult aspect of having a deaf child?

General Questions
132. From your experience, do you have any advice you could give other parents with deaf children?
133. What do you think the Chinese government could do to help families with deaf children?

Notes

CHAPTER TWO

1. In a survey in rural Hubei in 1981, women were asked why people wanted children: 51 percent said that they were needed as security in old age; 25 percent, that they were needed to continue the family line; 20 percent, to provide more labor; and only 3.5 percent, "for the sheer enjoyment and happiness" (Kane 1987, 186).

2. In *Stigma: Notes on the Management of Spoiled Identity* (1963), Goffman applies the term "passing" to the actions of individuals with stigmatizing characteristics who hide them in order to appear normal and therefore more socially acceptable.

3. But some parents do show spontaneous initiative. During a visit to a rural area near Nanjing in 1996, I met a group of parents with deaf children who had banded together to request that a teacher from a rehabilitation center in the city visit and tell them how to educate their children.

4. According to the 1990 census, 90 million people, or 8.3 percent of China's population, belong to fifty-five recognized ethnic groups. The largest group is the Tibetans, numbering 15.5 million. Chinese government policy toward the minorities officially has been to encourage preservation of minority languages and cultural heritage while supporting economic development; promoting education has been a priority (Kormondy 1995). Ethnic minority populations were not subject to birth control policies until the mid-1980s because their infant mortality rates had been very high in the 1950s and 1960s and because some groups had resisted government intervention (Kane 1987). Now family limitation is encouraged, but the regulations for minorities are more relaxed than for the majority Han Chinese population.

5. Arnold and Liu (1986) advocate efforts to eliminate discrimination against women in education and employment to eradicate ideas of male superiority so that son preference will be reduced.

6. These figures are based on information provided by local officials: in other words, if a daughter is born and the birth is not reported, the

sex ratio in that area will be raised erroneously. Girls whose birth is concealed risk losing out on schooling and other rights.

7. Underreporting of births, both by parents and by local officials, is a massive problem: Zeng Yi (1996) calculates it at between 25 and 28 percent in the early 1990s.

8. U.S. figures for the prevalence of mental retardation, defined as an IQ of 70 or below, are generally placed at about 3 percent of the population (Cleland 1978; Plog and Santamour 1980). It is not clear what definitions were used in the Chinese survey or how it was carried out. According to Kleinman and Lin (1981), the incidence of mental handicap in China is similar to that in the United States and other Western countries.

9. A similar line tends to be drawn in the United States as well; while women can choose to terminate their pregnancy when a fetal genetic defect or abnormality is detected, children born with disabilities, except in the most extreme cases, are helped to survive. Parents' wishes are respected in deciding for or against abortion; however, doctors' opinions may be the most significant factor in determining whether life support is withheld from newborn babies, as a study of infant deaths in a California hospital's intensive care unit concluded (cited in a disability rights newsletter; "Getting Rid of Disabled Infants" 1998).

10. The Eugenics Law was given a different name in the English translation to ward off protests from Western countries over the use of the word "eugenics." All quotations from the law are taken from the official English translation.

11. Infectious diseases include AIDS, gonorrhea, syphilis, and leprosy as well as "other infectious diseases medically considered to have adverse effects on marriage and reproduction"; mental diseases include schizophrenia, manic-depressive psychosis, and "other mental diseases of a serious nature."

12. However, recent research indicates that 50 to 80 percent of autosomal recessive congenital deafness may be due to mutation in the connexin 26 gene, which DNA analysis of a blood sample can identify (Estevil et al. 1998; Lench et al. 1998). The connexin 26 research has been carried out mainly on European sample groups: the prevalence of the mutation may vary in different populations (Reardon 1998) and data are not available yet for Chinese groups. The idea of genetic testing for deafness has been intensely controversial in the United States and in Britain, with critics worrying that genetic screening may be lead to pregnancies being terminated by hearing and deaf parents who seek to

control whether they have hearing or deaf children (Anna Middleton, conversation with author, 1998; Middleton, Hewison, and Mueller 1998).

13. In his paper presented at a National Deaf Children's Society Conference, Kent cites the relatively small number of abortions carried out in the United Kingdom on the grounds of genetic abnormality: 2,000 annually (180,000 pregnancies are terminated for nonmedical reasons).

14. One young psychology graduate told me that he is alive only because his older sister is deaf; when I saw him in 1996, his father was very distressed because the sister had insisted on marrying a deaf man and their baby son turned out to be deaf. In such circumstances the hearing child must feel increased pressure to fulfill family expectations.

15. From earliest childhood, food is powerfully associated with emotional comfort in the lives of Chinese people; eating good food in a bustling, noisy gathering of relatives and friends conveys a particularly strong sense of well-being and security.

16. In this study "egocentricity" is clearly regarded as a negative quality, yet a Western researcher might cast the same range of behavioral traits positively, as demonstrating "high self-esteem" or "independence."

17. In this study, the daily routines of children in kindergartens in America, Japan, and mainland China were videotaped: parents and teachers in each country were then asked to comment on the tapes. This reflexive methodology produced a wealth of insights.

CHAPTER THREE

1. In general, deaf children and deaf adults are put into the category "hearing-speech disabled," reflecting the fact that many deaf children do not acquire speech and also the cultural concept that hearing loss and inability to speak are a single entity.

2. Some parents in Western countries as well who are unable to accept or cope with a child with a disability give their child over to the care of the social services.

3. A similar disparity exists in the United States. The prevalence of hearing loss is greater at all ages when family income is lower and when individuals reside in a rural rather than a metropolitan area (Holt and Hotto 1994).

4. Western hearing parents also show both a preoccupation with ascertaining the cause of their child's deafness and the fear that it may be genetic. Meadow (1968) attributes this to parents' feelings of guilt:

they need to know whether they are responsible for their child's deafness, but if the deafness is found to be genetic in origin they fear being stigmatized as genetically imperfect.

5. The collection of letters (hereafter cited as LZH) written to Zhou Hong, principal of a rehabilitation center for deaf children and father of a deaf daughter, by parents of deaf children, is discussed at length in chapter 6; they have been numbered for ease of reference.

6. Women in rural China who give birth to daughters, rather than sons, are also liable to be blamed for producing an unwanted child (Davin 1995). To a lesser degree, Western mothers also are exposed to this attitude: Gregory points out that popular mother-and-baby books give advice on how to minimize the risk of having a disabled child, "with the corollary that if anything does go wrong the mother may feel somehow to blame" (1991, 124).

7. There is no term in common Chinese specifically for rubella. The word *fengzhen* is used, but it also means an allergic rash, particularly in response to cold harsh weather. This gap in vocabulary reflects and has perhaps also perpetuated the lack of recognition of rubella and its effects on the unborn child. (Doctors use the phrase *Deguo mazhen*, a literal translation of "German measles.")

8. Because the center enrolls children with significant residual hearing, there is a relatively high proportion with acquired deafness.

9. In 1996 Australian Hearing Services helped establish a two-year training program for audiologists at the Tongren Hospital in Beijing; a similar masters-level program is being set up at Peking Union Medical College with American support (Fangang Zeng, letter to author, 10 May 1997).

10. Sutton (1977) provides an analysis of the myth and speculates on what actually happened in Liaoyang.

11. Each implant costs $100, sometimes subsidized by the patient's work unit or by the CDPF. The surgery costs $20 and the hospital stay about $100 (F. Zeng 1995).

12. In mainstream schools teachers' pay and chances of promotion depend on the class average: any children with special needs are seen as threatening the class's test results. The 1990 Law for Disabled Persons mandates that mainstream schools should admit suitable disabled children, and schools are being pressured to accede to this.

13. Some large urban deaf schools have speech training classes for selected groups of students with sufficient residual hearing, or "oral classes" in which the teacher uses speech and sign simultaneously and students are required to use spoken language in the class; however, these still

take place in the overall context of a school curriculum taught mainly through sign-supported Chinese.

14. All translations of the 1990 law are from Sydenham 1993 (appendix pp. iv–xi).

15. It has been considered impractical to replace China's pictographic written language with *pinyin,* the romanized form of Chinese, because the language has so many homophones and because the many and very different regional dialects of spoken Chinese would have different written forms if spelled phonetically. However, all primary school children learn the roman alphabet and *pinyin* syllables in their first year at school to give them a sense of how words can be written phonetically.

16. This program has since been replaced by a three-year distance learning course better suited to training teachers from all over China.

17. The most famous of these exemplary models is Zhang Haidi, a young disabled girl in a wheelchair who managed to educate herself through her own efforts; she appeared frequently in newspaper articles, on television, and on propaganda posters in the mid-1980s (Landsberger 1995); see further discussion in chapter 4.

18. Parents of deaf children in Western countries also find it difficult to plan their child's education and cope with prejudice; however, in countries with more resources and better services for deaf children, these problems are likely to be less acute.

19. *Putonghua* means "common speech" or "standard speech," which implies that it is the norm. However, the State Language Work Committee plans to rename China's national dialect *tongyuhua*—"shared language" or "language in common"—to remove any suggestion of discrimination against the languages of China's ethnic minorities (Searl 1997).

20. Most researchers quote the figure for deaf children with deaf parents in the United States as around 10 percent (Schein 1989), although data from the 1984–85 Annual Survey of Hearing Impaired Children and Youth, cited by Schein, yield only 4 percent. In the United Kingdom, between 5 to 10 percent of deaf children have deaf parents (Llewellyn-Jones 1988; Miles 1988; Denmark 1989).

21. In the United States, Britain, and other Western countries, it is now usual to denote cultural deafness by capitalizing "Deaf"; the lowercase form is used to describe the audiological condition of hearing loss or those who by choice or history do not identify with the Deaf community. I have not followed this practice, primarily because, as I will argue, the cultural model seems to be largely absent from popular and

professional discourse in China (moreover, since Chinese characters cannot be capitalized, the convention is impossible to apply locally).

22. Of the eighty-four children enrolled in the CRR Center for Deaf Children in Beijing in 1995, five had deaf parents. In each of these families, the hearing grandparents communicated with the teachers at the center and had taken over responsibility for the children's education.

23. Yau and He's article on name signs provides a fascinating glimpse of children's life in a Chinese deaf school. At the school they studied, newly enrolled pupils were given their name signs by older pupils; following the practice in mainstream hearing society in China, these signs include the appellation "younger brother" or "younger sister."

24. In contrast, researchers of the Deaf community in the United States and the United Kingdom argue that membership must be *achieved:* "Membership in a deaf community is achieved through (1) *identification* with the deaf world, (2) *shared experiences* that come of being hearing impaired, and (3) *participation* in the community's activities. Without all three characteristics, one cannot be nor would one choose to be a member of a deaf community" (Higgins 1994, 23).

Chapter Four

1. The English words "speech" and "language" are represented in the Chinese professional literature by the single word *yuyan;* the conflation of the two concepts obscures the complexities of language acquisition and results in the teachers' overemphasis on speech production.

2. Eighty percent of deaf children live in rural areas (Xu Tinggui 1993); the 74.7 percent figure more recently offered by the Chinese Deaf Association reflects the steady expansion of the urban population ("Eastern Red" 1998). See also table 3.

3. Conversions are only approximate because of the changing value of Chinese currency and fluctuating exchange rates.

Chapter Five

1. The questionnaire specifically addressed these points—"At home, who communicates most with your child?" and "At home, who understands your child best?" (questions 87 and 88). In all cases the same person was named in both answers.

2. There were three classes in the rehabilitation center: the first class consisted of four children with good oral skills; the second class had six children with more severe hearing losses, who were between five and seven years old; and the third class consisted of four younger children, also with severe hearing losses, who were three and four.

3. Up until recently, state enterprises have been responsible for housing employees and their families; low rents take up only a fraction of people's income. But as the economy is undergoing reform, families are being encouraged to buy their own apartments.
4. "Deaf awareness," a term used in the United States and the United Kingdom, indicates the behavior of hearing people when interacting with deaf people that shows sensitivity to their communication requirements: for example, ensuring well-illuminated surroundings.
5. "Somatization," the experiencing of bodily symptoms in place of specific emotions, is a recognized and well-documented Chinese pattern of response to life events (Cheung 1995; Russell and Yik 1996). As Russell and Yik point out, from the Chinese perspective Westerners "psychologize" their emotions; they experience the impact of events psychologically and describe this experience using a vocabulary related to feelings and emotions.
6. The word the father uses here about his daughter, *canfei*, was employed up until the 1980s to mean "disabled"; it has since been officially replaced by the word *canji*, which is less pejorative. *Canfei* has strongly negative connotations of uselessness, like the English word "cripple"; this father is imagining his daughter as a useless, dependent burden.
7. One child was jaundiced at birth: the jaundice itself, or an underlying cause such as infection, could have damaged his hearing; or there might have been a genetic cause (though there was no family history of deafness).
8. This man, a close friend of the center's principal, is one of the very few deaf people in China to achieve qualification as a teacher of the deaf; he is bilingual in Chinese and Chinese Sign Language.
9. This points up a cultural difference; for example, Gregory (1976) records the experiences of English mothers having to deal with the embarrassed reactions of strangers who find out that their child is deaf or attempt to communicate with the deaf child.
10. In this family, the grandmother was the main respondent; but I was also able to discuss some questions with the deaf girl's mother through the senior teacher at the preschool, who knew sign language because she had once taught at the deaf school.
11. According to a survey carried out in March 1998, nearly all (362 out of 369) children attending Nanjing Deaf School had hearing parents (Callaway 1999).
12. As mentioned in chapter 2, I did find an example of mutual organization and self-help among a group of parents of deaf children in the

countryside who banded together to request a special teacher from the city to help them educate their children.

Chapter Six

1. As a convenient shorthand, from this point on in the chapter I refer to all the writers as "parents."
2. One way of coping is to refuse to discuss the child with outsiders; a Beijing university student told me that her aunt, who lived in the countryside and had two deaf sons, never spoke about them to people outside the family; she simply refused to answer when people asked her about them.
3. For detailed explanation of these traditional therapies, see chapter 3; all aim to restore health by stimulating and redistributing the flow of *qi* in the body to attain harmony.
4. According to her father, Tingting had several years of acupuncture treatment combined with courses of traditional Chinese herbs; apparently there was a slight improvement in her hearing by the time she was four years old.
5. As already noted, there is little distinction made, even in professional discourse, between a child learning to articulate words or sentences and acquiring mastery of language; parents emphasized speech, not language.
6. *Peng* means a "roc," a legendary bird of great size and power symbolizing a bright future.
7. She probably is from the countryside and does not have the residence documents that would enable her to get a secure job in an urban work unit. Temporary workers are not entitled to benefits such as accommodation, pensions, sick pay, and so on.
8. *Yuan* means a circle in Chinese; as a name, it suggests prosperity and good fortune.
9. Apsaras are mythical beings depicted in the famous Buddhist frescoes in the Dunhuang caves in Gansu Province.
10. The "iron tree" (*Cycas revoluta,* also known as sago cycas) blossoms very infrequently. An iron tree in blossom is a traditional Chinese metaphor for something that is rarely seen or hardly possible: in this case, a deaf child learning to speak.

Chapter Seven

1. When I met in 1996 with the family with deaf parents I had interviewed in 1994 (the hearing grandmother had been the respondent),

I noted some interesting changes in the family environment that perhaps, in part, reflected the positive effects of the experimental class. Previously depressed and uninvolved with her deaf daughter's education, the deaf mother now seemed much happier and spent some time each day signing storybooks with her. In addition, the deaf daughter had become much more extroverted and now had several hearing playmates in the neighborhood.

REFERENCES

Authors from mainland China are listed with the family name first and given name in full; Chinese authors from outside mainland China follow different styles, as preferred by the individual authors.

Abbreviation: *Zhongguo canji ren kangfu xiehui tingli yuyan kangfu zhuanye weiyuan hui di er jie xueshu nianhui lunwen huibian* (Proceedings of the Second Annual Conference of the Hearing and Language Rehabilitation Specialist Committee Members of the China Disabled People's Rehabilitation Association), held in Suzhou, has been abbreviated to *Suzhou lunwen huibian* (Suzhou Conference Proceedings) throughout.

"Amity Supports Laid-Off Blind Workers." 1998. *chinabrief* 1(3): 4.

An Xiaoxian. 1993. "Long'er jiazhang xuexiao shi shixian long'er zaoqi kangfu de yi ba yaoshi" (School for parents of deaf children is the key to the realization of deaf children's early rehabilitation). *Zhongguo long'er kangfu* (Rehabilitation of Deaf Children in China), no. 1: 27–29.

Arnold, Fred, and Liu Zhaoxiang. 1986. "Sex Preference, Fertility, and Family Planning in China." *Population and Development Review* 12(2): 221–46.

Baker, Hugh D. R. 1979. *Chinese Family and Kinship*. New York: Columbia University Press.

Balkany, Thomas, and Michal Luntz. 1998. "Diagnosis and Management of Sensorineural Hearing Disorders." In *Pediatric Otology and Neurotology,* ed. Anil K. Lalwani and Kenneth M. Grundfast, 397–403. Philadelphia: Lippincott-Raven.

Banister, Judith. 1984. *China's Changing Population*. Stanford: Stanford University Press.

"Banknotes: *2020* Vision Full of Markets." 1998. *China Development Briefing* 2(1): 19–21.

"Birth Planning in Sichuan Province, China." 1988. *Population and Development Review* 14(2): 369–75.

Bittles, Alan. 1994. "The Role and Significance of Consanguinity as a Demographic Variable." *Population and Development Review* 20(3): 561–84.

Bogdan, Robert, and Sari Knopp Biklen. 1992. *Qualitative Research for Education*. 2nd ed. Boston: Allyn and Bacon.

Bond, Michael Harris. 1991. *Beyond the Chinese Face: Insights from Psychology*. New York: Oxford University Press.

Bond, Michael Harris, and Kwang-kuo Hwuang. 1986. "The Social Psychology of the Chinese People." In *The Psychology of the Chinese People*, ed. Michael Harris Bond, 213–66. Hong Kong: Oxford University Press.

Breiner, Sander J. 1980. "Early Child Development in China." *Child Psychiatry and Human Development* 11(2): 87–95.

Burgess, Robin, and Zhuang Juzhong. 1996. *Dimensions of Gender Bias in Intrahousehold Allocation in Rural China*. London: London School of Economics, Suntory-Toyota International Centre for Economics and Related Disciplines.

Callaway, Alison. 1986. "Educating Deaf Children." *China Now* 116: 24–25.

———. 1998a. "All in the Family." *China in Focus*, summer, 18–19.

———. 1998b. "Chinese Government Gives Positive Lead." *British Deaf News*, February, 9.

———. 1999. "Considering Sign Bilingual Education in Cultural Context: A Survey of Deaf Schools in Jiangsu Province, China." *Deafness and Education International* 1(1): 34–46.

Canji ertong ziliao: Zhongguo canji ren chouyang diaocha xilie ziliao (Data on disabled children: Data from China's sample survey of disabled people). 1991. Beijing: Zhongguo shehui chubanshe.

Carino, Teresa. 1998. "Telling a Tale in More Ways Than One: An Experiment in Bilingual Education." *Amity Newsletter* 46(3): 4.

Carter, Anita E. 1911. *The School for Chinese Deaf: The Story of Our Deaf Girls*. Shanghai: Commercial Press.

———. 1938. *Sketch of the Life of Annetta Thompson Mills, Founder of the Chefoo School for the Deaf*. Chefoo: James McMullan.

Chai, Denise. 1992. "One Child Family Dream: Policy Makers' Nightmare." *China Now* 142: 8–10.

Chen Guiqin. 1993. "Long'er kangfu jigou bixu zhongshi jiazhang gongzuo" (Rehabilitation institutions for deaf children must pay great attention to work with parents). *Zhongguo long'er kangfu* (Rehabilitation of Deaf Children in China), no. 2: 30–31.

Chen Sheying. 1996. *Social Policy of the Economic State and Community Care in Chinese Culture: Aging, Family, Urban Change, and the Socialist Welfare Pluralism.* Aldershot, Hants.: Avebury.

Chen Suzhen. 1995. "Long'er jiating hanshou cunzai wenti ji duice" (Some problems in teaching deaf children's families through correspondence, and their solutions). In *Suzhou lunwen huibian* (Suzhou Conference Proceedings), 198–201.

Cheung, Fanny. 1995. "Facts and Myths about Somatization among the Chinese." In *Chinese Societies and Mental Health*, ed. Lin Tsung-yi, Tseng Wen-shing, and Yeh Eng-kung. New York: Oxford University Press.

Children and Women of China: A UNICEF Situation Analysis. 1989. Beijing: People's Education Press.

China Association of the Deaf. 1990. "Under the Umbrella of a National Federation for Disabled Persons." *World Federation of the Deaf News*, no. 4: 18–19.

China Statistical Yearbook (in Chinese: *Zhongguo tongji nianjian*). 1991. Beijing: China Statistical Publishing House.

———. 1994. Beijing: China Statistical Publishing House.

———. 1997. Beijing: China Statistical Publishing House.

"China Surveys the Handicapped." 1987. *Beijing Review*, 21–27 December, 7–8.

"Chinese Population Policy: A *People's Daily* Editorial." 1982. *Population and Development Review* 8(3): 633–35.

Ching C. C. 1982. "The One-Child Family in China: The Need for Psychosocial Research." *Studies in Family Planning* 13(6/7): 208–12.

Ching, Lucy. 1980. *One of the Lucky Ones.* Hong Kong: Gulliver Books.

Choi Sungkyu. 1995. "Cross-Cultural Attitudes toward Deaf Culture in a Multi- and Singular Cultural Society: A Survey of Residential School-Based Teachers for the Deaf Who Are Deaf and Hearing." Ed.D. diss., Ball State University. 1995. Abstract in *Dissertation Abstracts International* 56: 1734A.

Cleland, Charles Carr. 1978. *Mental Retardation: A Developmental Approach.* Englewood Cliffs, N.J.: Prentice-Hall.

Cleverley, John F. 1985. *The Schooling of China: Tradition and Modernity in Chinese Education*. Sydney: Allen and Unwin.

Croll, Elisabeth. 1983. *Chinese Women Since Mao*. London: Zed Books.

———. 1994. *From Heaven to Earth: Images and Experiences of Development in China*. London: Routledge.

———. 1995. *Changing Identities of Chinese Women: Rhetoric, Experience, and Self-Perception in Twentieth-Century China*. Hong Kong: Hong Kong University Press; London: Zed Books; Armonk, N.Y.: M. E. Sharpe.

Davin, Delia. 1976. *Woman-Work: Women and the Party in Revolutionary China*. Oxford: Clarendon.

———. 1987. "Gender and Population in the People's Republic of China." In *Women, State, and Ideology*, ed. Haleh Afshar, 111–29. London: Macmillan.

———. 1990a. "The Early Childhood Education of the Only Child Generation in Urban China." In *Chinese Education: Problems, Policies, and Perspectives*, ed. Irving Epstein, 42–65. New York: Garland.

———. 1990b. "'Never Mind If It's a Girl, You Can Have Another Try': The Modification of the One-Child Family Policy and Its Implications for Gender Relations in Rural Areas." In *Remaking Peasant China*, ed. Jorgen Delman, Clemens Stubbe Ostergaard, and Fleming Christiansen, 81–91. Aarhus: Aarhus University Press.

———. 1995. "China's Population Policy: Abusing or Protecting Human Rights." *China Review*, no. 5: 9–11.

Denmark, Clark. 1989. "Is English the First Language of Deaf Children?" In *Bilingualism—Teaching English as a Second Language to Deaf Children*. Proceedings of a conference held in Derby, 7–14 November. Middlesex: LASER.

The Development of the Undertakings of Disabled Persons in China. 1997. Beijing: China Disabled People's Federation.

Dikotter, Frank. 1992. *The Discourse of Race in Modern China*. Stanford: Stanford University Press.

———. 1996. "Throw-Away Babies: The Growth of Eugenic Policies and Practices in China." *Times Literary Supplement*, 12 January, 4–5.

———. 1998. *Imperfect Conceptions: Medical Knowledge, Birth Defects, and Eugenics in China*. London: Hurst.

Dimmock, Arthur. 1995. "Girdle." *British Deaf News* 26(2): 19.

"Eastern Red." 1998. *World Federation of the Deaf News* 11(2): 16–20.

Eisenburg, Louis, Harvey Taub, and Louis Dicarlo. 1974. "Acupuncture Therapy of Sensorineural Deafness: Evaluation Study." *New York State Journal of Medicine* 74(11): 1942–49.

"Empty Burden." 1987. In *Chinese Lives: An Oral History of Contemporary China,* by Zhang Xinxin and Sang Ye, ed. and trans. W. J. F. Jenner and Delia Davin, 293–94. London: Penguin.

Entrican, Sara. [1905?]. *The Story of the Chifu School.* Trenton, N.J.: Silent Worker.

Estevil, Xavier, Paolo Fortina, Saul Surrey, Raquel Rabionet, Salvatore Melchionda, Leonardo D'Agruma, Elaine Mansfield, Eric Rappaport, Nancy Govea, Montse Milà, Leopoldo Zelante, and Paolo Gasparini. 1998. "Connexin-26 Mutations in Sporadic and Inherited Sensorineural Deafness." *Lancet* 351: 394–98.

Fairbanks, David, Ellis Wallenburg, and Blair Webb. 1974. "Acupuncture for Hearing Loss: A Study of Patients Treated in Washington, DC." *Archives of Otolaryngology* 99: 395–401.

Falbo, Toni. 1982. "The One-Child Family in the United States: Research Issues and Results." *Studies in Family Planning* 13(6/7): 212–15.

Fletcher, Lorraine. 1987. *A Language for Ben: A Deaf Child's Right to Sign.* London: Souvenir Press.

Forecki, Marcia Calhoun. 1985. *Speak to Me!* Washington, D.C.: Gallaudet University Press.

Freeman, Norman, and Gustav Habermann. 1996. "Linguistic Socialization: A Chinese Perspective." In *The Handbook of Chinese Psychology,* ed. Michael Harris Bond, 79–92. Hong Kong: Oxford University Press.

Fu Weikang. 1975. *The Story of Chinese Acupuncture and Moxibustion.* Beijing: Foreign Languages Press.

Gao Chenbo. 1996. "Tan dui long haizi de jiating jiaoyu" (A discussion about the family education of deaf children). *Shandong Tejiao* (Special Education in Shandong), no. 1: 24–25.

Gao Chenghua. 1991. "Muqian long'er kangfu zhong yingdang yin wei zhuyi de ji ge wenti" (Several problems in the rehabilitation of deaf children that should be given more attention at the present time). *Zhongguo long'er kangfu* (Rehabilitation of Deaf Children in China), no. 1: 5–6.

Gao Ge, Stella Ting-Toomey, and William Gudykunst. 1996. "Chinese Communication Processes." In *The Handbook of Chinese Psychology,* ed. Michael Harris Bond, 280–93. Hong Kong: Oxford University Press.

Gates, Hill. 1993. "Cultural Support for Birth Limitation among Urban Capital-Owning Women." In *Chinese Families in the Post-Mao Era,* ed.

Deborah Davis and Stevan Harrell, 251–74. Berkeley: University of California Press.

Ge Chaomin. 1993. "Jiating long'er kangfu gongzuo shijian yu sikao" (The family rehabilitation of deaf children: Implementation, and reflections). *Zhongguo long'er kangfu* (Rehabilitation of Deaf Children in China), no. 1: 13–15.

"Getting Rid of Disabled Infants—The Slaughter Still Goes On." 1998. *Disability Awareness in Action* 66: 4.

Gittings, John. 1996. *Real China: From Cannibalism to Karaoke.* London: Simon and Schuster.

Goffman, Erving. 1963. *Stigma: Notes on the Management of Spoiled Identity.* Englewood Cliffs, N.J.: Prentice-Hall.

Goldin-Meadow, Susan, and Carolyn Mylander. 1998. "Spontaneous Sign Systems Created by Deaf Children in Two Cultures." *Nature* 391: 279–81.

Greenberg, Mark. 1994. "Preventive Interventions with Deaf Children." In *Keep Deaf Children in Mind: Current Issues in Mental Health,* ed. Carlo Laurenzi and Peter Hindley, 25–31. London: National Deaf Children's Society.

Greenberg, Mark, Carol Kusche, Ruth Gustafson, and Rosemary Calderon. 1984. "The PATHS Project: A Model for the Prevention of Psychosocial Difficulties in Deaf Children." In *Habilitation and Rehabilitation of Deaf Adolescents: Proceedings of the National Conference on the Habilitation and Rehabilitation of Deaf Adolescents, Wagoner, Oklahoma, April 17–20, 1984,* ed. Glenn B. Anderson and Douglas Watson. Washington, D.C.: National Academy of Gallaudet College.

Greenhalgh, Susan. 1986. "Shifts in China's Population Policy, 1984–86: Views from the Central, Provincial, and Local Levels." *Population and Development Review* 12(3): 491–515.

———. 1992. "The Changing Value of Children in the Transition from Socialism: The View from Three Chinese Villages." *Population Council Working Papers* no. 43.

Greenhalgh, Susan, and Li Jiali. 1993. "Engendering Reproductive Practice in Peasant China: The Political Roots of the Rising Sex Ratios at Birth." *Population Council Working Papers* no. 57.

Greenhalgh, Susan, Zhu Chuzhu, and Li Nan. 1993. "Restraining Population Growth in Three Chinese Villages: 1988–93." *Population Council Working Papers* no. 55.

———. 1994. "Restraining Population Growth in Three Chinese Villages: 1988–93." *Population and Development Review* 20(2): 365–95.

Gregory, Susan. 1976. *The Deaf Child and His Family.* London: Allen and Unwin.

———. 1991. "Challenging Motherhood: Mothers and Their Deaf Children." In *Motherhood: Meanings, Practices, and Ideologies,* ed. Ann Phoenix, Anne Woollett, and Eva Lloyd, 123–42. London: Sage Publications.

———. 1994. "The Developing Deaf Child." In *Keep Deaf Children in Mind: Current Issues in Mental Health,* ed. Carlo Laurenzi and Peter Hindley, 4–11. London: National Deaf Children's Society.

Gregory, Susan, Juliet Bishop, and Lesley Sheldon. 1995. *Deaf Young People and Their Families: Developing Understanding.* Cambridge: Cambridge University Press.

Gruffydh-Williams, Howard. 1962. "Leaves in an Eastern Wind: Part II." *Teacher of the Deaf* 60: 169–75.

Guo Xi. 1993. "Yao jin yi bu fangkuan 'yuyan zhengce'" (We must further relax the language policy). *Xiandai teshu jiaoyu* (Modern Special Education), no. 1: 10–11.

Guo Zaixiang. 1995. "Lun long'er jiazhang de kangfu yu peixun" (Discussion of the rehabilitation and training of the parents of deaf children). *Zhongguo long'er kangfu* (Rehabilitation of Deaf Children in China), no. 2: 15–16.

Haralambos, Michael, and Martin Holborn. 1991. *Sociology: Themes and Perspectives.* 3rd ed. London: Collins Educational.

Hawkes, Nigel. 1995. "Scientists Attack China over Selective Breeding." *Times* (London), 5 June, 11a.

Hesketh, Therese. 1996. "The Maternal and Child Health Care Law." Lecture at the Great Britain-China Centre, 15 Belgrave Square, London, 21 March.

Higgins, Paul. 1991. "Outsiders in a Hearing World." In *Constructing Deafness,* ed. Susan Gregory and Gillian M. Hartley. London: Pinter in association with the Open University.

Hillier, Sheila. M., and J. A. Jewell. 1983. *Health Care and Traditional Medicine in China, 1880–1982.* London: Routledge and Kegan Paul.

Hillier, Sheila. M, and Zheng Xiang. 1994. "Rural Health Care in China: Past, Present, and Future." In *China: The Next Decades,* ed. Dennis Dwyer. Harlow, Essex: Longman.

Hindley, Peter. 1994. "Child Psychiatry and Preventive Mental Health — with Deaf Children: A Contradiction in Terms?" In *Keep Deaf Children in Mind: Current Issues in Mental Health,* ed. Carlo Laurenzi and Peter Hindley, 41–45. London: National Deaf Children's Society.

Ho, David. 1986. "Chinese Patterns of Socialization: A Critical Review." In *The Psychology of the Chinese People*, ed. Michael Harris Bond, 1–37. Hong Kong: Oxford University Press.

———. 1996. "Filial Piety and Its Psychological Consequences." In *The Handbook of Chinese Psychology*, ed. Michael Harris Bond, 155–65. Hong Kong: Oxford University Press.

Holt, Judith A., and Sue A. Hotto. 1994. *Demographic Aspects of Hearing Impairment: Questions and Answers*. 3rd ed. Washington D.C.: Center for Assessment and Demographic Studies, Gallaudet University.

Hua Wenli. 1995. "Jiazhang zai long'er yuxun zhong de zuoyong bu ke hushi" (The role of parents in deaf children's language training should not be neglected). In *Suzhou lunwen huibian* (Suzhou Conference Proceedings), 195–96.

Huang Kaicheng. 1994. "Speech Therapy for Deaf Children and the Role of the Head of the Family in Extracurricular Instruction." *Special Children and Teachers' Research*, no. 2.

Hull, Terence. 1990. "Recent Trends in Sex Ratios at Birth in China." *Population and Development Review* 16(1): 63–83.

Jenner, William J. F. 1992. *The Tyranny of History: The Roots of China's Crisis*. London: Penguin.

Jiao Shulan, Ji Guiping, and Jing Qicheng. 1986. "Comparative Study of Behavioral Qualities of Only Children and Sibling Children." *Child Development* 57: 357–61.

Jiao Zhimin. 1995. "Shoujie long'er zaoqi kangfu jiaoyu dazhuan ban biye" (First intake of the university course in the early childhood education of deaf children graduates). *Zhongguo long'er kangfu* (Rehabilitation of Deaf Children in China), no. 4: 31.

Jiao Zhimin, Sun Xi, Guo Zhandong, Liang Wei, and Zhou Lijun. 1995. "Long'er shequ, jiating kangfu moshi de yanjiu" (Research on models for the community and family rehabilitation of deaf children). In *Suzhou lunwen huibian* (Suzhou Conference Proceedings), 202–5.

Johansson, Sten, and Ola Nygren. 1991. "The Missing Girls of China: A Demographic Account." *Population and Development Review* 17(1): 35–51.

Kane, Penny. 1987. *The Second Billion: Population and Family Planning in China*. Ringwood, Victoria: Penguin.

Kaptchuk, Ted J. 1983. *The Web That Has No Weaver: Understanding Chinese Medicine*. New York: Congdon and Weed.

Kent, Alistair. 1998. "The Ethics of Genetic Testing." Paper presented at the National Deaf Children's Society Conference on Pediatric

Audiology and Health Care: The Next Ten Years, 19 June, Birmingham, U.K.

Kessen, William, ed. 1975. *Childhood in China*. New Haven: Yale University Press.

King, Ambrose, and Michael Harris Bond. 1985. "The Confucian Paradigm of Man: A Sociological View." In *Chinese Culture and Mental Health*, ed. Tseng Wen-shing and David Y. H. Wu, 29–45. Orlando, Fla.: Academic Press.

Kleinman, Arthur, and Lin Tsung-yi. 1981. Epilogue of *Normal and Abnormal Behavior in Chinese Culture*, ed. Arthur Kleinman, and Lin Tsung-yi, 403–10. Dordrecht: Reidel.

Kormondy, Edward. 1995. "Minority Education, Cultural Preservation, and Economic Development in China." *Compare* 25(2): 161–78.

Kristof, N. 1993. "Chinese Turn to Ultrasound, Scorning Baby Girls for Boys." *New York Times,* 21 July, 1a, 6a.

Landsberger, Stefan. 1995. *Chinese Propaganda Posters: From Revolution to Modernization*. Amsterdam: Pepin Press.

Lane, Harlan. 1992. *The Mask of Benevolence: Disabling the Deaf Community*. New York: Knopf.

Lang, Raymond. 1998. "Empowerment and CBR? Some Issues Raised from the South Indian Experience." Paper presented at the U.K. Forum on Disability and Development, University of Leeds, 2 April.

Lee Yueh-Ting, Russ Kleinbach, Hu Pei-Cheng, Peng Zu-Zhi, and Chen Xiang-Yang. 1996. "Cross-Cultural Research on Euthanasia and Abortion." *Journal of Social Issues* 52(2): 131–48.

Lench, Nicholas, Mark Houseman, Valerie Newton, Guy Van Camp, and Robert Mueller. 1998. "Connexin-26 Mutations in Sporadic Nonsyndromal Sensorineural Deafness." *Lancet* 351: 415.

Lewin, Keith M., Angela W. Little, Xu Hui, and Zheng Jiwei. 1994. *Educational Innovation in China: Tracing the Impact of the 1985 Reforms*. Harlow, Essex: Longman.

Li Chunyu, and Guo Zaixiang. 1995. "Long'er jiating kangfu jiaoyu zongshu" (Summary of family rehabilitation of deaf children). In *Suzhou lunwen huibian* (Suzhou Conference Proceedings), 191–94.

Li Liqin. 1995. "Long jian he yi xunlian shiyan baogao" (Integration: A report on training experience). In *Suzhou lunwen huibian* (Suzhou Conference Proceedings), 181–83.

Li Ming. 1997. "Long'er kangfu jiaoxue fa de gainian wenti" (Conceptual issues and educational methods in the rehabilitation of deaf children).

Zhongguo long'er kangfu (Rehabilitation of Deaf Children in China) 6(1): 12–13, 18.

Li Shaozhu, Zhou Jing, and Guo Xi. 1993. *Long'er zaoqi kangfu jiaoyu: lilun yu fangfa* (Early rehabilitation education of deaf children: Theory and practice). Nanjing: Nanjing daxue chubanshe.

Li Xintian. 1985. "The Effect of Family on the Mental Health of the Chinese People." In *Chinese Culture and Mental Health,* ed. Tseng Wen-shing and David Wu, 85–93. Orlando, Fla.: Academic Press.

Li Yingui. 1993. "Yi ge long'er jiazhang de jue ze" (The choice of a deaf child's parent). *Zhongguo long'er kangfu* (Rehabilitation of Deaf Children in China), no. 3: 27–29.

Lian Yong. 1992. "Shilun long'er kangfu gongzuo de zhong 'jiazhang wenti' ji qi duice" (Discussion of the "parent problem" in deaf children's rehabilitation work, and countermeasures). *Zhongguo long'er kangfu* (Rehabilitation of Deaf Children in China), no. 4: 4–6.

"Life or Death Dilemma for Parents." 1999. Action Research press release, 29 March.

Liljestrom, Rita, Eva Noren-Bjorn, Gertrud Schyl-Bjurman, Birgit Ohrn, Lars H. Gustafsson, and Orvar Lofgren. 1982. *Young Children in China*. Trans. Tove Skutnabb-Kangas and Robert Philipson. Clevedon, Avon: Multilingual Matters.

Lin Tsung-yi, and Lin Mei-chen. 1981. "Love, Denial, and Rejection: Responses of Chinese Families to Mental Illness." In *Normal and Abnormal Behavior in Chinese Culture,* ed. Arthur Kleinman and Lin Tsung-yi, 387–401. Dordrecht: Reidel.

Liu Fudian. 1995. "Long'er jiazhang xinli qianxi" (Notes on the psychology of parents with deaf children). *Zhongguo long'er kangfu* (Rehabilitation of Deaf Children in China), no. 2: 12–14.

Liu Qian, Deng Yuancheng, Li Lin, and Lin Guizhen. 1982. "Evaluation of Acupuncture Treatment for Sensorineural Deafness and Deaf-Mutism Based on Twenty Years' Experience." *Chinese Medical Journal* 95(1): 21–24.

Liu Xin and Meng Sheng. 1992. "Jiazhang tan long'er jiaxiao" (Parents talk about deaf children's family education). *Zhongguo long'er kangfu* (Rehabilitation of Deaf Children in China), no. 1: 31.

Liu Xuezhong, Xu Lirong, Zhang Silin, and Xu Yin. 1993. "Prevalence and Aetiology of Profound Deafness in the General Population of Sichuan, China." *Journal of Laryngology and Otology* 107: 990–93.

———. 1994. "Epidemiological and Genetic Studies of Congenital Profound Deafness in the General Population of Sichuan, China." *American Journal of Medical Genetics* 53: 192–95.

Liu Yanxia. 1995. "Long you'er de renxing xingwei ji jiaozheng" (The willful behavior of deaf children and its correction). *Zhongguo long'er kangfu* (Rehabilitation of Deaf Children in China), no. 2: 11–12.

Liu Zhenxing. 1992. "Wo guo longren xianqu dui teshu jiaoyu de gongxian—yijian lun longren canyu longjiao shiye de yiyi ji qi zishen youshi" (The contributions to special education made by China's deaf pioneers—incorporating a discussion on the significance of deaf people's participation in deaf education and their particular strengths). *Nanjing teshi xuebao* (Nanjing Special Education Teachers' Journal), no. 2: 5–13.

———. 1993. "Cong Ru long liang ge ban xuesheng jiankuang tan pinkun diqu teshu jiaoyu de fazhan" (The development of special education in poor areas with reference to two deaf classes in Ruyang county). *Nanjing teshi xuebao* (Nanjing Special Education Teachers' Journal), no. 4: 11–13.

———. 1996. "Qian tan long ren canyu longxiao jiaoyu" (Notes on the participation of deaf people in deaf education). *Long'er jiating kangfu xinxi* (Deaf Children's Family Rehabilitation News). [Newsletter for parents of deaf children in Nanjing.]

Llewellyn-Jones, Miranda. 1988. "Bilingualism and the Education of Deaf Children." In *Educating the Deaf Child: The Bilingual Option*. Proceedings of a conference held in Derby, 14–28 October 1987. Kimpton, Middlesex: LASER.

Luo Qian. 1997. "A Developing Concern over the Disabled." *China Today* 46(5): 10–13.

Luterman, David. 1987. *Deafness in the Family*. Boston: College-Hill Press.

———. 1990. "Audiological Counseling and the Diagnostic Process." *American Speech-Language-Hearing Association (ASHA)* 32(4): 35–37.

LZH. Letters to Zhou Hong—see chapter 6.

Marschark, Marc. 1993. *Psychological Development of Deaf Children*. Oxford: Oxford University Press.

Martin, Diana. 1997. "Childbirth and Maternity among the Chinese of Hong Kong with the Aim of Showing How the Mix of Inherited and Modern Elements Are Selected to Adapt to Middle-Class Family Aspirations." Paper presented at the Joint East Asian Studies Conference, University of Durham, U.K., 2–4 April.

Martin, Frederick, Karen Abadie, and Denise Descouzis. 1989. "Counseling Families of Hearing-Impaired Children: Comparisons of the Attitudes of Australian and U.S. Parents and Audiologists." *Australian Journal of Audiology* 11(2): 41–54.

McNamara, Sheila Z. 1995. *Traditional Chinese Medicine.* London: Hamish Hamilton.

McNeill, Patrick. 1990. *Research Methods.* 2nd ed. London: Routledge.

Meadow, Kathryn P. 1967. "The Effect of Early Manual Communication and Family Climate on the Deaf Child's Development." Ph.D. diss., University of California, Berkeley.

———. 1968. "Parental Response to the Medical Ambiguities of Congenital Deafness." *Journal of Health and Social Behavior* 9: 299–309.

Meadow, Kathryn P., and Raymond Trybus. 1979. "Behavioral and Emotional Problems of Deaf Children: An Overview." In *Hearing and Hearing Impairment,* ed. Larry J. Bradford, and William G. Hardy, 395–403. New York: Grune and Stratton.

Mei Fusheng. 1998. "Shouyu zai longya ren wenhua jiaoyu zhong de diwei—longya ren xuyao shenme jiaoyu" (The place of sign language in deaf people's culture and education: What is needed in deaf people's education). Typescript.

Mencius. 1970. *Mencius.* Trans. D.C. Lau. Middlesex: Penguin.

Middleton, Anna, J. Hewison, and R. Mueller. 1998. "Attitudes of Deaf Adults toward Genetic Testing for Hereditary Deafness." *American Journal of Human Genetics* 63: 1175–80.

Miles, Dorothy D. 1988. *British Sign Language: A Beginner's Guide.* London: BBC Books.

Mills, Annetta T. 1910. *China through a Car-window: Observations on the Modern China, Made in the Course of a Four Months' Journey in Behalf of the Chinese Deaf: With Some Account of the School at Chefoo.* Washington, D.C.: Volta Bureau.

Milwertz, Cecilia Nathansen. 1997. *Accepting Population Control: Urban Chinese Women and the One-Child Family Policy.* Richmond, Surrey: Curzon.

Northern, Jerry L., and Marion P. Downs. 1991. *Hearing in Children.* 4th ed. Baltimore: Williams and Wilkins.

Northern, Jerry L., and S. Epstein. 1998. "Neonatal Hearing Screening: Early Identification." In *Pediatric Otology and Neurotology,* ed. Anil K. Lalwani and Kenneth M. Grundfast, 155–62. Philadelphia: Lippincott-Raven.

Oblau, Gotthard. 1993. "From Mute to Child Prodigy: Amity Gives Fresh Impetus to China's Special Education." *Amity Newsletter,* no. 26: 1–3.

———. 1994. "No Money for Huanghuatang Township Hospital: Funding Problems Cripple Rural Health Care." *Amity Newsletter,* no. 29: 4.

O'Brien, Anthony. 1995. Letter to the editor. *Times* (London), 13 June, 17e.

"On Population and Population Policy in China." 1983. *Population and Development Review* 9(1): 181–84.

"On Province-Level Fertility Policy in China." 1983. *Population and Development Review* 9(3): 553–61.

"Orphanage Row Prompts Training Cash." 1996. *China Development Briefing* 1(1): 4–5.

Palmer, Brian. 1990. "Equality of Educational Opportunity—and for the Deaf?" Inaugural lecture, University of Reading, U.K., 4 December.

Pan Longsheng. 1993. "Fahui jiazhang zai houxu jiaoyu zhong de zuoyong" (Developing parents' role in follow-up education). *Zhongguo long'er kangfu* (Rehabilitation of Deaf Children in China), no. 2: 31–32.

Parsons, Frances M. 1988. *I Didn't Hear the Dragon Roar.* Washington, D.C.: Gallaudet University Press.

Parving, Agnete. 1996. "Epidemiology of Genetic Hearing Impairment." In *Genetics and Hearing Impairment,* ed. Alessandro Martin, Andrew Read, and Dafydd Stephens. London: Whurr Publishers.

"'Paying Great Attention to Eugenics': A Chinese View." 1983. *Population and Development Review* 9(4): 756–61.

Pfeiffer, David. 1994. "Eugenics and Disability Discrimination." *Disability and Society* 9(4): 481–99.

Phillips, Michael. 1993. "Strategies Used by Chinese Families Coping with Schizophrenia." In *Chinese Families in the Post-Mao Era,* ed. Deborah Davis and Stevan Harrell, 277–305. Berkeley: University of California Press.

Piao Yongxin. 1984. "The Deaf and Sign Language in China." Paper presented at the International Sign Language Workshop, University of Bristol, U.K.

———. 1987. "China, People's Republic of." In *Gallaudet Encyclopedia of Deaf People and Deafness,* ed. John V. Van Cleve. New York: McGraw-Hill.

———, principal ed. 1992. *Zhongguo shouyu: jiaoxue fudao* (Chinese Sign Language: A study guide). Beijing: Huaxia chubanshe.

———. 1996. *Teshu jiaoyu cidian* (Dictionary of special education). Beijing: Huaxia chubanshe.

Plog, Stanley C., and Miles B. Santamour, eds. 1980. *The Year 2000 and Mental Retardation.* New York: Plenum Press.

Podmore, David, and David Chaney. 1974. "Family Norms in a Rapidly Industrialising Society." *Journal of Marriage and the Family,* May, 400–407.

Population Research Office, Anhui University. 1982. "A Survey of One-Child Families in Anhui Province, China." *Studies in Family Planning* 13(6/7): 216–21.

Poston, Dudley, and Yu Meiyu. 1985. "Quality of Life, Intellectual Development, and Behavioural Characteristics of Single Children in China: Evidence from a 1980 Survey in Changsha, Hunan Province." *Journal of Biosocial Sciences* 17:127–36.

Press, Billie. 1987. "Observation on Early Child Development and Education in the People's Republic of China." *Early Child Development and Care* 29: 375–89.

"Provincial Responses to Rising Fertility in China." 1987. *Population and Development Review* 13(2): 363–69.

Reardon, W. 1998. "Connexin 26 Gene Mutation and Autosomal Recessive Deafness." *Lancet* 351: 383–84.

"Recommendations of the National Institute on Deafness and Other Communication Disorders (NIDCD) Working Group on Early Identification of Hearing Impairment on Acceptable Protocols for Use in Statewide Universal Newborn Hearing Screening Programs." 1997. Document developed at workshop on Universal Newborn Hearing Screening, Chevy Chase, Md., 4–5 September.

Reed, Helen. 1995. "NDCS Deaf Children in Mind Project: Personal and Social Development Initiative." Project outline. London: National Deaf Children's Society.

Rinne, Mary Glenn. 1997. "Potential Barriers to Implementing a Bilingual/Bicultural Program for Deaf Children." *Sign Language Studies* 93: 327–55.

Robinson, Kathy. 1991. *Children of Silence: The Story of My Daughters' Triumph over Deafness.* Rev. ed. New York: Penguin.

Roeser, Ross, John Campbell, and Aram Glorig. 1975. "Acupuncture and Sensorineural Hearing Loss: Objective and Subjective Analyses." *EENT Monthly* 54: 16–20.

Rosen, Samuel. 1974. "Feasibility of Acupuncture as a Treatment for Sensorineural Deafness in Children." *Laryngoscope* 84(2): 2202–17.

"Rural Health: Basics Neglected for Services That Pay." 1997. *China Development Briefing,* no. 5: 5–9.

Russell, James, and Michelle Yik. 1996. "Emotion among the Chinese." In *The Handbook of Chinese Psychology,* ed. Michael Harris Bond. Hong Kong: Oxford University Press.

"Scandal of Austria's Forced Sterilisations." 1997. *Daily Mail,* 28 August.

Schein, Jerome D. 1989. *At Home among Strangers.* Washington, D.C.: Gallaudet University Press.

Searl, Alan. 1997. "National Dialect Renamed." *China in Focus,* winter, 7.

Shapiro, Jack. 1989. "China and the Spirit of Change. *Soundbarrier* 23: 23.

Shaw, Pauline. 1985. *The Deaf Can Speak.* London: Faber and Faber.

Shofield, Janet Ward. 1993. "Increasing the Generalizability of Qualitative Research." In *Social Research: Philosophy, Politics and Practice,* ed. Martyn Hammersley. London: Open University Press; Sage Publications.

Shu Zhilan. 1995. "Jianli jianquan long'er jiazhang hanshou gongzuo" (Strengthening and consolidating the work of teaching children's parents through correspondence). In *Suzhou lunwen huibian* (Suzhou Conference Proceedings), 197.

Snow, J. 1995. "Aminoglycoside Ototoxicity." *Hearing International* 4(2): 11.

Solomon, Richard H. 1971. *Mao's Revolution and the Chinese Political Culture.* Berkeley: University of California Press.

Spradley, Thomas S., and James P. Spradley. 1978. *Deaf Like Me.* New York: Random House.

"Statistics on Deafness and Hearing Disorders in the United States." 1998. Factsheet issued by the National Institute on Deafness and Other Communication Disorders (NIDCD) Information Clearinghouse, Bethesda, Md.

Stedt, Joseph, and Donald F. Moores. 1990. "Manual Codes on English and American Sign Language: Historical Perspectives and Current Realities." In *Manual Communication: Implications for Education,* ed. Harry Bornstein, 1–20. Washington, D.C.: Gallaudet University Press.

Stokoe, William, and Robbin Battison. 1981. "Sign Language, Mental Health, and Satisfactory Interaction." In *Deafness and Mental Health,* ed. Laszlo K. Stein, Eugene D. Mindel, and Theresa Jabaley, 179–94. New York: Grune and Stratton.

Stone, Emma. 1996. "A Law to Protect, a Law to Prevent: Contextualising Disability Legislation in China." *Disability and Society* 11(4): 469–83.

Sutton, Andrew. 1977. "Acupuncture and Deaf-Mutism — An Essay in Cross-Cultural Defectology." *Educational Studies* 3(1): 1–10.

Sydenham, Kate. 1993. "Approaching Childhood Disability in a Developing Socialist Nation." Undergraduate thesis, School of East Asian Studies, University of Durham, U.K.

Tang Xiaoquan. 1992. "Shi lun wo guo 'ba wu' long'er kangfu gongzuo fang'an de shishi" (The implementation of China's Eighth Five-Year Plan for the rehabilitation of deaf children). *Zhongguo long'er kangfu* (Rehabilitation of Deaf Children in China), no. 2: 2–5.

———. 1993. "Zai shou jie quan guo long'er kangfu shequ jiating moshi yantao hui shang de fayan" (Speech at opening session of the national conference on models for the social and family rehabilitation of deaf children). *Zhongguo long'er kangfu* (Rehabilitation of Deaf Children in China), no. 1: 6–9.

Tao Kuotai, Qiu Jinghwa, Li Baolin, Tseng Wenshing, Hsu Jing, and D. McLaughlin. 1995. "One-Child-Per-Couple Family Planning and Child Behaviour Development: Six-Year Follow-up Study in Nanjing." In *Chinese Societies and Mental Health*, ed. Lin Tsung-yi, Tseng Wenshing, and Yeh Eng-Kung, 78–92. New York: Oxford University Press.

Thomas, Felicity. 1998. "Perilous Waters." *China in Focus*, summer, 12–13.

Tobin, Joseph J., David Y. H. Wu, and Dana H. Davidson. 1989. *Preschool in Three Cultures: Japan, China, and the United States*. New Haven: Yale University Press.

Tyler, Richard, and He Ningji. 1990. "Audiology in China." *American Speech-Language-Hearing Association (ASHA)* 32(5): 40–42.

Wang Hua. 1988. "How Many Are Handicapped?" *China Daily*, 7 January, 4.

Wang Kai. 1995. "Wo yong qigong zhiliao erji de jingguo" (My experience of using *qigong* to cure deafness). *Zhongguo canji ren* (Disability in China), 1: 31.

Wang Yarong. 1992. "Long'er kangfu ying lizu yu jiating" (The rehabilitation of deaf children should gain a foothold in the family). *Zhongguo long'er kangfu* (Rehabilitation of Deaf Children in China), no. 1: 26–27.

Wang Youguo. 1995a. "Jiazhang a, qing ni zhe wei zhujue shangtai — qiantan long'er kangfu ji jiazhang de zuoyong" (Parents, you should play the main role — strengthening the role of parents in deaf children's rehabilitation). In *Suzhou lunwen huibian* (Suzhou Conference Proceedings), 188–90.

———. 1995b. "Long'er kangfu xuyao jiazhang peihe" (The rehabilitation of deaf children requires the cooperation of parents). *Zhongguo long'er kangfu* (Rehabilitation of Deaf Children in China), no. 2: 19–21.

Wei Jianing, A. Fourcin, and A. Faulkner. 1992. "Speech Pattern Processing for Chinese Listeners with Profound Hearing Loss." Paper presented at International Congress on Acoustics, September, Beijing.

"When Illness Strikes: Greater Risks and Less Protection for Rural People." 1994. *Amity Newsletter*, no. 29: 5.

White, Gordon, Jude Howell, and Shang Xiaoyuan. 1996. *In Search of Civil Society: Market Reform and Social Change in Contemporary China*. Oxford: Clarendon; New York: Oxford University Press.

"Work for the Deaf in China." 1994. Document obtained from China Association of the Deaf, May 1996.

Work Program for Disabled Persons during the Ninth Five-Year Plan Period, 1996–2000. 1996. Beijing: China Disabled People's Federation.

Wright, A., A. Forge, and B. Kotecha. 1997. "Ototoxicity." Chapter 20 of *Otology*, ed. John Boothe, 3:1–36. In *Scott-Brown's Otolaryngology*, 6th ed., gen. ed. Alan G. Kerr. Oxford: Butterworth-Heinemann.

Wu, David. 1985. "Child Training in Chinese Culture." In *Chinese Culture and Mental Health*, ed. Tseng Wen-shing and David Wu, 113–33. Orlando, Fla.: Academic Press.

———. 1996. "Chinese Childhood Socialization." In *The Handbook of Chinese Psychology*, ed. Michael Harris Bond, 143–54. Hong Kong: Oxford University Press.

Xu Qianren, Gu Baofeng, and Chen Xiaoping. 1995. "'Long' 'long' zhi bian" (A deaf boy changes into a dragon). *Zhongguo canji ren* (Disability in China) 3: 44–45.

Xu S. A., R. Dowell, and G. Clark. 1987. "Results for Chinese and English in a Multi-channel Cochlear Implant Patient." *Annals of Otology, Rhinology, and Laryngology* 96 (suppl. 128): 126–27.

Xu Tinggui. 1993. "Kaizhan yi jiating xunlian wei zhu de long'er shequ kangfu de jidian shexiang" (Some ideas on giving priority to family training in the social rehabilitation of deaf children). *Zhongguo long'er kangfu* (Rehabilitation of Deaf Children in China), no. 1: 25–26.

Xu Xiaoming, Wang Wei, Zhang Jianxing, Yang Jianmin, Bai Zhenning, and Liu Baoshan. 1995. "Henan Zhoukou diqu 98 ming long'er xianzhuang diaocha fenxi" (Survey of the current situation of 98 deaf children in Henan province, Zhoukou district). *Zhongguo long'er kangfu* (Rehabilitation of Deaf Children in China), no. 1: 23–25.

Yan Fuchu. 1979. "Tong yi jiazu lianmeisu erzhongdu jiu li baogao" (Streptomycin ototoxicity in one family: A report of nine cases). *Zhongguo erbiyanhouke zazhi* (Chinese Journal of Otorhinolaryngology) 14(1): 27–30.

Yang H., Kao H., and Wang W. 1980. "Survey of Only Children in Educational Institutes of Beijing City Districts." *China Youth Daily*, 2 October.

Yang Jianmin. 1995. "Zhoukou diqu 0–8 sui ertong qingdameisu zhi long 437 li fenxi" (Analysis of the cases of 437 children aged 0 to 8 years deafened by gentamycin in Zhoukou district). In *Suzhou lunwen huibian* (Suzhou Conference Proceedings), 19–20.

Yang Kuo-shu. 1986. "Chinese Personality and Its Change." In *The Psychology of the Chinese People*, ed. Michael Harris Bond, 106–70. Hong Kong: Oxford University Press.

———. 1996. "Psychological Transformation of the Chinese People as a Result of Societal Modernization." In *The Handbook of Chinese Psychology*, ed. Michael Harris Bond, 479–98. Hong Kong: Oxford University Press.

Yang Rongxian. 1995. "Fanfu shequ long'er jiating kangfu zhidao" (Overview of deaf children's family rehabilitation community guidance). Abstract. In *Suzhou lunwen huibian* (Suzhou Conference Proceedings), 251.

Yau Shun-chiu. 1987. "Chinese." In *Gallaudet Encyclopedia of Deaf People and Deafness*, ed. John V. Van Cleve. New York: McGraw-Hill.

———. 1996. "The Weight of Tradition in the Formation of the Name Signs of the Deaf in China." *Diogenes* 17: 55–65.

Yau Shun-chiu, and He Jingxian. 1989. How Deaf Children in a Chinese Deaf School Get Their Name Signs." *Sign Language Studies* 65: 305–22.

Yin Zhiyun, and Liu Fuyun. 1995. "Ba long'er yuxun gongzuo de zhongdian fang dao nongcun" (We should put emphasis on deaf children's language training work in the countryside). Abstract. In *Suzhou lunwen huibian* (Suzhou Conference Proceedings), 208.

Young, Alys. 1995. "Family Adjustment to a Deaf Child in a Bilingual Framework." Ph.D. diss., University of Bristol, U.K.

Young, Alys, J. Ackerman, and Jim Kyle. 1998. *Looking On: Deaf People and the Organisation of Services*. Bristol: Policy Press.

Young, Mary E., and André Prost. 1985. *Child Health in China*. World Bank Staff Working Papers no. 767. Washington, D.C.: World Bank.

Yu An-bang. 1996. "Ultimate Life Concerns, Self, and Chinese Achievement Motivation." In *The Handbook of Chinese Psychology,* ed. Michael Harris Bond, 227–46. Hong Kong: Oxford University Press.

Zeng, Fangang. 1995. "Cochlear Implants in China." *Audiology* 34: 61–75.

Zeng Yi. 1986. "Changes in Family Structure in China: A Simulation Study." *Population and Development Review* 12(4): 675–703.

———. 1996. "Is Fertility in China in 1991–92 Far Below Replacement Level?" *Population Studies* 50(1): 27–34.

Zeng Yi, Tu Ping, Gu Baochang, Xu Yi, Li Bohua, and Li Yongping. 1993. "Causes and Implications of the Recent Increase in the Reported Sex Ratio at Birth in China." *Population and Development Review* 19(2): 283–302.

Zhang Meijuan. 1996. "Wo jiao nu'er xue shuo hua" (I teach my daughter to speak). *Zhongguo long'er kangfu* (Rehabilitation of Deaf Children in China), no. 1: 28–29.

Zhang Mingliang. 1991. "Yu long'er jiazhang tantanxin" (Talking with deaf children's parents). *Zhongguo long'er kangfu* (Rehabilitation of Deaf Children in China), no. 1: 13.

Zhang Suping. 1992. "Jiazhang yao canyu long you'er de yuxun jiaoxue" (Parents should take part in the speech training teaching of deaf children). *Zhongguo long'er kangfu* (Rehabilitation of Deaf Children in China), no. 1: 29.

Zhongguo canji ren shiye "jiu wu" jihua gangyao yu peitao shishi fang'an (Outline program and set of implementation plans for China's disabled people in the Ninth Five-Year Plan). 1996. Beijing: Huaxia chubanshe.

Zhou Hong, and Zhou Tingting. 1990. *Cong Nu'er dao Shentong* (From mute girl to child prodigy). Harbin: Harbin chubanshe.

Zhou Youguang. 1980. "The Chinese Finger Alphabet and the Chinese Finger Syllabary." *Sign Language Studies* 28: 209–16.

INDEX

Page numbers followed by *t* indicate tables.

abortion: Chinese eugenics policies and, 28; in Great Britain, 279 n. 13; sex-selective, 22, 23–25; views of, 24
acupuncture: as treatment for deafness, 60–62, 63, 150; research on, 62
adenosine triphosphate (ATP), 63
adoption: of deaf children, 211–12; in traditional Chinese families, 12
adult illiteracy, 48
advocacy: parents of deaf children and, 33–34, 255
American Sign Language, 82
aminoglycoside antibiotics, 56–57, 148. *See also* ototoxic antibiotics
Amity Foundation, 5, 258
Amity Rehabilitation Center, 157
anger: family perceptions of, 136
Anhui Province Disabled People's Rehabilitation and Research Center, 105
Annual Survey of Hearing Impaired Children and Youth (Gallaudet University), 52–53
antibiotics: ototoxic, 52, 53*t*, 54, 55–57, 148
apartments, 126
ATP. *See* adenosine triphosphate
audiologists, 58, 280 n. 9
auditory training, 254
Australia, 67
Australian Hearing Services, 280 n. 9

bacterial meningitis, 54
Battison, Robbin, 112
behavior problems: family perceptions of, 136; parents' control strategies, 167–70
behind-the-ear (BTE) aids, 65
benevolence: Confucian concept of, 13
bilingual education: assessment in, 261–62; deaf education and, 85–86; defined, 260; sign language and, 1–2, 85–86, 258–62; tensions between hearing and deaf teachers, 262; viewed by rehabilitation professionals, 260–61
bilingualism: in spoken Chinese, 86–87
births: underreporting of, 278 n. 7
Bishop, Juliet, 112
blind persons: treatment within Chinese families, 17
brain stem evoked response (BSER), 58
breastfeeding, 37
British Deaf News, 63
British Sign Language, 82–83
BSER. *See* brain stem evoked response
BTE aids. *See* behind-the-ear aids
Buddhism: traditional views of disabled persons, 80

CAD. *See* China Association for the Deaf
canfei (disabled person), 283 n. 6
canji (disabled person), 283 n. 6
Carter, Anita, 79
CDPF. *See* China Disabled People's Federation

307

Central Document Seven, 22
Centre for Deaf Studies (Bristol University), 1, 258
Chefoo School, 68, 79, 80
Chen Guiqin, 120
Chen Minzhang, 26, 27
child care: family stresses about, 213–15
child-rearing: contemporary urban values and practices, 38–41; of deaf children, 46–47, 166–70; studies of only children, 41–43; traditional values and practices, 36–38
children: Cultural Revolution and, 15; in rural families, 16; single, studies of, 41–43; socialization in preschool, 43–45; in traditional Chinese families, 12; in urban families, 16. *See also* deaf children
children, spoiling of: characterized by rehabilitation professionals, 110; concerns for single children, 41, 42–43, 99; prevention, 189; school socialization and, 43; traditional child-rearing and, 37–38, 40–41
China: civil society in, 19–20; deaf education in, 68–72; employment quotas for disabled persons, 257; ethnic minorities in, 26, 277 n. 4; family planning policies, 20–35; food and, emotional significance of, 279 n. 15; government policies for disabled persons, 72–75, 108–9; initiatives for preschool-age deaf children, 75–78; language standardization in, 86–87, 115, 281 n. 19; medical services for deafness, 57–68; national publicity for parent exemplars, 115–17; official organization for deaf persons, 92; population distribution in, 48; prevalence of hearing loss and deafness in, 49–50; raising status of disabled persons in, 257–58; sex ratios at birth, 23, 50–51; surveys of deaf children, 4, 49–56; twentieth-century reforms, overview of, 13–16; unemployment in, 257; urban-rural disparities in, 48; views of disabled persons in, 79–81; Western criticism of eugenics in, 31; Western medicine and, 59–60
China Association for the Deaf (CAD), 89, 92
China Disabled People's Federation (CDPF), 57, 73, 74, 81
China Rehabilitation Research Center for Deaf Children, 32; cochlear implants and, 67; hearing aid use at, 66; initiatives for preschool-age children and, 76–77, 78; number of students with deaf parents, 282 n. 22; rejection of child-centered approaches, 121; school for parents at, 119
China Welfare Fund for the Handicapped, 73
Chinese, spoken: bilingualism in, 86–87; children's skills in, 177–79; Chinese sign languages and, 83; deaf children's understanding of, 174–75; standardization in, 86–87, 115, 281 n. 19. *See also* speech
Chinese, written: Chinese sign languages and, 88. *See also* writing
Chinese Communist Party, 14–15
Chinese families: child-rearing values and practices, 36–38; children in, 12; civil society and, 19–20; economic impact of disabled family members, 18; effects of twentieth-century reforms on, 13–16; hierarchy in, 13; housing conditions, 125–27; influence of Confucianism on, 12–13; male dominance in, 11; only children in, 40–43; poverty

and, 11–12; role of everyday speech in, 47; sleeping arrangements, 127; treatment of disabled family members, 16–19. *See also* families with deaf children; rural families; urban families; urban families with deaf children

Chinese Sign Language: in deaf schools, 71–72; development of, 82; standardization and, 82, 83, 87. *See also* sign language

Chinese Sign Language Reform Committee, 87

Ching, Lucy, 17, 80, 81

civil society: Chinese families and, 19–20

cochlear implants, 66–68, 223–24

collectives, 14, 15

communes, 14–15

communication at home: children's oral skills, 177–79; children's understanding of spoken Chinese, 174–75; Chinese perspectives on, 113–14; between deaf and hearing children, 165; in deaf families, 180; getting attention, 172; levels desired by parents, 182; modes of, 173–74; parents' and children's strategies in, 175–77; parents' concerns about, 193–94; parents' perception of, 171; parents' views of sign language, 180–83; recommendations to improve, 240, 255; relative value of reading, writing, and speech, 183–85; with signs or gestures, 170, 173–74, 179–80; traditional family hierarchies, 38; Western perspectives on, 111–13

community rehabilitation, 99–100

Confucianism: "five relationships," 12–13; influence on child-rearing values and practices, 36; traditional views of disabled persons and, 80

consanguineous marriages, 26–27

cooking: child safety and, 170

corporal punishment, 41, 168–69

counseling, 118; inadequacy of, 237

cousins, 163–64

Croll, Elisabeth, 15, 123, 124

Cultural Revolution, 15

Dai Mu, 92

Davidson, Dana H., 44

deaf awareness, 283 n. 4; cultural context and, 195

deaf children: access to preschool rehabilitation, 70, 107, 254; acupuncture treatment, 62; adoption of, 211–12; categorized as hearing-speech disabled, 279 n. 1; child-rearing practices, 46–47, 166–70; in the Chinese model of rehabilitation, 120–21; Chinese surveys of, 4, 49–56; cochlear implants and, 67; communication at home, 111–14, 171–85; communication with hearing children, 165; described in the letters to Zhou Hong, 204–7; diagnosis of deafness in, 143–44, 208–9; emotional problems and, 110–14; family structures and, 132–33; gesture language and, 179–80; government initiatives for, 75–78; grandparents and, 132–35; hearing aid use, 65–66, 76, 158–59, 237–38; housing conditions and, 126; mainstream schools and, 185–86, 191–92, 215–16, 227–28, 238–39, 255–57; name signs and, 282 n. 23; numbers of, 50; numbers with deaf parents, 88, 281 n. 20; oral skills of, 177–79; parents' emphasis on speech, 174–75, 183–84, 185, 216–17; parents' hopes and concerns for the future, 191–92, 215–17, 236; parents'

deaf children (*continued*)
rejection of, 32; parents' views of, 135–38, 154–56; preschool deaf education and, long-term impact of, 196–97; relationships with other children, 163–65; in rural regions, 282 n. 2 (*see also* rural families; rural populations/regions); safety issues and, 170; services for, 33–34; sex ratios, 50–51; sign language and, parents' views of, 180–83; sleeping arrangements, 127; socialization and, 46–47, 99; in social situations, 159–63; society's views of, 34–35, 79–80; study participants, characteristics of, 132; study participants, follow-up reports on, 195–96; understanding of spoken Chinese, 174–75; views of Western parents toward, 137, 142; Western studies on, 4. *See also* families with deaf children; urban families with deaf children

Deaf Children in Mind project (Britain), 113

deaf community: adult role models and, 91–92; China Association for the Deaf and, 92; deaf families and, 88–89; membership in, 282 n. 24; personal networks and, 89; role of deaf schools and welfare factories in, 89

deaf culture, 281–82 n. 21; adult role models and, 91–92; perspectives on, 90–91

deaf education: bilingual approaches to, 85–86, 258–62; children's progress in, parents' views of, 190–91; Chinese sign language and, 71–72, 82, 84–86; choosing nursery schools, 185–86; curriculum, 71; developing future approaches to, 262–65; fingerspelling in, 68; future of, 240–41; history of, 68–70; official description of methods in, 85; parents' advocacy and, 33–34; parents as teachers, 117–18, 186–87, 224–27; parents' involvement in, arguments for, 93–96; parents' meetings at school, 187–90; parents' responsibilities in, 114–15; rights of deaf persons to, 75; in rural and urban areas, 70, 71; traditional views of, 80. *See also* family rehabilitation; preschool rehabilitation

deaf families, 88–89; communication in, 180; family planning policies and, 35; numbers of, 281 n. 20

deaf-mutes, 233, 234, 236

deafness: causes of, 52, 53*t*, 54–57; changing cultural attitudes toward, 257–58; degrees of hearing loss, 52; described in the letters to Zhou Hong, 205–7; diagnosis of, 143–44, 208–9; images of health and illness, 231–33; images of muteness, 233–34; images of normality, 235–36; images of sound and soundlessness, 234–35; improving cultural attitudes toward, 240; medical services for, 57–68; parents' access to information about, 156–58, 239; parents' attitudes toward, 81, 137, 231–36, 238, 253; parents' perception of causes, 148–49; parents' previous experience of, 154–56; prevalence of, 49–50; sex ratios, 50–51; socioeconomic correlates in the U.S., 279 n. 3; treatments, 150–51 (*see also* treatments for deafness); urban-rural distribution figures, 51; in the U.S., causes and prevention of, 52–54. *See also* hereditary deafness

deafness screening programs, 239, 278–79 n. 12

deaf organizations, 92. *See also* parents' organizations/networks; support groups
deaf parents: communication with deaf children, 111–12; family planning policies and, 35; numbers with deaf children, 88, 281 n. 20; occupations of, 130
"deaf people's sign language," 83, 84
deaf persons: contemporary views of, 80–81; impact within Chinese families, 17; marriages between, 35; raising status of, 257–58; as role models in deaf culture, 91–92; services for, 33, 57–68; stigmatization of, 17; traditional views of, 79–80
deaf schools: access to, 70, 107, 254; Chinese sign language in, 71–72, 84–85; curriculum in, 71; deaf culture and, 90–91; future of, 240–41; history of, 68, 69–70; name signs for students, 282 n. 23; numbers of, 69–70; population characteristics, 70–71; role in deaf community, 89; in rural areas, 107; speech and oral classes in, 280–81 n. 13. *See also* preschool rehabilitation centers
deaf services: medical, 57–68; in urban areas, 33–34
deaf teachers: in bilingual classes, 258–60, 261; conflicts with hearing teachers, 262; declining numbers of, 72; as role models in deaf culture, 91; viewed by rehabilitation professionals, 260–61
Deng Pufang, 72–73, 81
denial of deafness, by parents, 103–4
desensitization treatment, 63
diagnosis: grandparents' response to, 146–48; inadequacy of support services during, 237; parents' responses to, 100–105, 142, 144–46, 209–12; parents' role in, 143–44, 208–9, 237; recommendations for improving, 254
Dictionary of Special Education (Piao), 85
disabilities: Chinese government policies on, 108–9; Chinese eugenics policies and, 25–31; economic impact on Chinese families, 18; preventive health-care and, 28–29; stigmatization of, 17
Disability in China (journal), 60, 116
disabled children: attitudes toward having, 30, 280 n. 6; eugenics policies and, 28–30, 278 n. 9; views of, 34–35
disabled persons: Chinese eugenics policies and, 25–31; Chinese terms for, 283 n. 6; contemporary views of, 80–81; economic impact on Chinese families, 18; government policies and, 72–75; raising status of, 257–58; stigmatization of, 17; traditional views of, 79–80; treatment within Chinese families, 16–19; U.S. medical policies and, 278 n. 9
discipline, 99, 166–70. *See also* child-rearing
disease: deafness viewed as, 232–33
doctors: serial consultations by parents, 58–59, 104–5, 149, 150, 237, 239–40
drugs: ototoxic, 52, 53*t*, 54, 55–57

ear, nose, and throat physicians, 58
early childhood intervention: arguments for parental involvement in, 93–96; Western opinions on, 96. *See also* preschool rehabilitation
education: grandparents' levels, 131; mainstreaming and, (*see* mainstreaming); parents' levels, 106, 129–30, 203–4; practices in pre-

education (*continued*)
  school, 43–45; rights of disabled persons to, 75; traditional views of, 38, 40. *See also* deaf education; mainstreaming; preschool rehabilitation
Eighth Five-Year Plan, 74, 76, 94
emotional problems: Chinese characterizations of, 110–11, 113–14; Western characterizations of, 111–13
employment: family conflicts with child care and, 213–14; links to rehabilitation success, 106–8; parents' hopes and concerns for their child, 191–92; quotas for disabled persons, 257
ethnic minorities, 26, 277 n. 4
eugenics policies: coercion and, 30; on consanguineous marriages, 26–27; criticisms of, 28–32; ethnic minorities and, 26; impetus for, 25, 28; involuntary sterilization and, 30–31; laws implementing, 25, 27–28; overview of, 25–26, 27–28; types of, 25
Europe: diversity of family life in, 194–95

families. *See* Chinese families; families with deaf children; rural families; urban families; urban families with deaf children
families with deaf children: adoption of deaf children, 211–12; communication in, 111–13, 171–85; conflicts and stresses, 213–15; dynamics within, 34; family structures, 132–33, 207–8; financial resources and, 241; hopes and concerns for their child's future, 191–93, 215–17, 236; rejection of deaf children, 32; second children and, 32–35; serial consultation of physicians, 58–59, 104–5, 149, 150, 237, 239–40; stresses in, 213–15; Western studies on, 4. *See also* deaf families; urban families with deaf children
family education: definition of, 97; one-child family policy and, 97–98; parental responsibilities in, 98–99
family planning policies: applied to deaf couples, 35; eugenic, 25–31; one-child policy, 20–25; second children and, 32–35; underreporting of births, 278 n. 7
family rehabilitation: arguments for, 93–96; concepts of family education in, 97–98; issues of language in, 115; parents' responsibilities in, 98–99, 114–15; in rural areas, 108–9
family structures, 132–33, 207–8
farming collectives, 14, 15
fathers: traditional child-rearing behaviors, 38
febrile illness, 52, 53*t*
female children: disabled, perceptions of, 34–35; infanticide and, 22, 23, 24; one-child family planning policy and, 21, 22, 23–25; sex-selective abortion and, 22, 23–25; in traditional Chinese families, 12; in urban families, 16, 21
female children, deaf: adoption of, 211–12; sex ratios, 50–51; traditional views of, 79
female infanticide: one-child family planning policy and, 22, 23, 24; in traditional Chinese families, 12
feudal practices: reform of, 13–14
filial piety, 36–37, 39
fingerspelling, 68
"five relationships, the," 12–13, 36
Five-Year Plan for Disabled People

(1988–93), 73–74, 75–76. *See also* Eighth Five-Year Plan; Ninth Five-Year Plan
Fletcher, Lorraine, 117
food: emotional significance of, 279 n. 15
From Mute Girl to Child Prodigy (Zhou and Zhou), 116
Fu Zhiwei, 92

Gao Chenghua, 96
Gao Lihua, 63
genetic diseases: categorization of, 29–30; Chinese eugenics policies and, 25–32. *See also* hereditary deafness
genetic screening, 278–79 n. 12
gentamycin, as cause of deafness, 54, 56
"gesture language," 83, 84
gestures, use of, 173–74, 179–80
grandparents: as caregivers, 132–33, 134; deaf child's relationships with other children and, 163–65; diagnosis of child deafness and, 146–48; educational levels of, 131; frequency of contact with deaf children, 133–34; occupations of, 132; previous experience with deafness, 155, 156; relationship with parents of deaf children, 215; as teachers, 134–35
Great Britain: abortions in, 279 n. 13; deaf community membership, 282 n. 24; genetic screening for deafness and, 278–79 n. 12; notions of parent-professional interactions, 119; numbers of deaf families in, 281 n. 20; parents' perceptions of deaf children, 137; programs for assisting parent-child communication, 112–13

Greenberg, Mark, 113
Gregory, Susan, 4, 82, 112, 174
guan (teacher authority), 44
guilt, 279–80 n. 4
Guo Xi, 100–101, 115

health care, 48
hearing aids, 65–66, 76; parents' reasons not to buy, 223; parents' responsibilities for, 114; parents' views of, 158–59, 222–23, 237–38
hearing loss: described in the letters to Zhou Hong, 205–7; socioeconomic correlates in the U.S., 279 n. 3
He Ningji, 65
herbal therapies, 62–63, 151
hereditary deafness: connexin 26 gene and, 278 n. 12; genetic testing and, 278–79 n. 12; incidence of, 52, 53*t*; parents' denial of, 54–55, 206
Hexagon Well Primary School (Nanjing), 6
home education, 186–87, 224–27. *See also* parents of deaf children: family rehabilitation responsibilities, preschool rehabilitation and
hong (persuasion), 41
housing conditions, 125–27
Huang Kaicheng, 117
Hua Wenli, 115

illiteracy rates, 48
income levels: of parents of deaf children, 130–31
infanticide. *See* female infanticide
infants: causes and prevention of deafness in, 52, 53–54; disabled, U.S. medical policies and, 278 n. 9
interviews: evaluating and generalizing results from, 7–10; issues of cultural bias and, 6–7; occupations of per-

interviews (*continued*)
sons interviewed, 6; parents' views of, 127–28; points of focus in, 122–23; preparations for, 3–5; process of, 5–6, 124–25; research goals for, 2–3; transcription and translation of, 128. *See also* questionnaires
intravenous therapy, 151, 152
involuntary sterilization policies, 30–31
iron tree, as metaphor for deaf child, 284 n. 10

Jenner, William, 19, 87

kanamycin, as cause of deafness, 56
Keller, Helen, 116
Kessen, William, 45
kindergarten: child socialization and educational practices in, 43–45; national curriculum, 44

land reform, 14–15
language development: implications for mainstreaming, 255–57; parents' lack of awareness about, 195; recommendations for, 255
language skills: parents' views of, 183–85
Law on the Protection of Disabled Persons (1990), 26, 74–75, 280 n. 12
Lei Feng, 116
letters to Zhou Hong, 241–52; analysis of, 8–9, 201–2; basic patterns of, 200–201; characteristics of writers, 9–10, 200, 202–4; on cochlear implants, 223–24; criteria for inclusion in analysis, 199–200; on deaf children, 204–7; on diagnosis of deafness, 208–12; on family conflicts and stresses, 213–15; on family structures, 207–8; geographical distribution of writers, 204, 205*t*;

on hearing aids, 222–23; on home education, 224–27; key issues in, 236–39, 241; on mainstreaming deaf children, 227–28; media coverage of Zhou Hong and, 198–99; parents' attitudes toward deafness in, 231–36; parents' hopes and fears described in, 215–17; parents' pursuit of treatments for deafness described in, 217–21; requests for help from parents, 228–31; on second children, 207–8; translation of, 201
Lian Yong, 106
Li Ming, 263–64
lipreading, 175
Li Shaozhu, 100–101
Liu Fudian, 101–2, 103–4, 107
Liu Qian, 62
Liu Xin, 110
Liu Yanxia, 110
Liu Zhenxing, 68, 91, 107
Li Yingui, 118
long (deafness), 233
longya ren (deaf-mute person), 233
longya xuexiao (deaf-mute school), 233

mainstreaming: critical issues in, 240; language development and, 255–57; Law on the Protection of Disabled Persons and, 280 n. 12; parents' hopes and concerns for, 191–92, 215–16, 227–28, 238–39
male children: deaf, sex ratios and, 50–51; in traditional Chinese families, 12; in urban families, 16
Mandarin Chinese, 86–87
Mao Zedong: Cultural Revolution and, 15; family planning policies and, 20
marriage: of deaf couples, 35
Marriage Law of 1950, 14
Marriage Law of 1981, 27

marriages, consanguineous, 26–27
Maternal and Child Health Care Law of 1995, 25, 27–28, 29, 30, 35
maternal illnesses, 52, 53*t*, 55, 148
medical services: cochlear implants, 66–68; costs of, 152; diagnostic, 58–59; hearing aids, 65–66; overview of, 57–58; parents' access to information about, 156–58, 239; parents' pursuit of cures, 153–54, 217–19, 237; reimbursements and, 152–53; serial consultations by parents, 58–59, 104–5, 149–50, 237, 239–40. *See also* support services; treatments for deafness
Mei Fusheng, 86
Mencius, 12–13
Meng Sheng, 110
meningitis. *See* bacterial meningitis
mental illness, 18–19
mental retardation: environmental causes of, 28; eugenics policies and, 25, 26, 28; involuntary sterilization policies and, 30–31; number of people with, 25; in the U.S., 278 n. 8
middle ear infections, 52, 53*t*, 54
Mills, Annetta, 68
Modern Special Education (journal), 115
moral training, 71
mothers: bearing unwanted children, 280 n. 6; in child rehabilitation, 107, 108; family stresses and, 213–15; maternal illnesses, 52, 53*t*, 55, 148; responsibilities in family rehabilitation, 114–15
moxibustion, 62
muteness, 233–34, 236

name signs, 282 n. 23
Nanjing Deaf School, 183, 258, 283 n. 11
Nanjing Normal University, 77

National Survey of the Disabled (China), 49–56
negative eugenics, 25
neomycin, 56
neonates. *See* infants
ni'ai (spoiling children), 37
Ninth Five-Year Plan, 57, 74; goals for deaf education, 70; goals for preschool-age deaf children, 76, 77–78; proposal for family rehabilitation guidance stations, 108–9
Normal School for Special Education (Nanjing), 72
normative bias, 124

occupations: of grandparents, 132; links to rehabilitation success, 106–7; of parents, 106–7, 130
one-child family planning policy: background to, 20–21; Central Document Seven, 22; compliance in urban and rural families, 21–22; effect of, on child's behavior, 41–43; eugenics and, 25, 30; exemptions to, 21, 32, 34; family education and, 97–98; increases in sex-selective abortion and female infanticide, 22, 23–25; parental expectations for children and, 101–2
orphanages, 31
ototoxic antibiotics: deafness and, 52, 53*t*, 54, 55–57, 148; eclectic therapies for, 63; natural reversibility of toxicity, 64

Pan Longsheng, 106–7
parent-child communication: Chinese perspectives on, 113–14; recommendations to improve, 240, 255; Western perspectives on, 111–13. *See also* communication at home
parents, Chinese: child-rearing practices and values, 36–41; in concepts

parents, Chinese (*continued*)
of family education, 97; corporal punishment and, 41; traditional notions of filial piety, 36–37. *See also* parents of deaf children
parents, Western: perceptions of deaf children, 137, 142
parents of deaf children: acquaintance with other deaf people, 154–56; advocacy of deaf interests, 33, 255; attitudes toward deafness, 81, 137, 231–36, 238, 253; authorship of letters to Zhou Hong, 200, 202–4; child-rearing practices, 166–70; children's language skills and, 183–85; children's progress in school and, 190–91; on cochlear implants, 223–24; communication at home, 111–13, 171–85; deaf awareness and, 126; diagnosis of deafness, role in, 143–44, 208–9, 237; educational levels, 106, 129–30, 203–4; family rehabilitation responsibilities, 98–99, 114–15; financial resources and, 241; gesture language and, 174, 179–80; grandparents and, 215; guilt and, 279–80 n. 4; hearing aids and, 66, 158–59, 222–23, 237–38; hereditary deafness and, denial of, 54–55, 206; hopes and concerns for their child's future, 191–93, 215–17, 236; income level and, 105, 130–31; knowledge of language development and, 195; in mainstream classrooms, 256; mainstreaming and, hopes and concerns for, 191–92, 215–16, 227–28, 238–39; as national exemplars, 115–17; occupations of, 130; parents' meetings at school and, 187–90; parents' organizations and, 20, 254–55, 277 n. 3, 283–84 n. 12; perceptions of causes of deafness, 148–49; perceptions of child's personality, 135–38, 154–56; personal accounts by, 5; preschool rehabilitation and, 93–96, 108, 109, 118–20, 119, 121; preschool rehabilitation success, socioeconomic correlations, 105–9; reaction to diagnosis of deafness, 100–105, 142, 144–46; rejection of their children, 32; requests to Zhou Hong for help, 228–31; safety issues and, 170; second children and, 32–35, 138–42; serial consultation of doctors, 58–59, 104–5, 149–50, 237, 239–40; sign language and, instruction in, 183, 260; sign language and, views of, 114, 180–83; social contacts and, 159–65; speech training and, 47, 64, 95, 221, 225–27, 237; as study participants, 9–10, 127–28, 193–94, 195–96; as teachers, 117–18, 186–87, 224–27; treatments for deafness, search for, 149–54, 156–58, 217–21, 237, 239–40; valuing children's ability to speak, 174–75, 183–84, 185, 216–17; Western characterizations of, 104–5
parents' organizations/networks, 20; recommendations for, 254–55; spontaneous, 277 n. 3, 283–84 n. 12; Western perspectives on, 7. *See also* support groups
parents' schools, 119
Parsons, Frances, 84
"passing" concept, 277 n. 2
PATH project. *See* Providing Alternative Thinking Strategies project
patriarchy, 11
Peking Union Medical College, 280 n. 9

People's Daily (newspaper), 25
Phillips, Michael, 17–18
Piao Yongxin, 83–84
pinyin, 115, 281 n. 15
positive eugenics, 25
poverty: Chinese families and, 11–12; Chinese perceptions of, 103
pregnancy and deafness, 52, 53*t*
preschool rehabilitation: access to, 70, 107, 254; children's progress in, parents' views of, 190–91; choosing nursery schools, 185–86; costs of and subsidies for, 108; counseling and, 118; critical issues in, 239–41; definitions and concepts of, 96; developing future approaches to, 262–65; educating parents about, 108, 109, 119; experimental bilingual class in, 258–62; family rehabilitation guidance stations, 108–9; goal of normalization in, 121; government policies and initiatives, 74–78; home education and, 186–87; long-term impact on children, 196–97; mothers in, 107, 108; parent exemplars and, 115–17; parents' access to information about, 156–58; parents' educational level and, 106; parents' employment and, 106–8; parents' income level and, 105; parents' involvement in, arguments for, 93–96; parents' meetings at school, 187–90; parents' views of, 109; practices in, 45; recommendations for improving, 254–57; relationships between parents, professionals and deaf children in, 118–21
preschool rehabilitation centers, 33; access to, 70, 107, 254; choosing, 185–86; costs of and subsidies for, 108; family rehabilitation guidance stations and, 108–9; government initiatives for, 76–78; hearing aid use by children and, 66, 76; long-term impact on children, 196–97; parents' access to information about, 156–58; relationships between parents, professionals, and deaf children in, 120–21; staff shortages and, 77. *See also* deaf schools
preschools, hearing: child socialization and educational practices in, 43–45; deaf children in, 185–86, 227–28 (*see also* mainstreaming); national curriculum, 44
preventive eugenics, 25
profound deafness: prevalence of, 49
Providing Alternative Thinking Strategies (PATH) project, 113
psychological problems: parents' concerns about, 193
putonghua (Mandarin Chinese), 86–87, 115, 281 n. 19

qigong, 60, 63, 151
Qigong and Science (magazine), 60
qi (vital force), 60, 63, 151
Qi Zhaolong, 116
qualitative studies: evaluating and generalizing results from, 7–10. *See also* interviews; questionnaires
questionnaires, 267–76; critique of, 123–24; normative bias and, 124; points of focus in, 122–23; preparation of, 123. *See also* interviews

Railway Medical College (Nanjing), 151
reading: Chinese terms for, 124; parents' valuing of, 184, 185
rehabilitation: community, 99–100; definition of, 3; social, 99. *See also* family rehabilitation; preschool rehabilitation

Rehabilitation of Deaf Children in China (journal), 96
rehabilitation professionals: characterization of children's emotional problems, 110–11; characterization of parental responses to diagnosis, 100–105; characterization of parents' views of rehabilitation, 109; parents who become, 117–18; views of bilingual education, 260–61; views of deaf teachers, 260–61; views of parent-child communication, 113–14
Robinson, Kathy, 117
rubella, 52, 53t, 54, 55, 280 n. 7
rural families: access to rehabilitation programs, 107; characteristics of, 16; consanguineous marriages and, 26–27; one-child family planning policy and, 21–22; second children and, 34; socioeconomic links to rehabilitation success, 105, 106
rural populations/regions: access to deaf schools and rehabilitation programs, 70, 107; causes of deafness in, 52; community rehabilitation in, 100; deaf children in, 282 n. 2; family rehabilitation guidance stations, 108–9; incidence of deafness in, 51; income levels in, 48; isolation of deaf persons in, 90

safety, 170
schizophrenia, 17–18, 19
school principals, 187–88, 189
schools: national curricula, 44; rights of disabled persons to, 75; socialization of children and, 43–45; socialization of deaf children and, 46, 47. *See also* deaf schools; mainstreaming; preschool rehabilitation centers
screening programs, 239, 278–79 n. 12

second children, 32–35; arguments against having, 138–42, 207–8
self-esteem, 111, 112
self-restraint, 36
self-sufficiency, 75
serial consultations: by parents, 58–59, 104–5, 149–50, 237; recommendations to control, 239–40
sex ratios, 23, 50–51
sex-selective abortion, 22, 23–25
sexual equality, 14
Sheldon, Lesley, 112
Shen Yulin, 86
shoushi (sign or gesture), 173
shouyu (sign language), 84, 180
sign language: in bilingual education, 1–2, 85–86, 258–62; grammar of, 83, 84; parents' instruction in, 183, 260; parents' views of, 114, 180–83; Piao Yongxin on, 83–84; recommendations for home use, 240; standardization and, 82, 83, 86–87; teachers' views of, 71–72; as used by deaf people, 83, 84, 86, 87; written Chinese and, 88. *See also* Chinese Sign Language
sign language, informal: arguments to include in deaf education, 86; bilingual education and, 260; in communication at home, 173, 179–80; as gesture language, 83, 84; prevalence and richness of, 87–88; teachers' views of, 71–72
Sign Language Reform Committee, 82, 83
sleeping arrangements, 127
social institutions: Chinese families and, 19
socialization: deaf children and, 46–47, 99; in preschool, 43–45
social rehabilitation, 99
sound and soundlessness, 234–35
speech: children's skills in, 177–79; in

Chinese families, 47; in communication at home, 173, 174; deaf children's understanding of, 174–75; parents' valuing of, 174–75, 183–84, 185, 216–17, 238. *See also* Chinese, spoken
speech training: in deaf schools, 280–81 n. 13; parents and, 47, 64, 95, 221, 225–27, 237; recommendations for, 254; in rehabilitation, 76; viewed as treatment for deafness, 153
spoiling children. *See* children, spoiling of
sterilization, involuntary, 30–31
stigmatization, 17, 277 n. 2
Stokoe, William, 112
streptomycin, as cause of deafness, 56
stress, in family, 213–15
supplementary education, 187
support groups: parents' meetings at school and, 189–90. *See also* parents' organizations/networks
support services: inadequacy of, 237; recommendations for, 239, 240. *See also* medical services
surveys of deaf children, 4, 49–56

Tang Xiaoquan, 94–95, 114
teachers, hearing: Chinese sign language and, 71–72, 84–85; conflicts with deaf teachers, 262; grandparents as, 134–35; lack of deaf awareness, 126; parents as, 117–18, 186–87, 224–27; practices in preschool, 44–45; shortages in rehabilitation centers, 77; training of, 71, 72. *See also* deaf teachers
temper tantrums, 136, 169–70
Tibet/Tibetans, as minority group, 26, 277 n. 4
ting hua (listening), 38, 47
Tobin, Joseph, 44

toilet training, 37
Tongren Hospital (Beijing), 280 n. 9
tongyuhua (Mandarin Chinese), 281 n. 19
traditional medicine, 59–64, 150, 151
traffic: child safety and, 170
treatments for deafness: acupuncture, 60–62, 150; assessments of, 152; costs of, 152, 219–21; effects of, 221; herbal, 62–63, 151; intravenous, 151; massage therapy, 151; parents' access to information about, 156–58, 239; parents' pursuit of cures, 153–54, 217–19, 237; parents' requests to Zhou Hong regarding, 229–31; *qigong*, 60, 63, 151; reimbursements for, 152–53; speech training viewed as, 153; traditional medicine, 59–64; Western medicine, 59–60. *See also* medical services
Tyler, Richard, 65

ultrasounds: sex-selective abortions and, 23–24
unemployment, 257
United Nations Children's Fund (UNICEF), 31, 49, 50
United States: deaf community membership, 282 n. 24; diagnosis of hearing loss in, 58; diversity of family life in, 194–95; genetic screening for deafness and, 278–79 n. 12; involuntary sterilization policies and, 30–31; notions of parent-professional interactions, 119; numbers of deaf families in, 281 n. 20; perspectives on parent-child communication, 111–13; prevalence of mental retardation in, 278 n. 8; socioeconomic correlates with hearing loss, 279 n. 3

urban families: characteristics of, 15–16; child-rearing practices and values, 38–41; compliance with one-child family planning policy, 21; female children in, 21
urban families with deaf children: access to information about treatments for deafness, 156–58; diagnosis of deafness and, 142–48; family structures, 132–33, 207–8; grandparents and, 132–35; hearing aids and, 158–59; hopes and concerns for their child's future, 191–93, 215–17, 236; housing conditions, 125–27; issues of control and safety, 165–66; issues of cultural context and, 194–95; language development, lack of awareness of, 195; perceptions of the causes of deafness, 148–49; perceptions of deaf children, 135–38; preschool rehabilitation and, 185–91; previous experience of deafness, 154–56; second children and, 32–34, 138–42; serial consultation of doctors, 149–54; sleeping arrangements, 127; social contacts, responses and reactions to, 159–65; socioeconomic status, 129–32; as study participants, 193–94, 195–96
urban populations/regions: causes of deafness in, 52; deaf community in, 89; deaf education and, 70, 71; incidence of deafness in, 51; income levels in, 48

vitamin B, as treatment for deafness, 63

Wallenburg, Ellis, 62
Wang Hua, 49
Wang Yarong, 95, 116
wan xi shao (one-child family planning policy), 20–25
Wan Xuanrong, 116–17
Webb, Blair, 62
welfare factories, 89, 257
welfare services, 16
Western medicine: in China, 59–60
women: bearing unwanted children, 280 n. 6; reasons for having children, 277 n. 1; twentieth-century reforms and, 13–15
writing: in communication at home, 173, 174; parents' valuing of, 184, 185
Wu, David Y. H., 44
wu lun ("five relationships"), 12–13, 36

Xiaomei Ke, 57

yabaa (mutes), 233
Yang Jianmin, 56
Yang Kuo-shu, 38–39
Yau Shun-chiu, 90
Young, Alys, 121, 137
yuan, 284 n. 8
yuyan (speech, language), 282 n. 1

Zeng, Fangang, 67, 90
Zeng Yi, 23–24
Zhang Haidi, 116, 281 n. 17
Zhang Mei-juan, 117
Zhou Enlai, 86–87
Zhou Hong, 2, 5; advocacy of therapies for deafness, 60, 63–64; letters to, 198–99 (*see also* letters to Zhou Hong); national publicity as a parental exemplar, 116–17, 198; requests for help from parents, 228–31; why parents seek his advice, 118
Zhou Jing, 100–101
Zhou Tingting, 116, 198, 284 n. 4